fourth edition

APPLETON & LANGE REVIEW OF GENERAL PATHOLOGY

Edison Catalano, MD
Professor of Pathology
University of Medicine and Dentistry
Robert Wood Johnson Medical School at Camden
Cooper Hospital/UMC
Camden, New Jersey

Chief
Department of Pathology
Cooper Health System
Camden, New Jersey

Kanwaljeet Sandhu

Appleton & Lange Reviews/McGraw-Hill
Medical Publishing Division

New York   Chicago   San Francisco   Lisbon   London   Madrid   Mexico City   Milan
New Delhi   San Juan   Seoul   Singapore   Sydney   Toronto

Appleton & Lange Review of General Pathology, Fourth Edition

1234567890 VHVH 987654321

ISBN 0-07-138995-4

Notice

Medicine is an ever-changing science. As new research and clinical experience broaden our knowledge, changes in treatment and drug therapy are required. The author and the publisher of this work have checked with sources believed to be reliable in their efforts to provide information that is complete and generally in accord with the standards accepted at the time of publication. However, in view of the possibility of human error or changes in medical sciences, neither the author nor the publisher nor any other party who has been involved in the preparation or publication of this work warrants that the information contained herein is in every respect accurate or complete, and they are not responsible for any errors or omissions or for the results obtained from use of such information. Readers are encouraged to confirm the information contained herein with other sources. For example and in particular, readers are advised to check the product information sheet included in the package of each drug they plan to administer to be certain that the information contained in this book is accurate and that changes have not been made in the recommended dose or in the contraindications for administration. This recommendation is of particular importance in connection with new or infrequently used drugs.

This book was set in Palatino by Circle Graphics.
The editors were Catherine Wenz Johnson and John M. Morriss.
The production supervisor was Catherine Saggese.
The cover designer was Elizabeth Pisacreta.

Von Hoffmann Graphics was printer and binder.

This book is printed on acid-free paper.

Library of Congress Cataloging-in-Publication Data

Catalano, Edison.
    Appleton & Lange review of general pathology / Edison Catalano.—4th ed.
        p. ; cm.
    Rev. ed. of: Appleton & Lange's review of general pathology / Martin Gwent Lewis,
Thomas K. Barton, 3rd ed. c1993.
    Includes bibliographical references and index.
    ISBN 0-07-138995-4 (alk. paper)
        1. Pathology—Examinations, questions, etc. I. Title: Review of general pathology.
II. Title: Appleton and Lange review of general pathology. III. Lewis, Martin Gwent.
Appleton & Lange review of general pathology. IV. Title.
    [DNLM: 1. Pathology—Examination Questions. QZ 18.2 C357a 2003]
    RB119 .L485 2003
    616.07'076—dc21
                                                                2002067174

Contents

Preface

This book provides a format for review and revision of general pathology and both practice and self-assessment of knowledge required for the successful approach to examinations such as the United States Medical Licensing Examination.

It is not in any way intended to be a replacement for standard and more extensive and comprehensive textbooks of pathology. Rather, this is intended as a supplement to be used with the understanding that it is not an introduction to pathology but a book to be used by students who have already completed courses in pathology and read the more extensive texts.

At the end of the book, a practice test is presented so that readers can test their abilities and knowledge in the style and time frame that will be expected of them in the performance of the actual examination. Answers and explanations are also provided with the practice test, as are some hints and advice on the best method of approaching such an examination from a practical point of view.

Illustrated photographic questions are also included in each chapter. A separate chapter devoted entirely to such photographic questions is also provided to give practice and experience. This particular approach is being used more and more frequently in a number of professional examinations in pathology.

Finally, in addition to reviewing pathology and practicing examination techniques, it is hoped that readers will be stimulated to a greater study of pathology with particular emphasis on its clinical application.

General pathology or the general principles of disease is not the province of medical students or medical practitioners alone, but is also important to students of science, particularly those entering careers in biomedical research. It is hoped that these exercises will be a value to all who study disease for whatever reason.

Acknowledgments

This book is dedicated to my wife, Lilia, our children, Fabrizio and Andrea; my mother, Amelia; my sister, Rosa, and in loving memory of my father, Domingo and my brother, Ariel.

I would also like to thank Sherri Glemser, my executive assistant, for her dedication and tireless hours of work, and Bill Reed for his technical support.

Introduction

If you are planning to prepare for the United States Medical Licensing Examination (USMLE) Step 1, then this book is designed for you. Here, in one package, is a pathology review resource with over 1100 examination-type multiple-choice questions with referenced explanations for each answer.

This introduction provides specific information on the USMLE Step 1, information on question types, question-answering strategies, and various ways to use this review.

THE UNITED STATES MEDICAL LICENSING EXAMINATION STEP 1

The United States Medical Licensing Examination Step 1 is a 1-day computerized examination consisting of approximately 400 questions to test your knowledge in the basic sciences. It contains multiple-choice questions organized within three dimensions. Each dimension is weighted; however, the projected percentages for these dimensions are subject to change from exam to exam. The three dimensions are: (a) system; (b) process; and (c) organizational level. The application materials illustrate the percentage breakout, and offer you a detailed content outline to aid you in your review.

Question Formats

The style and presentation of the questions have been fully revised to conform with the United States Medical Licensing Examinations. This will enable you to familiarize yourself with the types of questions to be expected, and provide practice in recalling your knowledge in each format. Following the answer to each question, a reference to a particular and easily available text is provided for further reference and reading.

Each of the chapters contains single-best answer multiple-choice questions. In some cases, a group of two or three questions may be related to a situational theme. In addition, some questions have illustrative material (e.g., line illustrations of anatomy) that require understanding and interpretation on your part. Moreover, questions may be of three levels of difficulty: rote memory, memory question that requires more understanding of the problem, and a question that requires both understanding and judgment. In view of the fact that the USMLE Step 1 is moving toward the judgment, critical-thinking type question, we have attempted to write this review with this emphasis.

One Best Answer—Single Item Question. This is the most popular question format in most examination. It generally contains a brief statement, followed by five options of which only ONE is entirely correct. The options on the USMLE are lettered A, B, C, D, and E. Although the format for this question type is straightforward, the questions can be difficult, because some of the distractors may be partially right. The instructions you will see for this type of question will generally appear as below:

DIRECTIONS (Question 1): Each of the numbered items or incomplete statements in this section is followed by answers or by completions of the statement. Select the ONE lettered answer or completion that is BEST in each case.

An example of this question type is:

1. An obese 21-year-old woman complains of increased growth of coarse hair on her lip, chin,

chest, and abdomen. She also notes menstrual irregularity with periods of amenorrhea. The most likely cause is

    (A) polycystic ovary disease
    (B) an ovarian tumor
    (C) an adrenal tumor
    (D) Cushing's disease
    (E) familial hirsutism

In the question above, the key word is "most." Although ovarian tumors, adrenal tumors, and Cushing's disease are causes of hirsutism (described in the stem of the question), polycystic ovary disease is a much more common cause. Familial hirsutism is not associated with the menstrual irregularities mentioned. Thus, the most likely cause of the manifestations described can only be "(A) polycystic ovary disease."

Answers, Explanations, and References

In each chapter of this book, the question sections are followed by a section containing the answers, expla-

---

STRATEGIES FOR ANSWERING ONE BEST ANSWER–SINGLE ITEM QUESTIONS

1. Remember, only one choice can be the correct answer.
2. Read the question carefully to be sure that you understand what is being asked. Pay attention to key words such as "most" or "least."
3. Quickly read each choice for familiarity. (This important step is often not done by test takers.)
4. Go back and consider each choice individually.
5. If a choice is partially correct, tentatively consider it to be incorrect. (This step will help you eliminate choices and increase your odds of choosing the correct answer.)
6. Consider the remaining choices, and select the one you think is the answer. At this point, you may want to scan quickly the stem to be sure you understand the question and your answer.
7. If you do not know the answer, make an educated guess. Your score is based on the number of correct answers, not the number you get incorrect. **Do not leave any blanks.**
8. The actual examination is timed for an average of 60 seconds per question. It is important to be thorough to understand the question, but it is equally important for you to keep moving.

---

nations, and references to the questions. This section (a) tells you the answer to each question; (b) gives you an explanation/review of why the answer is correct, and background information on the subject matter; and (c) tells you where you can find more in-depth information on the subject matter in other books and/or journals. We encourage you to use this section as a basis for further study and understanding.

If you choose the correct answer to a question, you can then read the explanation (a) for reinforcement and (b) to add to your knowledge about the subject matter (remember that the explanations usually tell not only why the answer is correct, but also why the other choices are incorrect). **If you choose the wrong answer** to a question, you can read the explanation for a learning/reviewing discussion of the material in the question. Furthermore, you can note the reference cited (e.g., *Rubin and Farber, p. 1405*), look up the full source in the References at the end of the section (e.g., Rubin E, Farber JL. *Pathology.* Philadelphia: Lippincott, 1999), and refer to the pages cited for a more in-depth discussion.

SPECIFIC INFORMATION ON THE STEP 1 EXAMINATION

The official source of all information with respect to the United States Medical Licensing Examination Step 1 is the National Board of Medical Examiners (NBME), 3930 Chestnut Street, Philadelphia, PA 19104. Established in 1915, the NBME is a voluntary, nonprofit, independent organization whose sole function is the design, implementation, distribution, and processing of a vast bank of question items, certifying examinations, and evaluative services in the professional medical field. Please contact the NBME or visit the USMLE web site (www.usmle.org) for information on exam registration and scoring.

CHAPTER 1

Cell Injury and Death

The chief point in this application of Histology and Pathology is to obtain a recognition of the fact, that the cell is really the ultimate morphological element in which there is any manifestation of life, and that we must not transfer the seat of real action to any point beyond the cell.
—Rudolph Virchow (1858)

There are basic responses of cells to various forms of insult. Injury is produced by physical, chemical, microbial, immunologic, or even genetic means; the effects of ionizing radiation have been selected to be discussed in depth in this chapter. With injury, there is stress on the dynamic nature of the cells' response to injury (i.e., the ability of cells to adapt to varying levels of injury). Characteristic morphologic alterations of a degenerative nature arise in response to sublethal injury, with sequential changes in both morphology and biochemistry.

When the ability of cells to regulate their metabolism is exceeded by excessively large, persistent, or unusual forms of injury, the process of necrosis is initiated. The characteristic morphologic changes of cell death and the underlying biochemical basis are examined in this chapter, and comparison is made between methods of coping with widespread tissue injury and normal physiologic processes involving cell replacement. Emphasis is placed on the effects of inflammation and repair, which various forms of cell death initiate.

Detailed treatment of radiobiology and radiation pathology is aimed at familiarizing the reader with the basic forms of ionizing radiation and the major syndromes that may be initiated by various absorbed doses. The organs and cells most at risk are indicated.

BASIC FACTS AND CONCEPTS

Many forms of injuries result in a series of adaptive processes on the part of the cell that returns the cell to a state of equilibrium with its environment. Some stimuli cause such drastic changes that a return to the normal steady state is impossible, and a series of irreversible changes leads to cell death (Figure 1–1).

Subsequent additional events following these forms of necrosis include saponification, mummification, calcification, ossification, and acute inflammation and resulting fibrosis in some cases (see Chapter 2). Table 1–1 provides a more detailed summary of the main features, and Table 1–2 shows a comparison between the varieties of cell injury and responses. Figure 1–2 is a schematic representation of a typical mammalian cell.

ABNORMAL ACCUMULATION OF VARIOUS SUBSTANCES WITHIN CELLS

There are two basic types of accumulation: (a) excess of substances normal to the particular cell, and (b) abnormal substances, and three basic mechanisms: (a) decrease in normal metabolic removal, (b) inability to metabolize the substance, and (c) deposition of abnormal exogenous substance in which the cell has no mechanism to metabolize it.

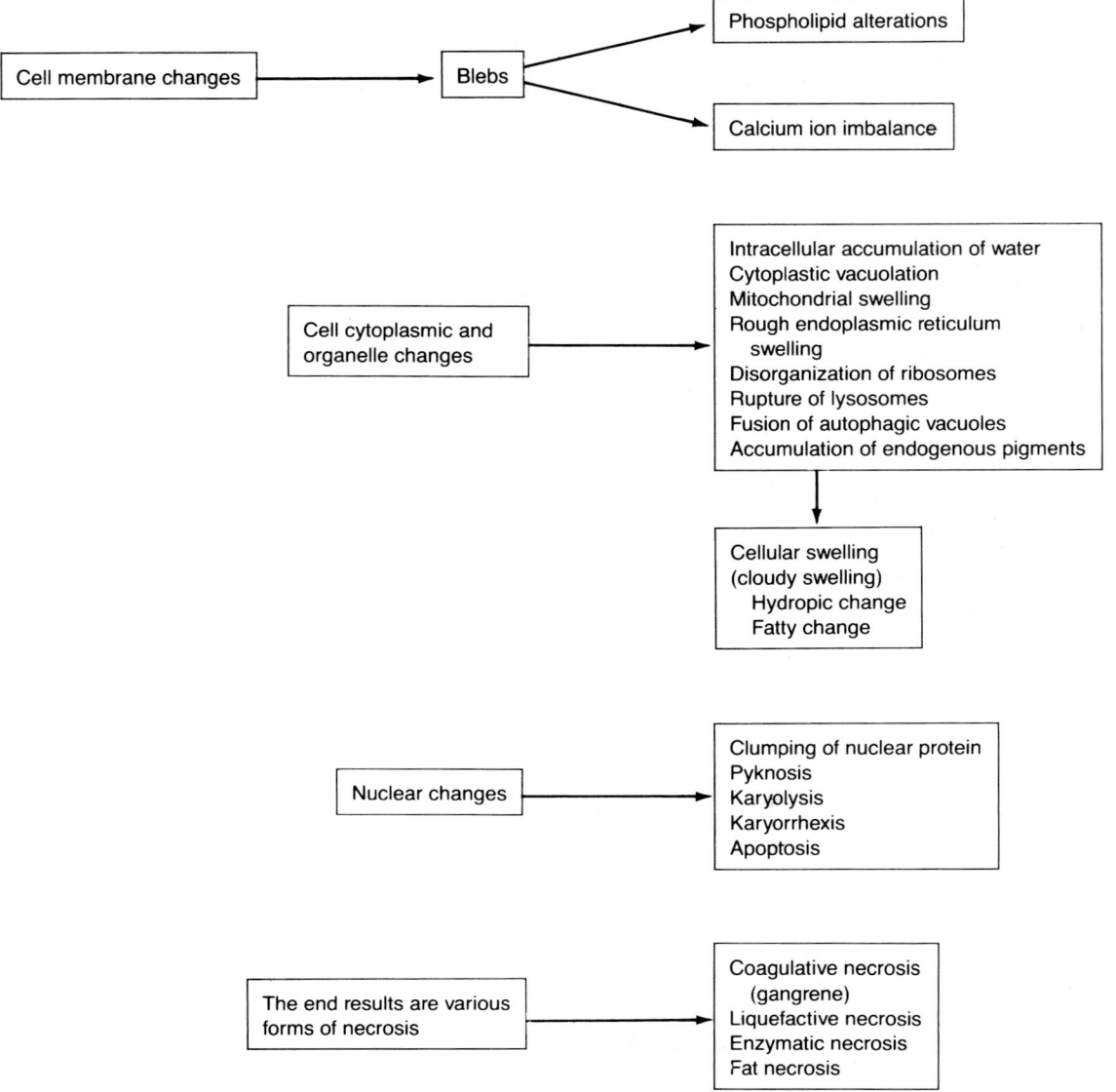

Figure 1–1. Types and modes of change follow irreversible damage to cells.

Table 1–1. SALIENT FEATURES OF CELL INJURY AND DEGENERATION

Condition	Microscopic Findings
Hydropic degeneration	Accumulation of intracellular fluid. Cells have a pale appearance of cytoplasm with distortion of nucleus. Cytoplasm is less granular than usual. Typically seen in proximal tubules of kidney
Hyaline degeneration	Homogeneous pink and ground-glass appearance, often the blurring hyaline obliteration of nuclear structure. Seen typically in small blood vessels or in the islets of Langerhans in diabetes
Fatty degeneration	Accumulation of lipids gives cells an empty appearance because of removal of lipids during normal processing of tissue. Seen typically in liver cells in response to a variety of insults
Amyloid deposition	Pink-staining material with a smudge-out appearance. Seen typically in interstitial tissue in spleen, liver, and the like or in the glomeruli of the kidney
Colliquative necrosis	Amorphous material, often bluish staining because of the nuclear protein present. Seen in an abscess and in brain infarcts where the staining is complicated by lipid
Fat necrosis	Breakdown of fat cells with a pale-staining appearance. Often complicated by deposition of calcium salts (staining dark blue) or alkaline change (saponification)
Dystrophic calcification	Deposition of calcium salts in tissues secondary to previous degenerative changes. As mentioned, fat necrosis may be one such predisposing abnormality

Table 1–2. COMPARISON OF VARIOUS FORMS OF CELL INJURY AND DEGENERATIONS

Condition	Degeneration	Infiltration	Breakdown of Cells	Inflammatory Response	Attraction of Calcium Salts
Hyaline degeneration	Yes	Yes	Not usually	Late or infrequent	Variable
Hydropic degeneration	Yes	No	No	No	No
Fatty degeneration	Yes	No	Late	Usually not or late	No
Amyloidosis	Yes	Yes	Variable or secondary response to pressure	Yes	
Colliquative necrosis	Yes	Yes	Yes	Yes	Variable
Fat necrosis	Yes	Yes	Yes		Yes

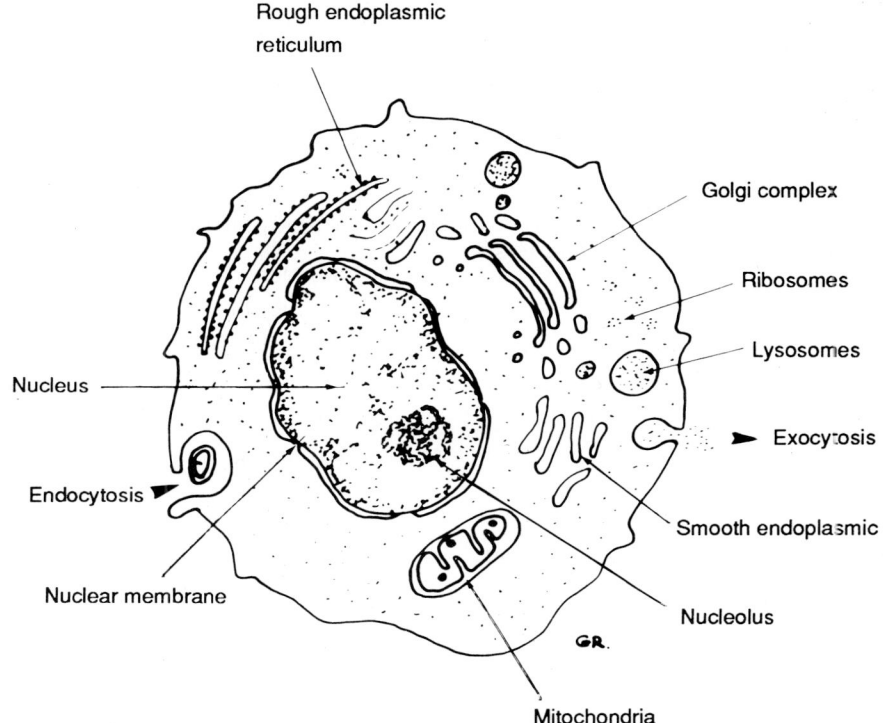

Figure 1–2. This is a schematic representation of a typical mammalian cell with the more important organelles, structures, and physiologic processes labeled.

Questions

DIRECTIONS (Questions 1 through 34): Each of the numbered items or incomplete statements in this section is followed by answers or by completions of the statement. Select the ONE lettered answer or completion that is BEST in each case.

1. Autolysis involves which organelle system as a major factor?

   (A) Golgi complex
   (B) nucleus
   (C) rough endoplasmic reticulum (RER)
   (D) lysosomes
   (E) nucleolus

2. Liquefaction, or colliquative necrosis, is seen especially in

   (A) lungs
   (B) kidney
   (C) brain
   (D) heart
   (E) liver

3. Gas gangrene is a form of necrosis associated with

   (A) mycotic infections
   (B) emphysema
   (C) tuberculosis
   (D) infections with *Clostridium*
   (E) muscle trauma

4. Atrophy in the thyroid epithelium in Hashimoto's disease results from

   (A) autoimmunity
   (B) pituitary malfunction

   (C) malnutrition
   (D) pressure caused by adjacent neoplasm
   (E) excessive thyroid-stimulating hormone (TSH)

5. Mitochondria contain enzymes involved in

   (A) activation and synthesis of some amino acids
   (B) glycolysis
   (C) oxidative phosphorylation
   (D) fatty acid synthesis
   (E) phosphogluconate pathway

6. The unit of exposure for health physics purposes is

   (A) roentgen equivalent physical (rep)
   (B) roentgen equivalent mammal (rem)
   (C) curie
   (D) relative biologic effectiveness (rbe)
   (E) microcurie

7. The cell type most likely to be damaged by ionizing irradiation is

   (A) glial cell
   (B) erythrocyte
   (C) intestinal crypt cell
   (D) melanocyte
   (E) cartilage

8. The most likely cause of death following exposure to 700 rads is

   (A) bone marrow syndrome
   (B) central nervous system (CNS) syndrome
   (C) gastrointestinal syndrome

(D) respiratory failure

(E) skin exfoliation

9. In distinguishing necrosis from apoptosis, what would be the most salient feature?

(A) bacterial infection

(B) viral infection

(C) normal development

(D) fungal infection

(E) ischemic injury

10. In the bone marrow syndrome, the most significant cause of nonterminal anemia is

(A) frank hemorrhage

(B) leakage from the circulation

(C) lysis of circulating erythrocytes

(D) deficiency of erythropoiesis

(E) leukemic transformation

11. In death resulting from the gastrointestinal syndrome, the mean survival time is measured in

(A) hours

(B) days

(C) weeks

(D) months

(E) years

12. The main cellular target for the action of radiation is

(A) DNA

(B) cell membrane

(C) mitochondria

(D) ribosomes

(E) lysosomes

13. Councilman bodies present in the livers of patients with viral hepatitis are an example of

(A) apoptosis

(B) atrophy

(C) metaplasia

(D) hyperplasia

(E) necrosis

14. Which of the following radiations is most penetrating to human tissue?

(A) alpha

(B) beta

(C) gamma

(D) x-ray

(E) protons

15. Which of the following radiations is most damaging to human tissue, given equal penetration?

(A) alpha

(B) beta

(C) gamma

(D) x-ray

(E) protons

16. Indicate the type of changes seen in the prostatic epithelium as a result of castration.

(A) dysplasia

(B) atrophy

(C) metaplasia

(D) hyperplasia

(E) necrosis

17. Indicate the most common changes in the thymus after administration corticoid steroids.

(A) atrophy

(B) hypoplasia

(C) apoptosis

(D) metaplasia

(E) necrosis

18. Which of the following lists of tissue is in the correct order of radiosensitivity?

(A) red cell precursors, neurons, lymphocytes, muscle fibers, small intestinal epithelial cells, fibroblasts, keratinocytes

(B) lymphocytes, red cell precursors, intestinal epithelial cells, neurons, keratinocytes, fibroblasts, muscle fibers

(C) intestinal epithelium, neurons, lymphocytes, fibroblasts, muscle

(D) neurons, muscle, fibroblasts, lymphocytes, keratinocytes

(E) keratinocytes, muscle, neurons, red cell precursors, fibroblasts

19. Apoptosis is different than necrosis because of

    (A) enzyme activation
    (B) nuclear fragmentation
    (C) breakdown of RNA
    (D) does not elicit inflammation
    (E) changes in the plasma membrane structure

20. As a normal development of tissues, the cell death is considered a phenomenon of

    (A) liquefactive necrosis
    (B) fat necrosis
    (C) autolysis
    (D) apoptosis
    (E) caseous necrosis

21. Name the organelle that intervenes in the regulation of intracellular Ca²⁺ by sequestration.

    (A) rough endoplasmic reticulum
    (B) Golgi complex
    (C) nucleus
    (D) lysosomes
    (E) mitochondrion

22. Which of the following microscopic descriptions is most characteristic of hyaline degeneration?

    (A) homogeneous ground-glass, pink-staining appearance in cells
    (B) accumulation of lipids in cells
    (C) presence of calcium salts with destruction of cellular detail
    (D) pyknotic densely stained nucleus
    (E) total amorphous appearance with no cell membrane discernable

23. The pigment known as lipofuscin (wear and tear) is originated from

    (A) intracellular lipid peroxidation
    (B) melanin metabolism
    (C) heterophagy
    (D) iron oxidation
    (E) glycogenolysis

24. Which of the following cellular responses to injury is the most reversible?

    (A) amyloid deposition
    (B) fat necrosis
    (C) colliquative necrosis
    (D) hydropic change
    (E) apoptosis

25. Which of the following cell changes associated with injury is most likely to be accompanied by disruption of the cell membrane?

    (A) cloudy swelling
    (B) hydropic change
    (C) apoptosis
    (D) coagulative necrosis
    (E) pyknosis

26. Dry gangrene is best described microscopically by

    (A) enzymatic fat necrosis
    (B) coagulative necrosis
    (C) swelling of RER
    (D) cell membrane blebs
    (E) caseous necrosis

27. In glycogen storage disorders, which of the following causes is most accurate?

    (A) accumulation of abnormal amounts of a normal substance
    (B) deposition of exogenous abnormal substance in the cells
    (C) deposition of abnormal amounts of lipid in the cells
    (D) deposition of mucopolysaccharides in the cells
    (E) accumulation of immunoglobulin in the cells

28. Indicate an early reversible cell injury change.

    (A) intramitochondrial calcium precipitation
    (B) nuclear fragmentation
    (C) fatty change

(D) plasma membrane rupture

(E) cytoplasmic hypereosinophilia

29. Which of the following is the most common process that may stimulate acute inflammation?

(A) dysplasia

(B) necrosis

(C) metaplasia

(D) apoptosis

(E) autolysis

30. Which of the following is most likely to result in calcium salt deposition in the tissues affected?

(A) amyloid change

(B) hyaline degenerative change

(C) colliquative necrosis

(D) fat necrosis

(E) hydropic change

Questions 31 through 33. (Refer to Figure 1–3.)

31. The area numbered 1 represents

(A) mitochondrion

(B) nucleolus

(C) Golgi complex

(D) lysosome

(E) RER

32. The area numbered 6 represents

(A) smooth endoplasmic reticulum

(B) nucleus

(C) polyribosomes

(D) mitochondrion

(E) Golgi complex

33. The area numbered 7 represents

(A) mitochondrion

(B) Golgi complex

(C) nuclear membrane

(D) polyribosomes

(E) RER

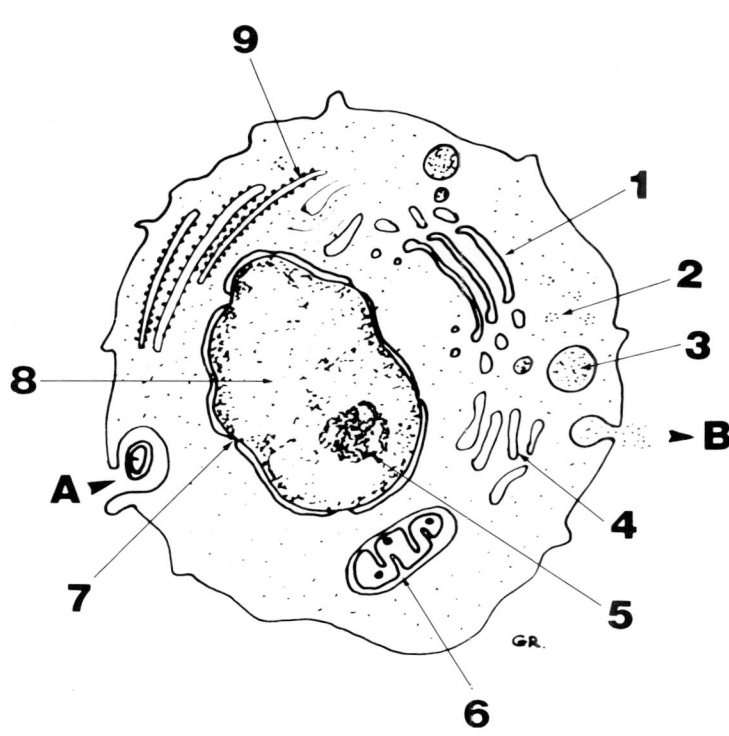

Figure 1–3. This is a schematic representation of a typical mammalian cell with the more important organelles and structures indicated by the numbers 1 through 9, and two physiologic processes labeled A and B.

DIRECTIONS (Questions 34 through 88): Each group of items in this section consists of a list of lettered options followed by a set of numbered words or phrases. For each numbered word or phrase, select the ONE lettered option that is most closely associated with it. Each lettered option may be selected once, more than once, or not at all.

Questions 34 through 37

(A) curie
(B) rad
(C) roentgen
(D) roentgen equivalent mammal (rem)

34. Unit of absorbed dose

35. Unit of dose equivalent (absorbed dose × quality factor)

36. Unit of activity (3.7×10^1 nuclear transformation/sec)

37. Unit of exposure for x-rays or gamma rays

Questions 38 through 40

(A) whole body exposure to 10,000 rads
(B) whole body exposure to 3,000 rads
(C) whole body exposure to 700 rads

38. Vomiting

39. Seizures

40. Diarrhea

Questions 41 through 45

(A) fatty degeneration
(B) cloudy swelling
(C) coagulation necrosis
(D) caseous necrosis
(E) fibrinoid necrosis

41. The liver after carbon tetrachloride uptake

42. Choline deficiency

43. Loss of tissue architecture, with a cheesy appearance and consistency

44. Reduction in both oxidative phosphorylation and mitochondrial activity

45. Classically seen in blood vessels, with loss of architecture and incorporation of plasma proteins into the vessel wall

Questions 46 through 48

(A) heterophagy
(B) pyknosis
(C) autophagy
(D) karyolysis
(E) exocytosis

46. Envelopment of damaged endogenous cellular elements and their digestion in the lysosomal system

47. Digestion in the lysosomal system of exogenous substances entering the cell through endocytosis

48. Cellular discharge of particular matter too large to diffuse through the cell membrane

Questions 49 through 52

(A) cloudy swelling
(B) karyorrhexis
(C) residual body
(D) saponification
(E) liquefaction necrosis

49. Salts deposited in necrotic fatty tissue

50. Lysosomal inclusion bodies

51. Reversible cellular change

52. Nuclear fragmentation

Questions 53 through 56

(A) caseous necrosis
(B) fat necrosis
(C) coagulation necrosis
(D) liquefaction necrosis
(E) dilation of the endoplasmic reticulum

53. Expected changes in the kidney after complete occlusion of the renal artery

54. Expected changes in the cerebral cortex after occlusion of the middle cerebral artery

55. Expected changes with infection by tubercle bacilli

56. Reversible cellular change

Questions 57 through 60

(A) melanin
(B) lipofuscin
(C) hemosiderin
(D) bilirubin
(E) ceroid

57. Increased content in tissues is termed "jaundice"

58. Lipochrome yellow–brown pigment that increases with aging

59. Aggregates of ferritin micelles

60. Brown–black pigment formed by the oxidation of tyrosine

Questions 61 through 64

(A) ribosomes
(B) mitochondria
(C) primary lysosomes
(D) cell membrane
(E) centriole

61. Major site of oxidative phosphorylation and energy production

62. Major site of protein synthesis

63. Intracellular bodies that organize mitotic division

64. Intracellular bodies containing hydrolytic enzymes necessary for the digestion of endogenous and exogenous substances

Questions 65 through 68

(A) Councilman bodies
(B) psammoma bodies
(C) Gandy–Gamna bodies
(D) Civatte bodies
(E) glycogen bodies

65. Intracellular accumulations seen with Pompe's disease

66. Apoptosis seen with lichen planus

67. Apoptosis seen with infectious or toxic hepatitis

68. Splenic scars containing calcium and hemosiderin

Questions 69 through 72

(A) single exposure of 25 rads
(B) single exposure of 150 rads
(C) single exposure of 250 rads
(D) single exposure of 800 rads
(E) single exposure of 1,250 rads

69. Acute cerebral syndrome, 100% mortality

70. Acute hematopoietic syndrome, 20–50% mortality

71. No short-term effects, 0% mortality

72. Acute radiation syndrome, 0% mortality

Questions 73 through 76

(A) fibrinoid necrosis
(B) gangrenous necrosis
(C) enzymatic fat necrosis
(D) gummatous necrosis
(E) liquefactive necrosis

73. Frequently seen with acute pancreatitis

74. Frequently seen with syphilitic infections

75. Frequently seen with autoimmune disorders

76. Frequently seen with ischemic distal extremities

Questions 77 through 80

(A) cytokeratin
(B) factor VIII
(C) HMB-45
(D) desmin
(E) glial fibrillary acid protein

77. Intermediate filament present in astrocytes

78. Intermediate filament present in all epithelial cells

79. Intermediate filament present in smooth muscle cells

80. Coagulation protein present in endothelial cells

Questions 81 through 84

(A) Mallory body
(B) neurofibrillary tangle
(C) vimentin
(D) ankyrin
(E) pinocytosis

81. Cell membrane protein

82. Increased with Alzheimer's disease

83. Increased with alcoholic liver disease

84. Intermediate filament present in all mesenchymal cells

Questions 85 through 88

(A) inhibits cellular respiration
(B) protects protein synthesis
(C) inhibits cell division
(D) protects against radiation
(E) binds to protein sulfhydrals
(F) free radical formation
(G) protects mitochondria
(H) protects cytoskeleton

85. A 36-year-old male smelter experiences an accidental lethal exposure to mercuric gas. At autopsy, his kidneys were swollen and demonstrated coagulative necrosis of the proximal tubular epithelial cells. What is the primary site of cellular injury occurring in mercury poisoning?

86. A 19-year-old commits suicide by ingesting sodium cyanide. At autopsy, the characteristic findings of acute cyanide poisoning are present including a pervasive almond-like smell and acute hemorrhagic gastritis. By what method does cyanide poison cells?

87. A 44-year-old is found to have an increased serum uric acid, increased urinary uric acid excretion, recurrent attacks of acute arthritis, and tophi. A diagnosis of gout is made. One of the medicines prescribed for the patient is colchicine. How does colchicine exert its beneficial effect?

88. A 54-year-old male janitor is cleaning a soiled carpet with carbon tetrachloride in an enclosed room. He develops malaise, nausea, stomach pains, and convulsions. Several days later he dies. At autopsy there is marked fatty change in the liver, acute renal tubular necrosis, and cerebral edema. The cause of death is believed to be acute carbon tetrachloride poisoning. What is the primary mode of cellular injury in carbon tetrachloride poisoning?

Answers and Explanations

1. **(D)** The lysosome system within the cell is a complex interaction and balance between endocytosis and pinocytosis and the primary lysosome system associated with the phagosomes versus the secondary lysosome and autophagosome side of the mechanism, which leads to exocytosis. This is summarized schematically in Figure 1–2. Although the Golgi apparatus and the RER contribute to this balance, it is the lysosome system itself with its release of hydrolases together with increased intercellular acidity that most favors tissue digestion and leads to autolysis rather than merely the accumulation of materials in the cells. (*Chandrasoma and Taylor, pp. 16–17*)

2. **(C)** Liquefaction, or colliquative necrosis, is also important in one of the complications of acute inflammation (Chapter 2). It is the breakdown of tissue as a result of severe injury resulting in a semifluid consistency. The degree of this type of necrosis in a particular tissue is partly determined by the inherent nature of the tissue concerned. The brain, which is in an almost semifluid state, is more easily broken down, and the lipid content added to the breakdown of the cellular components produces a particular kind of necrosis. Lungs, kidney, liver, and heart, which have a more solid cellular composition, undergo a different type of necrosis, and liquefaction is much rarer in these tissues (Table 1–2). (*Chandrasoma and Taylor, p. 17*)

3. **(D)** Gas gangrene is a form of tissue necrosis in which the underlying factor is ischemia, which leads to the necrosis. There is a superimposed production of gas, which is the by-product of anaerobic organisms that proliferate in the ischemic anaerobic conditions produced. The classic gas-producing organisms are *Clostridium* species. A mycotic infection is one in which a fungus is superimposed on a variety of different forms of tissue injury. Emphysema is a mechanical destructive process of the lung. Tuberculosis may produce caseous necrosis (Chapter 2), but this is distinctly different from that of gas gangrene. Muscle trauma in and of itself will not produce this phenomenon, but necrotic dead muscle following tissue trauma may be complicated by gas gangrene if clostridial organisms are introduced into the tissue (Tables 1–1 and 1–2). (*Cotran et al., pp. 368–369*)

4. **(A)** Hashimoto's disease is an autoimmune disease in which the thyroid epithelium is damaged, leading to an atrophic or hypofunction of the thyroid gland. Pituitary malfunction may cause secondary changes in the thyroid, and malnutrition may result in some abnormalities. Pressure caused by an adjacent neoplasm may cause local problems. None of these, however, causes the diffuse destruction of the gland seen in Hashimoto's disease. Excess TSH, in fact, usually is secondary to the gland no longer functioning, and, therefore, the negative feedback control from TSH is altered but has nothing to do with initiation of the disease as far as can be determined. (*Rubin and Farber, pp. 1171–1172*)

5. **(C)** The process of oxidative phosphorylation is a very important and vital step in energy production and transfer in most cells and is the function of the mitochondria and mitochondrial enzymes. The mitochondria have additional enzymatic functions. They also are involved in protein synthesis but not in the actual production

of amino acid and fatty acid synthesis. Phospho-gluconate pathways are of much less importance except under certain pathologic conditions in which lipid may accumulate as a result of mal-functioning of the mitochondrial mechanisms. *(Cotran et al., pp. 6–7)*

6. **(B)** The unit of exposure used for health physics purposes in humans is the rem. All types of radi-ation have different propensities to interact with tissue and, therefore, have different rbe. The amount of radiation times its characteristic rbe equals its rem (radiation × rbe = rem). Such a cal-culation allows standard comparison of exposure for different types of radiation. The rep is not used for biologic systems. Other units, including curie and microcurie, are measurements of emis-sion and are not used under these circumstances except in isotope work. *(Cotran et al., p. 425)*

7. **(C)** Intestinal epithelium, with its rapid turn-over, is the most sensitive, particularly the crypt cells, which are responsible for the continuous regeneration of the epithelium (Table 1–3). In general terms, the higher the turnover rate of the cells, the more likely they are to be radiosensi-

Table 1–3. RELATIVE SENSITIVITIES OF DIFFERENT CELL TYPES OF IRRADIATION

Cell Type	Radiosensitivity
Bone marrow Lymphoid Germ cells (testis, ovaries) Intestinal epithelium	Very sensitive
Epididymal and adnexal cells of skin Pharyngeal or esophageal Urothelium Gastric mucosa	Sensitive
Glial cells of CNS Connective tissue Endothelial Growing cartilage	Moderately sensitive
Mature cartilage and bone Mucous and serous glands Pulmonary Renal Hepatic Pancreatic Endocrine	Low sensitivity
Muscle Ganglion Neurons	Very low sensitivity

tive. The glial cell has a particularly moderate sensitivity. The erythrocyte (mature), being a non-nucleated cell, has virtually no effect except in very high doses of radiation. The melanocyte is very sensitive to ultraviolet radiation but not ionizing radiation to the same extent, and carti-lage cells have a relatively low sensitivity except in growing cartilage, which is moderately sensi-tive. *(Rubin and Farber, pp. 338–340)*

8. **(A)** High doses of whole body irradiation in the range of 10,000 rads usually can cause sud-den death thought to be from damage to all the systems, particularly the CNS. The gastrointes-tinal syndrome, in which the gastrointestinal tract is damaged, usually is an intermediate effect. The relatively lower doses of less than 1,000 rads usually cause destruction of the bone marrow, with the concomitant effects of aplas-tic anemia. This is, therefore, a more prolonged rather than a sudden cause of death (Tables 1–3 and 1–4). *(Rubin and Farber, pp. 338–340)*

9. **(C)** Apoptosis (program cell death) is a mor-phologic pattern of cell injury that is now ac-cepted as a distinctive and important mode of cell death. This cell death is an ongoing pheno-menon in multicellular organisms that occur in the healthy state and constitutes a balanced cell renewal of the organism. Apoptosis then consti-tutes a phenomenon in the normal development of the individual. A distinction between apopto-sis and necrosis is possible, because necrosis occurs in different circumstances in life, in-cluding aging. *(Cotran et al., pp. 18–21)*

10. **(D)** Nonterminal anemia is usually the result of deficiency in erythropoiesis and is the most significant in terms of bone marrow damage. Although frank hemorrhage and leakage from the circulation may occur as a complication of other aspects or irradiation (eg, the effects on the gastrointestinal tract; Table 1–4), this usu-ally is not a direct effect of the bone marrow. Lysis of the circulating erythrocytes can occur but requires enormous doses of irradiation, since mature erythrocytes can survive until they are deleted by natural events. It is the inability to replenish these erythrocytes that causes the non-terminal anemia of the bone marrow syndrome. Leukemic transformation is a very long-term

Table 1–4. RADIATION EFFECTS

Tissue or Organ	Acute Radiation Effects	Chronic or Delayed Radiation Effects
Lung	Pulmonary edema and swelling of alveolar cells	Intestinal fibrosis, alveolar fibrosis, ischemic changes
Gastrointestinal tract	Death of small intestinal mucosa with widespread ulceration	Tortuosity of blood vessels, relative ischemia and submucosal fibrosis, chronic ulceration and strictures
Kidney	Acute proximal tubular necrosis with intestinal edema	Sclerosing of blood vessels, glomerular sclerosis, tubular ischemia and atrophy

effect in those individuals who survive the radiation. *(Rubin and Farber, p. 339)*

11. **(B)** The gastrointestinal syndrome following irradiation is a result of complete destruction of the sensitive, rapidly regenerating epithelium of the small intestine. There are protracted and violent diarrhea and loss of fluid. Death usually ensues in a matter of days and certainly within a week (Questions 8 through 10 and Tables 1–3 and 1–4). The central nervous system (CNS) syndrome, with death within a matter of minutes to hours, results from massive irradiation. The more protracted forms of irradiation effects that last weeks, months, or years are related to bone marrow and the more chronic effects of irradiation. *(Rubin and Farber, p. 339)*

12. **(A)** The main cellular target for the action of radiation is DNA and the alteration of cellular division. Although massive doses of irradiation can cause damage to cell membrane, mitochondria, ribosomes, and indirectly the cytosome, these are not as characteristic as the effect on DNA, which is the cause of most of the cellular abnormalities in postirradiation syndromes. *(Cotran et al., pp. 426–427)*

13. **(A)** Apoptosis can occur secondary to certain viral diseases. Councilman bodies are one example of apoptosis in which the dead hepatocytes appear to be shrunken, pyknotic, and intensively eosinophilic. The Councilman bodies contain fragmented nuclei. There is no evidence of inflammation around the Councilman bodies. Atrophy, hyperplasia, metaplasia, and necrosis are not resulting in Councilman bodies formation. *(Cotran et al., pp. 18, 19)*

14. **(C)** Electromagnetic radiations in the gamma range are more penetrating than x-rays, since they are of a higher energy (shorter wave length). Alpha and beta are particulate radiations and are, therefore, less penetrating, as are protons (Table 1–5). *(Chandrasoma and Taylor, pp. 171–173)*

Table 1–5. SUMMARY OF EFFECTS OF IONIZATION IRRADIATION

Type of Ionization Irradiation	Tissue Penetration
X-rays	High (measured in feet)
Gamma rays	High (measured in feet)
Beta rays	Low (measured as 1.0 mm–1 cm)
Alpha rays	Very low (measured as <1.0 mm)
Protons	Intermediate (between gamma and beta)
Neutrons	High (measured in feet)

15. **(A)** Alpha particles have the highest linear energy transfer. They dissipate their energy in the shortest distance and are, therefore, the most damaging per unit length of penetration. Compare this with Question 14 and Table 1–5. *(Chandrasoma and Taylor, pp. 171–173)*

16. **(B)** After castration there is atrophy of the epithelial lining of the acinar glands of the prostate. Histologically, the acini are smaller, and the epithelial cells become flattened with decreased secretory activity. These changes are secondary to the lack of hormonal stimulation. *(Rubin and Farber, p. 952)*

17. **(C)** Death of immune cells, both B and T lymphocytes, after cytokine depletion, as well as deletion of autoreactive T cells in the developing thymus, is seen in apoptosis. The loss of lymphocytes in the thymus after glucocorticoid administration has also been proved in different research studies, secondary to apoptosis. *(Cotran et al., pp. 18, 19)*

18.   **(B)** The correct order of sensitivity of these tissues is lymphocytes followed by red cell precursors, intestinal epithelial cells, neurons, keratinocytes, fibroblasts, and finally muscle fibers (Tables 1–3 and 1–4). *(Chandrasoma and Taylor, pp. 171–175)*

19.   **(D)** During apoptosis, histological cellular changes occur. Some of them could be appreciated under the light microscopy, but many of them must be seen with electron microscopy. There is cell shrinkage, chromatin condensation, and formation of cytoplasmic blebs and apoptotic bodies. Phagocytosis of the apoptotic cells occur by adjacent healthy cells, either parenchymal cells or macrophages. Plasma membranes are thought to remain intact during the apoptosis until the last stages. One of the most important changes to consider in apoptosis is the failure of the apoptotic cells to elicit an inflammatory reaction, and this contrasts with cell necrosis. *(Cotran et al., pp. 18–23)*

20.   **(D)** Apoptosis by definition is programmed cell death that occurs in normal tissues. Therefore, apoptosis can be distinguished from autolysis, fat necrosis, liquefactive necrosis, or caseous necrosis. *(Cotran et al., pp. 18–23)*

21.   **(E)** The regulation of intracellular calcium and concentration is regulated by the mitochondria. None of the organelles listed in the answer of this question participate in the calcium regulation or sequestration. Moreover, it has been demonstrated that during reperfusion of irreversibly injured cells, large influx of calcium ions occur. An excess of calcium ions is known to induce loss of mitochondrial function, and it may be that the inability to reverse mitochondrial dysfunction reflects the flooding of the cells with calcium, rather than being a consequence of the mitochondrial abnormalities themselves. *(Rubin and Farber, pp. 5, 6)*

22.   **(A)** Hyaline degeneration is a complex series of cellular events. It has a particular appearance microscopically, with its ground-glass, pink-staining appearance and intact cell membrane. The accumulation of lipids, the presence of calcium salts, or the amorphous appearance of the cell with no discernible membranes as seen in amyloid are distinctly different. The pyknotic nucleus is not a characteristic of hyaline degeneration (Tables 1–1 and 1–2). *(Cotran et al., p. 45)*

23.   **(A)** Lipofuscin pigment granules represent an undigested material that results from intracellular lipid peroxidation. The enzymes in the lysosomes are capable of degrading most proteins and carbohydrates, but some lipids remain undigested. Lysosomes with undigested debris may persist within the cells as residual bodies or maybe extruded. Lipofuscin represents these granules. Actually, lipofuscin is the result of autophagy, which is a phenomenon involving the removal of damaged organelles during the cell injury and the cellular remodeling of differentiation, and it is particularly pronounced in cells undergoing atrophy induced by nutrient deprivation or hormonal involution. *(Cotran et al., p. 25)*

24.   **(D)** Hydropic change with the accumulation of materials in the cytoplasm can be altered if the stimulus is stopped. Amyloid deposition is a permanent state. Fat necrosis, with death of the cell, clearly is not reversible, neither is colliquative necrosis. Apoptosis is a phenomenon in which the cell nucleus becomes condensed, and the cell membrane and cytoplasmic contents condense around the nuclear material, forming densely staining bodies known as apoptotic bodies. This, again, clearly is not a reversible situation. *(Rubin and Farber, pp. 3–5)*

25.   **(D)** The process of necrosis results in the final rupture of the cell and release of its contents into the surrounding media. Cloudy swelling, noted in Question 24, is reversible because the cell membrane remains viable. Pyknosis and apoptosis are nuclear events that are not reversible but in which the cell membrane remains intact and is, therefore, distinctly different from coagulation necrosis. *(Cotran et al., pp. 8–15)*

26.   **(B)** Swelling of the RER and cell membrane blebs are early changes in cell injury and may even be reversible (Tables 1–6 and 1–7). Fat necrosis and caseous necrosis are characteristically seen in certain tissues, such as fat, or are related to damage by the tubercle bacillus in the case of caseous necrosis. In coagulative necrosis,

Table 1–6. COMPARISON OF MAIN SEQUENCES IN CELL DAMAGE PRODUCED BY CHEMICAL (TOXIC) AND ISCHEMIC INJURY

	Phase I	Phase II	Phase III
Chemical injury (carbon tetrachloride)			
— Endoplasmic reticulum	Lipid Peroxidation ——————————————————————→		Debris
	Membrane damage		
→ Polysomes ———————————————	Protein synthesis ————→	Fatty change	
Mitochondria			
→ Cell membranes ———————————	Alteration in sodium-potassium ——→ balance	Cell swelling	
→ Lysosomes ———————————————————————————→		Cell swelling	
→ Cell sap ———————————————————————————————→		Alteration in pH	
→ Nucleus ———→			Clumping of chromatin
			└→ Karyolysis
			└→ Debris
Ischemic injury			
→ Endoplasmic reticulum ———————————————————————→		Dilatation with detachment of polysomes and decrease in protein synthesis ————→	Debris → Myelin forms
→ Mitochondria ———————————————————————→		Swelling and loss of enzymes ——→	Flocculation
Decreased respiration			└→ Debris
			└→ Myelin forms
— Cell membranes ———→			Release of cell enzymes CPK[a] SGOT SGPT
Alteration in sodium-potassium balance			
→ Lysosomes ———→			Increased permeability Release of hydrolases
→ Cell sap ——————————————	Increased glycosis	Decrease in pH	
→ Cell nucleus ———————————————————————————→		Clumping of nuclear protein ——→	Karyolysis
			└→ Debris
			└→ Myelin forms

[a] CPK, creatine phosphokinase; SGOT, serum glutamic-oxaloacetic transaminase; SGPT, serum glutamic-pyruvic transaminase.

Table 1–7. SUMMARY OF ACCUMULATION OF INTRACELLULAR MATERIAL

Type of Substance		Typical Disorder Produced	Typical Cells Involved
Lipids		Fatty change	Liver Heart
Proteins		Hyaline droplets Immunoglobulin (Russell bodies)	Proximal renal tubules Plasma cells
Glycogen		Glycogen storage diseases Diabetes mellitus	Liver, heart, muscle, renal Liver, renal tubules, heart, islet
Complex substances Lipid, carbohydrates Mucopolysaccharides		Gaucher's disease Tay–Sachs disease Niemann–Pick disease	Heart, liver kidney Cells of CNS, Reticuloendothelial cells
Pigments		Lipofuscin Melanin	Liver, heart Skin, tumors, macrophages
	Endogenous	Hematin Hemosiderin	
		Hematin Bilirubin Homogentisic acid	Skin, connective tissue, cartilage
	Exogenous	Carbon ?	Histiocytes Macrophages

which is in some respects most similar to caseous necrosis, this is an ischemic event and related to the loss of blood supply. Gangrene characteristically is the result of this with a superimposed bacterial or fungal infection. *(Chandrasoma and Taylor, pp. 16–19)*

27. **(A)** Glycogen storage disorders result from a variety of causes. There is accumulation of abnormal amounts of glycogen, which is a normal substance, and, therefore, this does not represent an exogenous amount of abnormal material or the deposition of lipids or mucopolysaccharides or immunoglobulins. There is a variety of reasons for glycogen to be stored abnormally in these cells (Table 1–7). *(Cotran et al., pp. 41–42)*

28. **(C)** In reversible cell injury, two of the most prominent and early findings are fatty change as well as cellular swelling. The cellular swelling is a result of the cells of maintaining ionic and fluid homeostasis. The fatty change is seen in sublethal cell injury characterized by toxic, metabolic, or hypoxic injuries. It is possible to demonstrate fatty change in the cells that are forming vacules in the cytoplasm, rather small, or as large as the entire cell. These are most commonly seen in hepatocytes, as well as myocardial cells. In reversible cell injury, the most important changes are: (1) plasma membrane alterations; (2) mitochondrial changes; (3) dilatation of the endoplasmic reticulum; and (4) nuclear alterations. *(Cotran et al., p. 15)*

29. **(B)** Necrosis refers to a spectrum of morphologic changes that follow cell death in living tissue, largely resulting from the progressive degradative action of enzymes of the lethally injured cells. The morphologic changes seen in necrosis are the result of two processes: (1) enzymatic digestion of the cells; and (2) denaturation of proteins. Different types of necrosis has been described such as coagulative necrosis, liquefactive necrosis, caseous necrosis, fat necrosis, and gangrenous necrosis. Whatever the terminology used for describing the gross appearance of the necrosis, all of them develop a migration of inflammatory cells (polymorphonuclear cells) that are responding to the substances produced on the necrotic area. *(Cotran et al., pp. 15–20)*

30. **(D)** When necrosis of fat cells occurs, the resultant pH changes and the formation of lipid soaplike materials are highly attractant to calcium ions, and calcium deposition is, therefore, a very characteristic phenomenon. In amyloid degeneration, hyaline degeneration, and hydropic change, no such calcium deposition is seen. Colliquative necrosis has in common with fat necrosis the disruption of cells and the breakdown and liquefaction of tissue. If this does not involve predominantly fat cells, calcium deposition is less likely (Tables 1–6 and 1–7). *(Cotran et al., pp. 17, 18)*

31–33. These questions recall information concerning recognition of organelles in the cytoplasm of cells (Figure 1–2). *(Darnell et al., pp. 109–115)*

31. **(C)** This refers to the Golgi complex.

32. **(D)** The mitochondria are depicted.

33. **(C)** Number 7 refers to the nuclear membrane.

34–37. **(34-B, 35-D, 36-A, 37-C)** These questions concern definitions of various radiobiologic units. *(Chandrasoma and Thomas, p. 177)*

38–40. **(38-A, 39-A, 40-B)** Whole body exposure to 10,000 rads is likely to produce a very rapid onset of severe central nervous system damage along with damage to multiple other systems. This will produce seizures and vomiting because of cerebral edema and raised intercranial pressure. Vomiting could also occur as a result of whole body irradiation to 700 rads, as can diarrhea, because the effect on the gastrointestinal tract may produce both. Whole body exposure to 700 rads is more likely to produce the later-onset clinical manifestations of bone marrow syndrome, which would not be applicable in these alternatives. Whole body exposure to 3,000 rads would certainly produce the gastrointestinal syndrome and severe diarrhea (Table 1–4). *(Chandrasoma and Taylor, pp. 170–177)*

41–45. **(41-A, 42-A, 43-D, 44-B, 45-E)** Fatty degeneration can occur as a result of damage to the polysomes and mitochondria, particularly in toxic injury as seen in carbon tetrachloride poisoning of the liver. Choline deficiency may produce abnormal mitochondrial changes characteristic of fatty change and also further abnormal accumulation of fat because of deficient lipid metabolism in the liver cells. The picture of caseous necrosis is typically that of a loss of architecture with necrosis, with an appearance of a cheesy consistency. This usually is associated with necrosis associated with the lipid materials liberated from the tubercle bacillus. Cloudy swelling may occur as a result of both oxidative phosphorylation and mitochondrial and decreased activity but is a somewhat earlier change than that seen in fatty change in the same cells. A certain amount of overlap may occur. Fibrinoid necrosis is a breakdown of small blood vessels in which fibrin and other plasma proteins leak into the vessel wall and are trapped in the process, giving rise to a smudged-out and hyalinized appearance of the blood vessel walls (Figure 1–2, Tables 1–1, 1–2, and 1–7). The term "fibrinoid" is used to denote a fibrin-like staining characteristic that is not necessarily all fibrin. *(Cotran et al., pp. 15–19)*

46–48. (46-C, 47-A, 48-E) Primary lysosomes are membrane-delimited structures containing a diverse mixture of hydrolytic enzymes. Fusion of a primary lysosome with membrane-bound exogenous material is called "heterophagy." The fusion of a primary lysosome with endogenous cellular material is called "autophagy." The enzymes within the primary lysosome are synthesized in the rough endoplasmic reticulum and packaged into vesicles in the Golgi structures. These enzymes are capable of accelerating the dissolution of most endogenous (DNA, RNA, proteins, lipids, and carbohydrates) cellular, components as well as destroying exogenous materials, such as bacteria or viruses. The residual bodies are inclusions within the lysosomal vesicles composed of particular remnants that remain after autophagy or heterophagy. The residual bodies may be discharged from the cell through a process termed "exocytosis." In exocytosis, the cell membrane of the phagosome fuses with that of the outer cell membrane, liberating the contents of the phagosome out into the extracellular space (Figure 1–4). *(Cotran et al., pp. 25–27)*

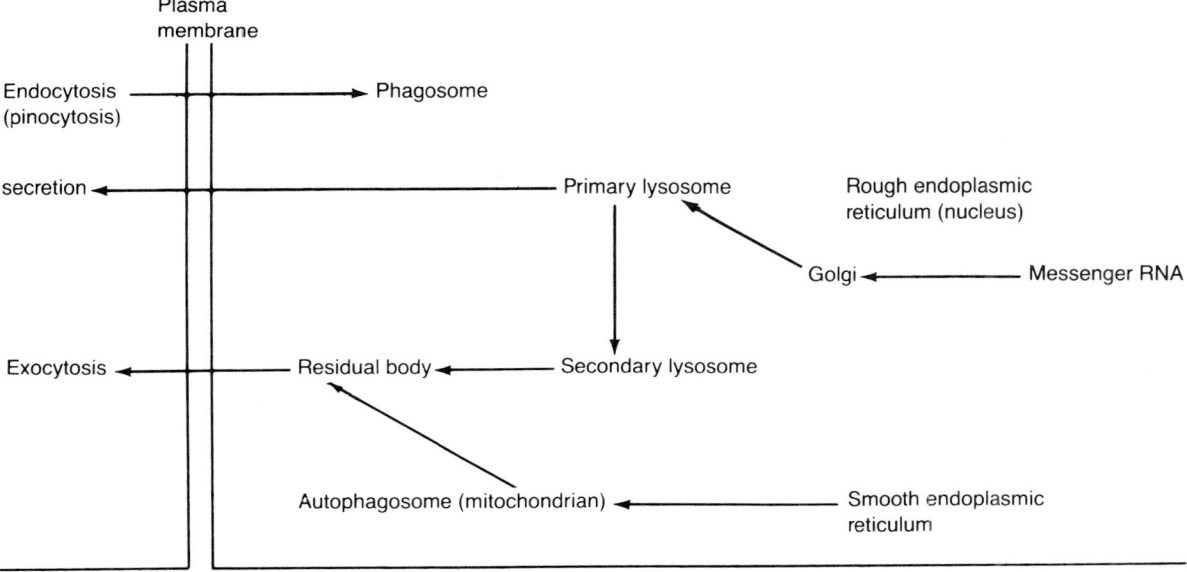

Cellular Accumulations: Result from an imbalance between endocytosis of materials, and their metabolism, and by-products removal through secretion or exocystosis. This also applies to normal by-products of cell organelle turn-over and replacement (autophagy).

Apoptosis: This is a form of cell death without disruption of the plasma membrane. The cell simply shrinks about the condensed nucleus forming a dense staining body called an apoptotic body which may then be phagocytized by macrophages. The result is cell deletion without rupture of the cell contents into the surrounding tissues. This method of aging in tissues, and deletion of cells is seen in a wide variety of circumstances and is being increasingly recognized as an important mechanism also seen in neoplasms.

Figure 1–4. The lysosomal system.

49–52. (49-D, 50-C, 51-A, 52-B) Saponification is the process of converting fats into alkali salts. Saponification is commonly seen in areas of fat necrosis with subsequent calcium deposition, such as recurrent chronic pancreatitis. Pancreatitis releases the enzyme lipase into the adjacent fatty tissues, breaking down triglycerides to free fatty acids and glycerol. The fatty acids complex with plasma calcium to form soaps. Residual bodies are the insoluble debris which remain in secondary phagolysosomes after enzymatic oxidation. They are eventually discharged from the cell by the process of exocytosis (Figure 1–4). Cloudy swelling is an early reversible cellular change caused by alterations of the plasma membrane's ability to maintain the energy-dependent sodium pump with subsequent disordered cell water homeostasis. In cloudy swelling, there is expansion of the cytoplasm, endoplasmic reticulum, and mitochondrium by an inflow of extracellular and intracellular water. Karyorrhexis is an irreversible change indicating death of the cell. Karyorrhexis is typified morphologically by progressive dissolution and disappearance of the nucleus. The nuclear dissolution is due to lysosomal enzymes, such as ribonuclease, which are liberated intracellularly during states of irreversible cell injury (Table 1–8). *(Rubin and Farber, pp. 13–16; Chandrasoma and Taylor, pp. 5–7, 15–17)*

53–56. (53-C, 54-D, 55-A, 56-E) Coagulation necrosis is most commonly caused by sudden cessation of blood flow to such organs as the heart, kidney, or spleen. Histologically, there is lack of staining in the affected tissues by routinely used hematoxylin and eosin dyes. This lack of dye uptake results in a characteristic faded ghost-like image of the normal architecture when the coagulated tissue is examined microscopically. Infarctions of the cerebral cortex, such as those following an occlusion of the middle cerebral artery, usually result in liquefaction necrosis. As the name implies, there is gross softening and rapid liquefaction of the brain tissue. The liquid tissues are composed of necrotic debris, numerous phagocytic microglial cells, a lack of granulation tissue, and an absence of collagen deposition. Infection by tubercle bacilli produces caseous necrosis and multinucleate Langhans' giant cells in individuals with intact delayed hypersensitivity. Dilation of the endoplasmic reticulum is a reversible cellular change. Other reversible cellular changes include cloudy swelling, fatty infiltration, ribosomal detachment, cytoplasmic blebs, and vacuole formation (Table 1–8). *(Chandrasoma and Taylor, pp. 15–18; Darnell et al., pp. 12–16)*

57–60. (57-D, 58-B, 59-C, 60-A) Various pigments are found in cells in both normal and pathologic conditions. Bilirubin is formed in the reticuloendothelial system through the normal catabolism of the hemoglobin porphyrin ring present in senescent erythrocytes. Newly formed bilirubin is then transported from the reticuloendothelial system into the liver. Once in the liver, bilirubin is conjugated and excreted into the bile. Additional chemical alterations allow bilirubin to exit the body in urine (urobilinogen) or feces (stercobilinogen). A significant increase in the serum bilirubin is termed "jaundice." Jaundice may result from increased erythrocytic destruction (hemolysis), decreased uptake by the liver (hepatitis), or biliary tract obstruction (stones). Lipofuscin is a "wear-and-tear" pigment also called "lipochrome." It is found in the cytoplasm of many cells throughout the body, particularly with aging, malnutrition, or chronic disease. Hemosiderin is an aggregation of ferritin micelles. The iron molecules of hemosiderin impart a brownish-yellow hue to involved tissue. Hemosiderin is normally found in the histiocytes of the reticuloendothelial system. States of increased hemosiderin deposition are termed "hemosiderosis." Hemosiderosis may be either hereditary

Table 1–8. STRUCTURAL CHANGES IN CELL INJURY AND DEATH

Reversible Cell Injury	Irreversible Cell Injury
Blebs in cell membrane	Defects in cell membranes
Intramembraneous aggregations	Cell membrane myelin figures
Generalized cytoplasmic swelling	
Endoplasmic reticulum swelling	Lysosomal autolysis and rupture
Mitochondrial swelling with small densities	Endoplasmic reticulum rupture
Clumping of nuclear chromatin	Mitochondrial swelling with large densities
Detachment of ribosomes	Pyknosis, karyorrhexis, karyolysis
	Rupture of ribosomes

or acquired. Melanin is formed through the oxidation of tyrosine. Melanin pigment is brown–black and formed in melanosome organelles present in melanocytes. Once synthesized, melanin may be passed through melanocytic dendrites into adjacent keratinocytes. Melanin has a protective effect against actinic damage. (*Cotran et al., pp. 24–26, 42; Chandrasoma and Taylor, pp. 7–12*)

61–64. (61-B, 62-A, 63-E, 64-C) Reversible and irreversible cellular injuries may be morphologically correlated with corresponding alterations in the organelles, nucleus, cytoplasm, and cell membrane (Table 1–8). The cellular organelles each have distinct functions. The ribosomes are the site of protein synthesis as amino acid building blocks are strung together over the RNA template. Primary lysosomes are membrane-bound organelles containing hydrolytic enzymes. The primary lysosomes fuse with foreign or endogenous material to form phagolysosomes. The mitochondria are the major site of oxidative phosphorylation and energy production. Centrioles are intracellular organelles whose primary function is in organizing mitosis and chromosomal disjunction. The Golgi apparatus organelle packages enzymes into membrane-delimited structures. (*Cotran et al., pp. 25–29*)

65–68. (65-E, 66-D, 67-A, 68-C) Pompe's disease is a hereditary glycogen storage disease (glycogenoses). Affected individuals are unable to metabolize fully glycogen because of a lack of the acid maltase enzyme. As a result, glycogen bodies accumulate in muscle cells throughout the body leading to cardiac failure in the infantile form of the disease. Apoptosis is the atrophic disappearance or dropping out of individual cells. In severe liver damage, such as with yellow fever or viral hepatitis, the apoptotic cells are called Councilman bodies. Civatte bodies are apoptotic cells from the basal epidermal layers seen with the dermatologic disorder of lichen planus. Both Councilman and Civatte bodies share a similar morphology being eosinophilic, anucleate, shrunken, and measuring about 10 microns in diameter. The Gandy–Gamna bodies are large (0.4 to 1.0 cm) multi-

cellular collections of hemosiderin, scar tissue, and calcium in the spleens of individuals with portal hypertension and splenomegaly. (*Rubin and Farber, pp. 780–782, 1101–1102, 1226–1229, 1409, 1431–1433*)

69–72. (69-E, 70-C, 71-A, 72-B) Ionizing radiation is divided into particulate and waveform radiation. Alpha particles have minimal skin penetration potential and have a mass number of four. Beta particles can penetrate human tissue to a depth of about 1 cm and have negligible mass. X-rays and gamma rays are both waveform, nonparticulate radiations with high energies and deep tissue penetration abilities. An acute dose of 25 rads would produce no significant immediate effects. An exposure of 150 rads would produce an acute radiation syndrome with a 2- to 8-week latency period and the clinical features of nausea, vomiting, malaise, and fatigue. A single 250 rads exposure would produce a hematopoietic radiation syndrome with a latency period of 1 to 2 weeks and clinical symptoms of leukopenia and thrombocytopenia. An acute dose of 800 rads would produce a gastrointestinal radiation syndrome with a 1- to 14-day latency and clinical features of diarrhea, fluid loss, electrolyte imbalance, and gastrointestinal mucosal necrosis. A dose of 1,250 rads would result in a cerebral syndrome characterized by ataxia, convulsions, delirium, coma, and death within 2 days. (*Chandrasoma and Taylor, pp. 171–177*)

73–76. (73-C, 74-D, 75-A, 76-B) Cell death invariably results in necrosis. Different body sites and different pathologic processes may influence the morphologic pattern of necrosis. Acute pancreatitis, for example, may produce enzymatic fat necrosis characterized by the death of adjacent fat cells and enzymatically catalyzed (lipase) decomposition of triglycerides into free fatty acids. The released fatty acids then combine with calcium to form soaps (saponification). Syphilitic infections typically produce gummatous necrosis attributable to cell-mediated hypersensitivity to the infecting organisms. Most autoimmune disorders can cause fibrinoid necrosis characterized by acellular, strongly eosinophilic alterations in target organs. Gangrenous necrosis is a type of coagulative necrosis. It is common in the distal extremities of individuals with ischemia. The ischemic tissue dies and then becomes black, hard, and shrunken (dry gangrene). If there is superimposed bacterial infection, the tissue may liquefy or suppurate (wet gangrene). *(Cotran et al., pp. 15–19, 362–365)*

77–80. (77-E, 78-A, 79-D, 80-B) A number of intermediate cytoplasmic filaments are present in the cytoskeleton of cells. Cells usually synthesize only one or two kinds of intermediate filaments. For example, desmin is produced by smooth muscle cells, astrocytes make glial fibrillary acid protein, neurofilament is made by neurons, vimentin is found in mesenchymal cells, and mesothelial cells synthesize both keratin and vimentin. These filaments can serve as markers to identify the cell of origin in undifferentiated tumors. For example, undifferentiated carcinomas (malignant tumors of epithelial cells) will usually retain the ability to manufacture cytokeratin. By demonstrating the presence of cytokeratin in a tumor cell, we can usually assume that it arose from an aberrant epithelial cell line. In the practice of surgical pathology, a battery of several filaments are tested together as a panel. Most testing uses an immunologic method with a visible peroxidase endpoint (immunoperoxidase method). *(Cotran et al., pp. 27, 28)*

81–84. (81-D, 82-B, 83-A, 84-C) The cytomembrane skeleton of most cells contains the structural proteins of ankyrin and spectrin. In some cells, such as erythrocytes, the hereditary absence of membrane skeleton proteins may lead to deformed cells and hemolytic anemia. Intermediate filaments are present in the cytoplasm of cells. Different types of cells have different intermediate filaments. For example, vimentin is present in all mesenchymal cells, desmin in smooth muscle cells, and cytokeratin in epithelial cells. Mallory bodies, intracellular cytoplasmic eosinophilic inclusions, are usually seen scattered in hepatocytes of individuals with alcoholic liver disease. The Mallory bodies, also termed "alcoholic hyaline," are fibrillary degenerative concretions derived from the

cell's cytoskeleton and contain the intermediate filament cytokeratin. Neurofibrillary tangles are seen with increased frequency in the cerebral neurons of Alzheimer's patients. They appear in the cytoplasm as agyrophilic complexes of interwoven paired helical protein filaments. *(Cotran et al., pp. 27, 28; Chandrasoma and Taylor, pp. 649–651, 933–935)*

85.   (E) Mercury poisons cells by binding to the sulfhydryl moieties present in proteins. This binding usually inactivates a wide variety of enzyme systems throughout the cell via occupation of the enzymatic active site or by steric hindrance of the active site. Most accidental mercury poisonings are encountered in the mining or chemical industries. Inhalation is the usual route of poison exposure. Once inhaled, mercury is preferentially distributed to the kidneys. Binding to the sulfhydral groups of the proximal tubular cells results in cell death that displays a coagulative necrosis pattern. In lower doses, mercury intoxication exhibits principally neuropsychiatric features. *(Rubin and Farber, pp. 330, 331)*

86.   (A) Cyanide poisons by inhibiting cellular respiration. Cyanide irreversibly binds to the enzyme cytochrome oxidase, the final enzyme in the respiratory chain, blocking respiration and oxygen-dependent energy production. Fatal intoxication can occur with the ingestion of only 0.1 mg of sodium cyanide. Most poisonings are suicidal in nature. However, some accidental intoxications result from exposure during the refining of gold and during laetrile therapy. *(Rubin and Farber, p. 328)*

87.   (C) Colchicine inhibits cellular division. Colchicin is an alkaloid found in the seeds of the meadow saffron. Increased quantities of uric acid, a purine catabolite, is found in most individuals affected with gout, and therapies are directed at reducing serum and urinary concentrations of uric acid. Colchicine is prescribed for patients with gout in an attempt to reduce cellular mitosis and uric acid production. The clinical spectrum of gout usually includes podagra, tophus formation, and renal crystal deposition. Other antigout therapeutic agents used may include analgesics, anti-inflammatory drugs, and allopurinol (xanthine oxidase inhibitor). *(Rubin and Farber, p. 1405)*

88. **(F)** Carbon tetrachloride damages cells through the formation of active-free radicals. Carbon tetrachloride is converted into toxic-free radicals by the smooth endoplasmic reticulum's mixed-function oxidase system. This system is designed to inactivate lipid soluble drugs. Once the formation of active-free radicals is begun, the reaction becomes autocatalytic with rapid destruction of the endoplasmic reticulum, dissociation of polyribosomes, and cytoplasmic lipid accumulation. The cells of the liver, brain, and kidneys are prominently affected. *(Cotran et al., p. 15)*

REFERENCES

Chandrasoma P, Taylor CR. *Concise Pathology,* 3rd ed. Norwalk, CT: Appleton & Lange, 1998.

Cotran RS, Kumar V, Robbins SL. *Robbins Pathologic Basis of Disease,* 6th ed. Philadelphia: Saunders, 1999.

Darnell J, Lodish M, Baltimore I. *Molecular Cell Biology,* 2nd ed. New York: Scientific American Books, 1990.

Rubin E, Farber JL. *Pathology.* Philadelphia: Lippincott, 1999.

CHAPTER 2

Inflammation, Healing, and Repair

I consider inflammation as an increased action of that power which a part naturally possesses; and in healthy inflammation at least, it is probably attended with an increase in power; but in inflammations which terminate in mortification there is no increase in power, but on the contrary a diminution of it.

—John Hunter (1794)

A central area in general pathology is covered extensively in this chapter. It is important to be able to identify the cardinal signs of inflammation and to understand the underlying mechanisms that produce these signs. The importance of an essentially vascular and microvascular response of the tissue to any injury must be appreciated, and the sequential events that result from injury must be understood.

The importance of fluid production in inflammation, including the differences between exudates and transudates (Table 2–1) is of considerable importance, and some understanding of the various chemical mediators of inflammation and their link with the complement system, and potentially with coagulation, should be appreciated. A good understanding of the processes of inflammation per se will permit evaluation of localized inflammatory response, with its own peculiarities, at any given site.

The various complications of the inflammatory response should be understood—the formation of pus, the abnormalities of the vasculature, and the production and manifestations of chronic inflammation that are related to the process of healing and repair. Although healing and repair are inevitable events after any injury in which inflammation has taken place, the degree of resolution with or without the formation of scar tissue depends on various factors, including complications. In addition, the relationship between acute inflammation, healing and repair, and chronic inflammation should be understood.

ACUTE INFLAMMATION

Basic Facts

Acute inflammation is an inevitable response of living vasculature to any injurious stimulus; a necessary precursor to healing and repair.

Cardinal Signs

- **Redness.** Increase in blood flow with stagnation and engorgement of blood vessels
- **Swelling.** Perivascular exudation of protein-rich fluid, the degree depending on the localization of the process and the severity of the response
- **Heat.** Variable, depending on increase in vascularity and proximity to body surfaces
- **Pain.** Complicated interaction of the physical and chemical components of the process
- **Loss of function.** Variable, depending on the site, severity, and extent

The process of acute inflammation is an extension and prolongation of the response to injury illustrated by the triple response of Lewis, as shown in Figure 2–1.

- **Chemical medication.** The controlled and regulated mechanism of enhancement of progressive incremental leukocytosis and phagocytosis
- **Systemic effects.** Include fever, increased erythrocyte sedimentation rate (ESR), and leukocytosis

Summary of Patterns and Modes of Acute Inflammation

- **Serous.** Collection of exudate in the simplest form of acute inflammation, often representing the earliest type of exudative process, with few leukocytes present

Table 2–1. COMPARISON OF CHARACTERISTICS OF DIFFERENT TYPES OF EFFUSIONS (FLUIDS FROM BODY CAVITIES)

| | Transudate | Exudate due to inflammation | | |
		Early or Mild	Moderate–Severe	Severe Suppurative
Protein	Low	Moderate	High, with fibrinogen	Very high, with fibrinogen and fibrin
Specific gravity	Low	Medium	High	High
Cellularity	Very low	Low	Moderate PMNs[a] a few monocytes	Many PMNs with toxic changes, dying and dead bacteria, RBCs[b] in some cases
Coagulability	No	Usually no	Yes	Variable, depending on enzymes released

[a] PMN, polymorphonuclear leukocyte.
[b] RBC, red blood cell.

- **Fibrinous.** Exudation of fluid rich in fibrinogen, which on contact with body linings and surfaces deposits strands of fibrin
- **Catarrhal.** The process of inflammation involving mucus-secreting surfaces in which the fibrin and protein exudate is mixed with mucus
- **Suppurative.** Purulent exudate, containing fibrin and numerous neutrophils
- **Membranous (pseudomembranous).** A type of catarrhal inflammation with formation of a pseudomembrane exudate adherent to the underlying surface

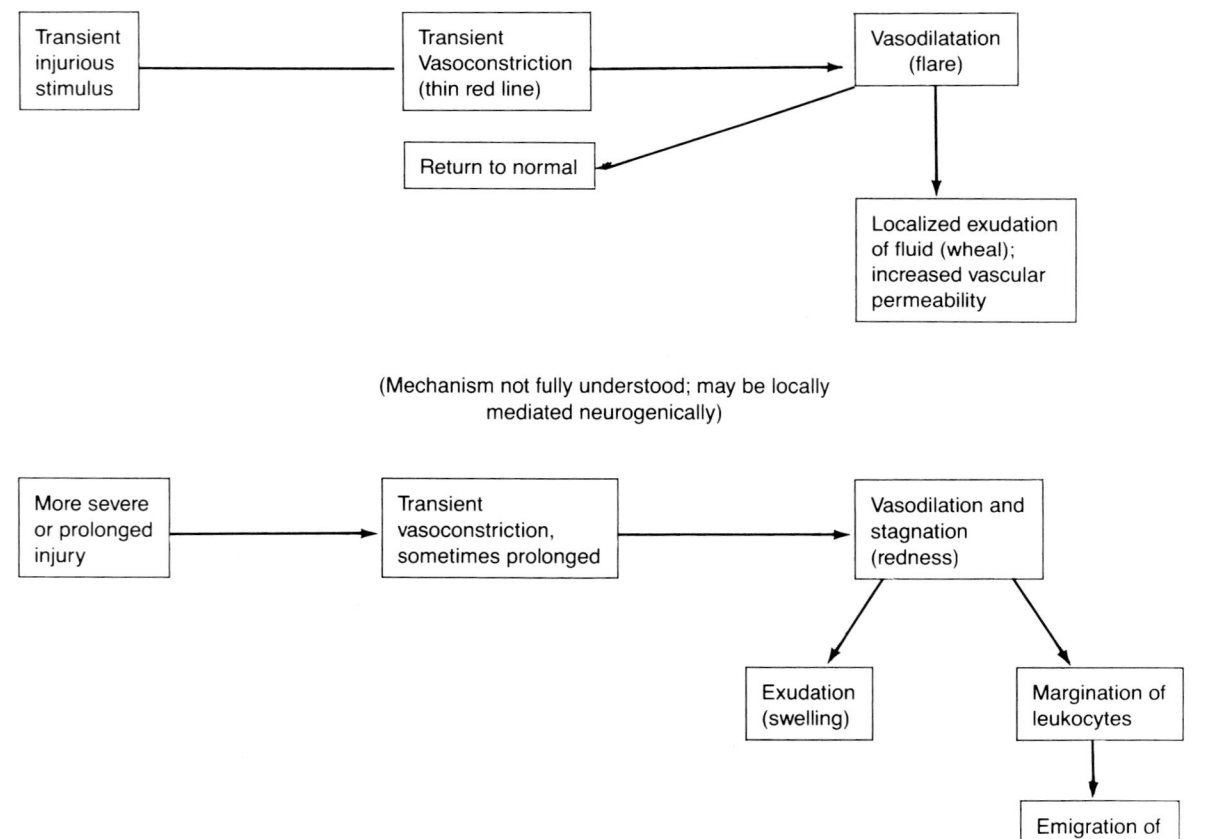

Figure 2–1. Triple response to injury (Lewis).

- **Hemorrhagic.** Severe inflammatory exudate associated with damage to capillaries and consequent diapedesis and hemorrhage of red cells

Further Modifications According to Type and Site
- **Effusions—body cavities.** Serous, fibrinous, purulent
- **Cellulitis—connective tissue.** If breakdown of tissue occurs, allows spread of exudate
- **Abscess.** Localized collection of dead and dying organisms and leukocytes with liquefaction necrosis of tissue
- **Ulceration.** Loss of continuity of surface of a tissue or organ, usually epithelial
- **Empyema.** A form of suppurative inflammation with collection of pus in the pleural cavity

Systemic Expression and Recognition in Acute Inflammation
- Fever
- Increased white blood cell count (leukocytosis) with increased proportion of band neutrophils (left shift)
- Elevated ESR
- Increased level of C-reactive protein in serum

CHRONIC INFLAMMATION

Basic Facts and Definitions
Chronic inflammation is a prolonged proliferative cellular response to injury, which may appear de novo or as a consequence of an initial acute inflammatory response (Figures 2–2 and 2–3).

Characteristic Features
An accumulation in the tissues of lymphocytes, plasma cells, and monocytes and macrophages in various combinations. The end result is the production of collagen by stimulated fibroblasts. The appearance is often that of a combination of attempts at healing and repair in the presence of continued inflammatory response (Table 2–2).

Summary of Patterns and Modes of Chronic Inflammation
- **Chronic serous.** The persistence of serous exudation in a body cavity, usually with presence of varying numbers of lymphocytes
- **Chronic fibrous.** The continuation of injury and inflammatory response in the presence of attempts at healing, with resultant increased fibrosis, with variable numbers of lymphocytes

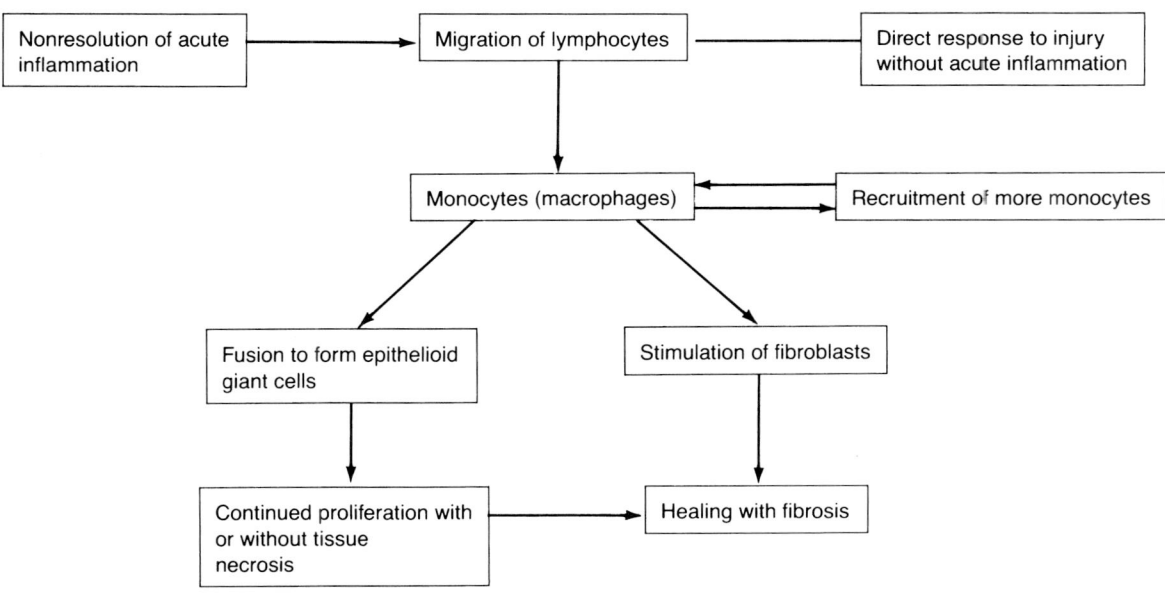

Figure 2–2. Schematic summary of sequential events in chronic inflammation.

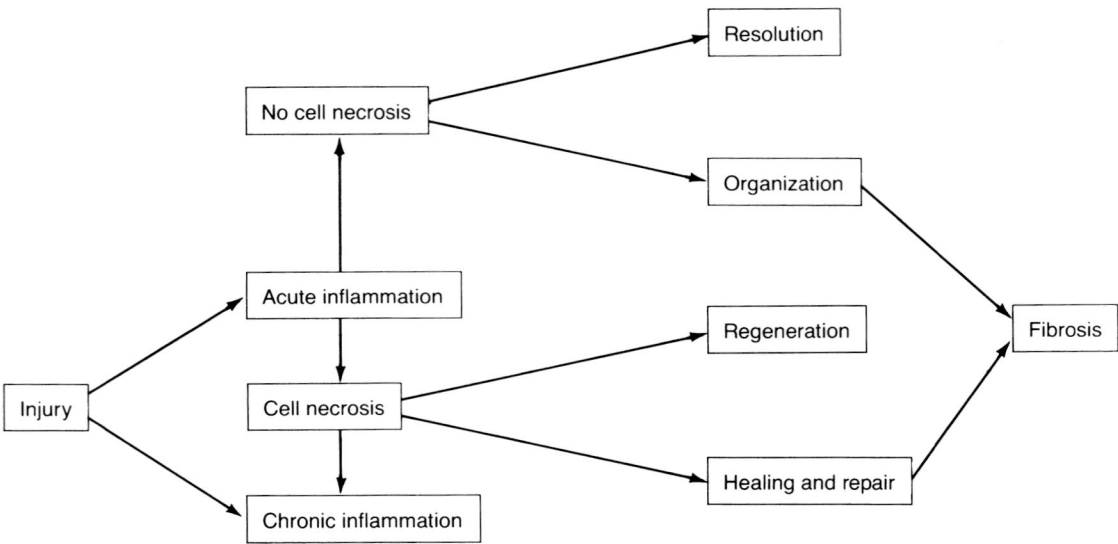

Figure 2–3. Summary of possible responses in injury.

- **Chronic suppurative.** The response to large collections of pus (abscesses) that do not resolve or drain, present typically at the surrounding fibrous encapsulated areas
- **Granulomatous.** Characterized by the formation of granulomas, nodular proliferative lesions composed of monocytes forming sheets of cells (epithelioid histiocytes, some fusing to form multinucleated giant cells) surrounded by lymphocytes and fibroblasts, sometimes with areas of necrosis, such as caseation necrosis (as

in tuberculosis) or gummatous necrosis (as in syphilis)

HEALING AND REPAIR

Definition
Healing is the replacement of lost tissue with collagen (scar tissue). This cannot be achieved by resolution or regeneration.

Table 2–2. COMPARISON OF MAIN FEATURES OF ACUTE AND CHRONIC INFLAMMATION

	Acute Inflammation	Chronic Inflammation
Duration	Usually transient (hours to days), a rapid series of responses to injury (hours to days)	More slowly evolving, usually following acute inflammation that has not subsided (weeks to months)
Main tissue changes	Vascular response with increased permeability and exudation of proteinaceous fluid rich in fibrinogen	Increased collagen formation and proliferative vascular changes (e.g., endarteritis obliterans in long-standing cases) not exudative
Characteristic cells	Polymorphonuclear leukocytes and occasional eosinophils (short-lived cells, recruited by chemotactic mediators)	Lymphocytes, monocytes, plasma cells, macrophages, including multinucleated giant cells (long-lived cells, recruited by chemotactic mediators)
Mediators	Sequential release of substances effecting vascular changes and chemotaxis	Products of inflammatory cells that further recruit other cells (including fibroblasts)
Usual outcome	Resolution with or without regeneration, or healing by repair with some fibrosis; may proceed to suppurative or chronic inflammation	Usually results in fibrosis and varying degrees of tissue replacement, rather than resolution or regeneration

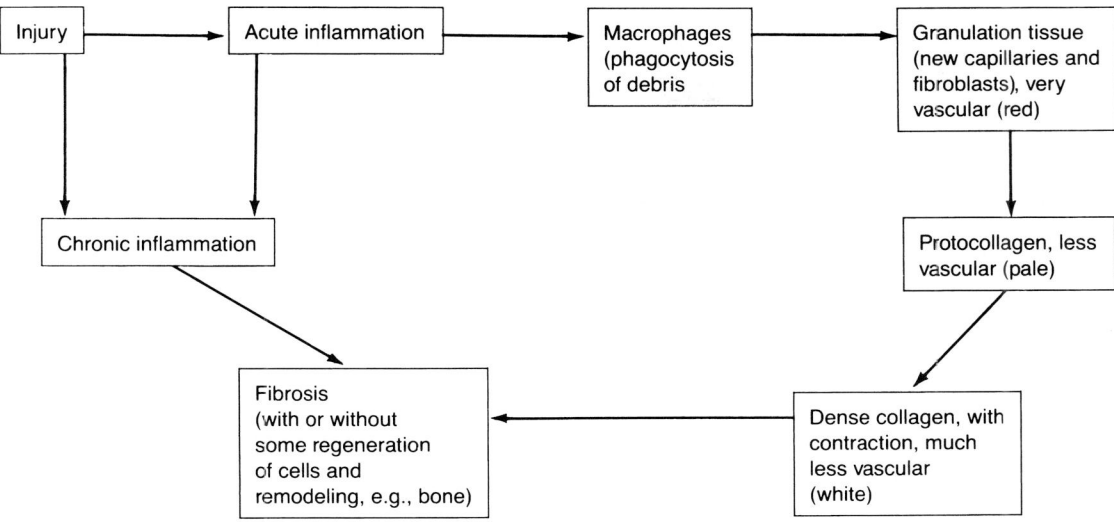

Figure 2–4. Summary of salient features and events in healing and repair.

Basic Facts

A summary of salient features and events in healing and repair is shown in Figure 2–4.

Summary of Patterns and Modes of Healing and Repair

- **Primary union.** Wound healing by first intention
- **Secondary union.** Wound healing by second intention

The basic events are the same, but the amount of granulation and, thus, scar tissue is greater in secondary union.

- **Fibrosis.** Fibrosis is the usual outcome of successful healing, but may result in lesions, some examples of which are shown in Table 2–3. In some severe cases, eventual superimposed calcification or ossification may occur

Table 2–3. EXAMPLES OF DETRIMENTAL ASPECTS OF HEALING BY FIBROSIS IN TISSUES AND ORGANS

Tissue or Organ	Detrimental Aspects of Healing
Lung	Peribronchial fibrosis and bronchiectasis Interstitial pulmonary fibrosis
Pleura	Pleural fibrosis and adhesions
Heart	Ventricular aneurysm formation due to replacement of necrotic myocardial wall by scar tissue
Pericardium	Constrictive pericarditis Pericardial adhesions
Peritoneum	Adhesions and fibrous bands (may cause intestinal obstruction)
Joints	Fibrosis, adhesions (may result in ankylosis)
Stomach	Fibrous stenosis of pyloris (following healing of gastric ulcer)
Brain	Gliosis (may cause hydrocephalus)

Questions

89. The cardinal sign(s) of acute inflammation is (are)

    (A) redness
    (B) swelling
    (C) heat
    (D) pain
    (E) all of the above

90. The manifestation of redness in acute inflammation is most likely the result of

    (A) edema of the tissues
    (B) margination of white blood cells in blood vessels
    (C) thrombosis of blood vessels
    (D) dilation of blood vessels
    (E) fibrin deposition in tissues

91. The cardinal sign of swelling associated with acute inflammation results from

    (A) arteriolar constriction
    (B) arteriolar dilatation
    (C) venous obstruction
    (D) outpouring of protein-rich fluid into tissues
    (E) proliferation of fibroblasts

92. Which of the following is most characteristic of a transudate?

    (A) increase in hydrostatic pressure
    (B) fluid with low specific gravity
    (C) fluid that does not clot on standing
    (D) little or no fibrinogen
    (E) all of the above

93. Which of the following is (are) most associated with an exudate?

    (A) altered vascular permeability
    (B) fluid with high specific gravity
    (C) fluid that clots on standing
    (D) presence of fibrinogen in the fluid
    (E) all of the above

94. Fluid removed from the peritoneal cavity has the following characteristics: high specific gravity, clots spontaneously on standing, turbid and yellow in color, contains fibrinogen. Which of the following does this most fully represent?

    (A) transudate caused by high portal vein pressure
    (B) transudate caused by right heart failure
    (C) exudate caused by peritoneal inflammation
    (D) fluid associated with starvation or protein loss
    (E) hemorrhage caused by ruptured aortic aneurysm

95. Pain associated with acute inflammation is thought to be caused by

    (A) pressure effects of exudate fluid
    (B) histamine
    (C) serotonin
    (D) kinins
    (E) all of the above

96. Which of the following are considered chemical mediators in the inflammatory response?

    (A) histamine
    (B) serotonin
    (C) kinins
    (D) prostaglandins
    (E) all of the above

97. Which type of inflammation commonly is characterized by collections of dead and dying polymorphs, dead and dying bacteria, and necrosis of tissue, all of which form a turbid or thick fluid in tissues?

    (A) catarrhal inflammation
    (B) phlegmonous inflammation
    (C) cellulitis
    (D) abscess formation
    (E) granulomatous inflammation

98. Which of the following events in acute inflammation occurs first?

    (A) phagocytosis
    (B) stasis
    (C) margination of leukocytes
    (D) emigration of leukocytes
    (E) lymphadenitis

99. Inflammation is best defined as

    (A) a reaction of the microcirculation in tissue to injury
    (B) a form of edema
    (C) chemotaxis of white cells to bacteria
    (D) a form of abnormal cell growth
    (E) cellular changes resulting in injury

100. Mediators of vascular permeability are thought to achieve their effects by

    (A) increased intravascular hydrostatic pressure
    (B) decreased intravascular hydrostatic pressure
    (C) contraction of endothelial cells and venules
    (D) dissolving capillary basement membrane
    (E) binding serum albumin to tissue

101. The immediate transient phase of vascular permeability in most types of tissue injury is mediated by

    (A) complement
    (B) Hageman factor
    (C) anaphylatoxin
    (D) histamine
    (E) serum albumin

102. Which of the following is most important in the early or exudative phase of acute inflammation?

    (A) lymphokines
    (B) leukotriene B_4
    (C) histamine
    (D) prostaglandin D_2
    (E) interleukin I

103. Indicate a cell that can undergo mitosis.

    (A) hepatocyte
    (B) cardiac myocyte
    (C) metamyelocyte
    (D) neuron
    (E) neutrophil

104. Which of the following substances is the best to REDUCE the effects of acute inflammation?

    (A) histamine
    (B) prostaglandin D_2
    (C) bradykinin
    (D) aspirin
    (E) eosinophilic chemotactic factor of anaphylaxis

105. Which cell types are most characteristic of tissue with acute inflammation?

(A) plasma cells
(B) foreign body giant cells
(C) Langhans' giant cells
(D) lymphocytes
(E) polymorphonuclear leukocytes

106. Which cell types are most commonly seen in tissue undergoing chronic inflammation?

(A) eosinophil leukocytes
(B) mast cells
(C) polymorphonuclear leukocytes
(D) lymphocytes
(E) platelets

107. The features, edema, presence of fibrin, dilatation, and vascular engorgement, are characteristic of

(A) chronic inflammation
(B) early acute inflammation
(C) suppurative inflammation
(D) late wound healing
(E) granulation tissue

108. The features, monocytes, giant cells, fibroblasts, and lymphocytes, are characteristic of

(A) acute inflammation
(B) granulation tissue
(C) wound healing
(D) chronic inflammation
(E) suppuration

109. The predominant cell seen in an inflammatory response to staphylococcal infection is

(A) lymphocyte
(B) monocyte
(C) eosinophil
(D) mast cell
(E) polymorphonuclear leukocyte (PMN)

110. The predominant cell seen in inflammation resulting from viral infection is

(A) lymphocyte
(B) mast cell
(C) eosinophil
(D) polymorphonuclear leukocyte
(E) plasma cell

111. The predominant cell seen in an inflammatory response to protozoal parasites is

(A) lymphocyte
(B) polymorphonuclear leukocyte
(C) eosinophil
(D) plasma cell
(E) mast cell

112. The predominant cell seen in an inflammatory response to *Salmonella typhi* is

(A) plasma cell
(B) polymorphonuclear leukocyte
(C) monocyte
(D) mast cell
(E) eosinophil

113. Granulation tissue is characterized by

(A) proliferation of new capillaries with fibroblasts and new collagen formation
(B) giant cells and fibroblasts
(C) giant cells and lymphocytes
(D) giant cells, plasma cells, and lymphocytes
(E) neutrophils and necrotic tissue

114. The periphery of a hematoma is infiltrated by new capillaries, fibroblasts, and collagen; this process is described as

(A) lysis of the clot
(B) organization of the hematoma
(C) recanalization
(D) embolization
(E) thrombosis

115. Which of the following are complications of acute inflammation?

(A) suppuration
(B) abscess formation
(C) scar formation
(D) organization with adhesions between mesothelial surfaces
(E) all of the above

116. The proper formation of collagen in a healing wound requires

(A) high levels of adrenocortical hormones
(B) cholesterol
(C) vitamin C
(D) vitamin D
(E) vitamin K

117. The modified form of granulation tissue containing new bone seen around a healing fracture is called

(A) involucrum
(B) laminated bone
(C) fibrocartilage
(D) callus
(E) periosteal new bone

118. After injury with loss of cells, which of the following is (are) most likely to regenerate most completely?

(A) neurons of the central nervous system (CNS)
(B) liver parenchymal cells
(C) skeletal muscle
(D) heart muscle
(E) neurons of the retina

119. Acute inflammatory exudate and saponification occur in

(A) stromal fatty infiltration
(B) fatty metamorphosis
(C) enzymatic fat necrosis
(D) fatty change
(E) cloudy swelling

120. Which of the following best describe granulation tissue?

(A) collagen and giant cells
(B) fibroblasts and macrophages
(C) capillary buds and fibroblasts
(D) capillary buds and lymphocytes
(E) fibroblasts and giant cells

121. By definition granulation tissue most typically contains

(A) fibroblasts and blood vessels
(B) multinucleated giant cells
(C) activated macrophages (epithelioid cells)
(D) lymphocytes and plasma cells
(E) acellular, dense collagen

122. What factor is responsible for inducing angiogenesis?

(A) vascular endothelial growth factor (VEGF)
(B) platelet derived growth factor
(C) epidermal growth factor
(D) transforming growth factor-beta
(E) gamma interferon

123. Hemorrhage in an acute inflammatory reaction is best explained by

(A) fibrinolysis
(B) release of leukocyte lysosomal enzymes
(C) damage to blood vessels
(D) production of lymphokines
(E) release of chemical mediators of vascular permeability

124. The development of tensile strength in a healing wound depends primarily on

(A) contraction of the scar
(B) collagen content of the wound
(C) ascorbic acid content of the scar
(D) appearance of capillary sprouts
(E) level of keloidogenic factor

125. Of the following events that are part of the acute inflammatory response, which would occur THIRD in correct sequence?

(A) vascular dilatation
(B) local hemoconcentration and slowing of blood flow
(C) margination of white blood cells
(D) emigration of white blood cells
(E) increased vascular permeability

126. When there is extensive tissue loss and the reparative process is delayed, it may result in

    (A) dysplasia
    (B) disordered architecture from regeneration
    (C) scar formation
    (D) neoplastic transformation
    (E) physiologic atrophy

127. In a histological section of an acute inflamed area the predominant cell would be

    (A) heart failure cells
    (B) macrophages
    (C) Langhans giant cells
    (D) lymphocytes
    (E) neutrophils

Questions 128 through 130. (Refer to Figure 2–5.)

128. The cells are

    (A) plasma cells
    (B) peritoneal macrophages
    (C) polymorphonuclear leukocytes (PMN)
    (D) lymphocytes
    (E) malignant cells

129. The most appropriate description of the condition is

    (A) chronic peritonitis
    (B) tuberculous peritonitis
    (C) carcinomatous peritonitis
    (D) acute peritonitis
    (E) ascites

130. The most likely source of the reaction is

    (A) ovarian carcinoma
    (B) carcinoma of the stomach
    (C) tuberculosis of the intestine
    (D) ruptured appendix
    (E) heart failure

Questions 131 through 133. (Refer to Figure 2–6.)

131. Which type of reaction does this represent?

    (A) acute suppurative inflammation
    (B) granulomatous inflammation
    (C) subacute inflammation
    (D) granulation tissue
    (E) chronic inflammation

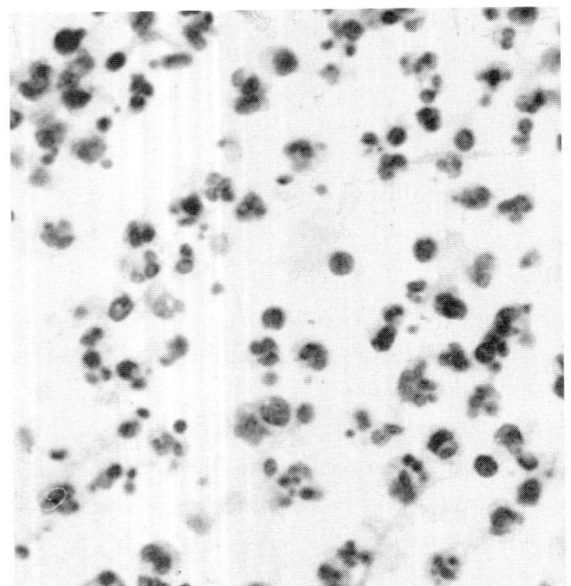

Figure 2–5. Microscopy of fluid removed from the peritoneal cavity.

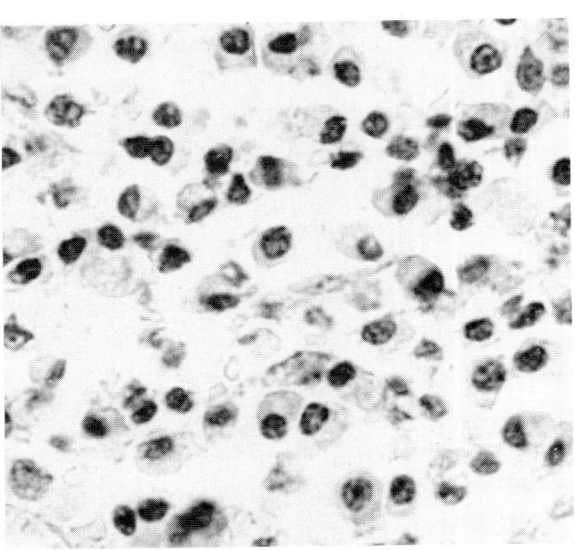

Figure 2–6. High-power photomicrograph of cells seen in a firm, painless skin nodule.

132. Which laboratory investigation is likely to be the most useful diagnostically?

(A) gram stain
(B) stain for acid-fast bacteria
(C) examination of fresh tissue by darkfield illumination
(D) stain for fungi
(E) culture of tissue on blood agar

133. The most likely diagnosis, assuming one of the above techniques to be positive, is

(A) cat-scratch fever
(B) measles
(C) staphylococcal lymphadenitis
(D) tuberculosis lymphadenitis
(E) primary chancre of syphilis

Questions 134 through 136. (Refer to Figure 2–7.)

134. This most likely represents

(A) malignant lymphoma
(B) secondary carcinoma
(C) granulomatous inflammation
(D) acute inflammation
(E) healing by first intention

135. A stain for microorganisms would most likely show

(A) gram-positive cocci in clusters
(B) gram-negative bacilli
(C) Feulgen-positive inclusions for viruses
(D) acid-fast bacilli (Ziehl–Neelsen stain)
(E) malignant cells

136. What is the most likely diagnosis?

(A) tuberculosis
(B) syphilis
(C) gonorrhea
(D) *Trichinella spiralis*
(E) staphylococcal abscess

Questions 137 and 138. (Refer to Figures 2–8 and 2–9.)

137. The features are most consistent with

(A) acute inflammatory exudate
(B) chronic granulomatous inflammation
(C) scar tissue
(D) neoplastic transformation
(E) necrosis of tissue

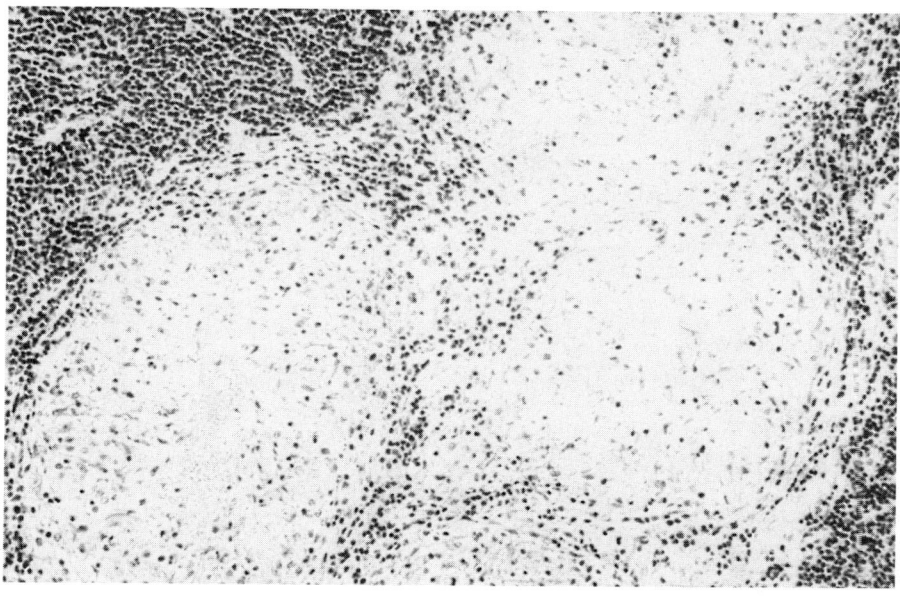

Figure 2–7. Photomicrograph of a lymph node biopsy.

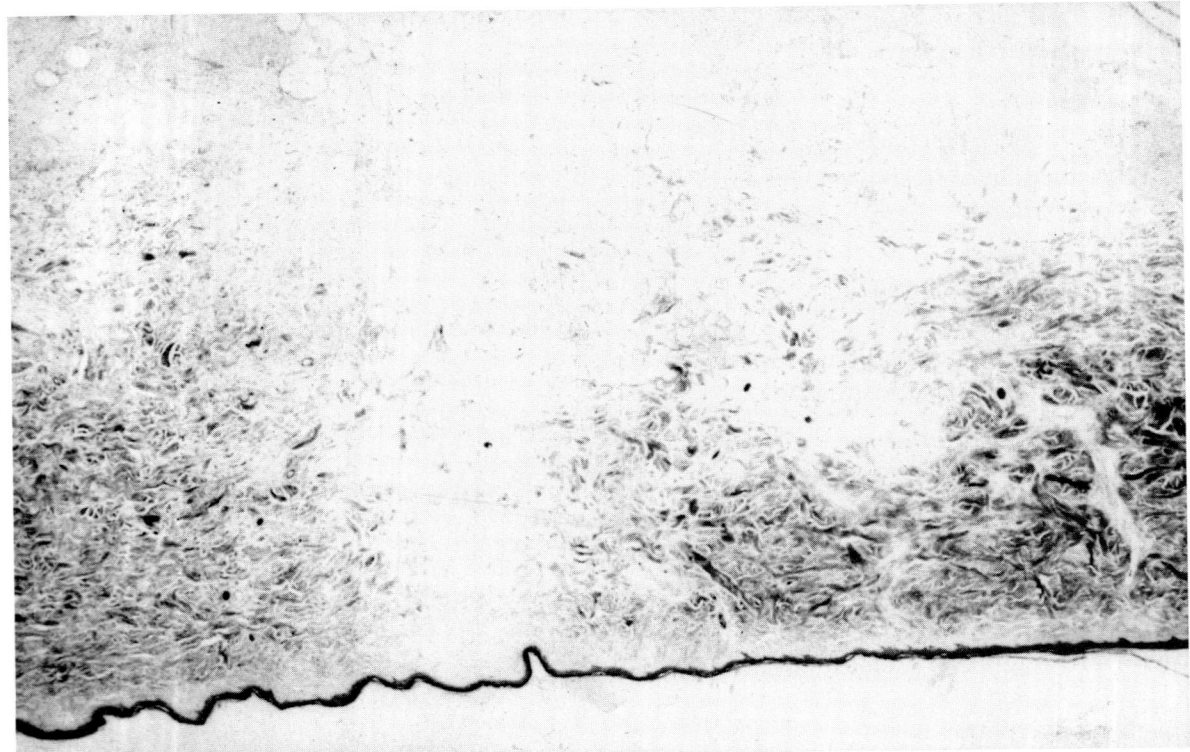

Figure 2–8. Low-power magnification of skin.

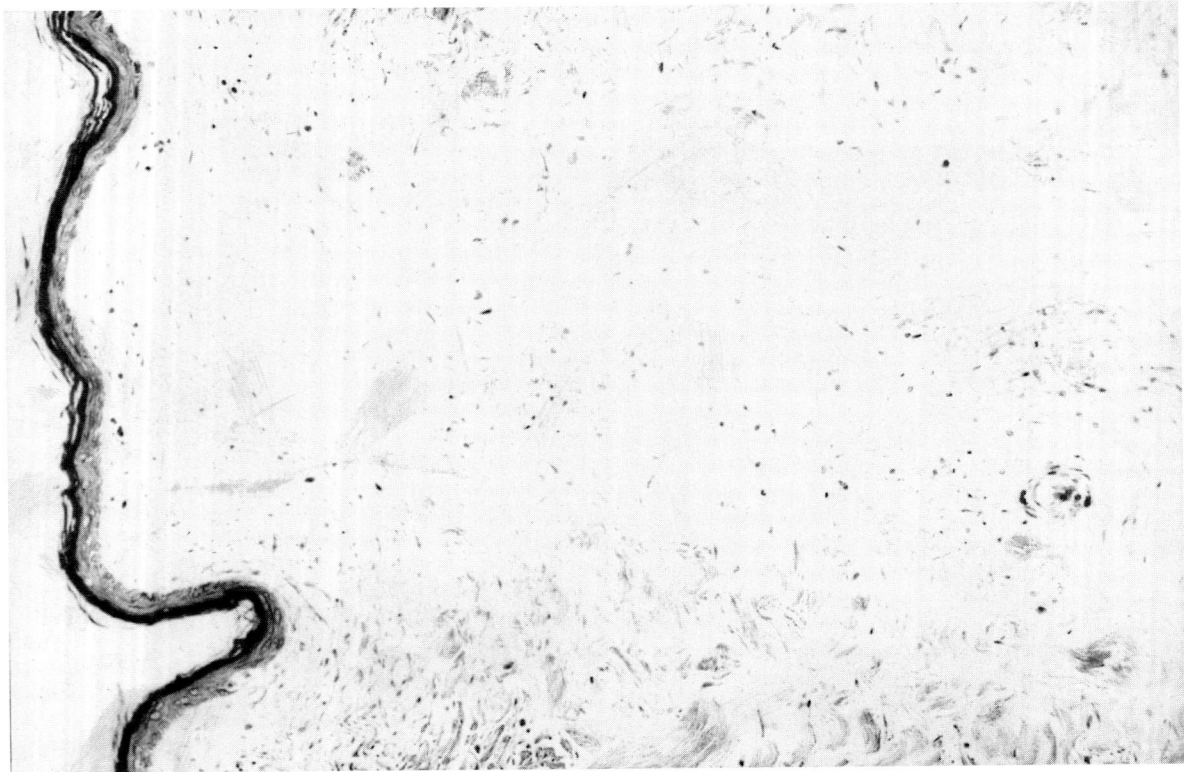

Figure 2–9. High-power magnification of skin.

138. Which is the best description of the features demonstrated?

(A) healing scar in skin
(B) tuberculosis of the skin
(C) abscess of the subcutaneous tissue
(D) foreign body granuloma of skin
(E) malignant melanoma of skin

DIRECTIONS (Questions 139 through 193): Each group of items in this section consists of a list of lettered options followed by a set of numbered words or phrases. For each numbered word or phrase, select the ONE lettered option that is most closely associated with it. Each lettered option may be selected once, more than once, or not at all.

Questions 139 through 144

(A) polymorphonuclear leukocytes (PMN)
(B) eosinophils
(C) basophils
(D) plasma cells
(E) monocytes

139. Abscess formation

140. Immunoglobulin synthesis

141. Giant cell formation

142. Edge of recent infarct

143. Bronchial wall in asthmatic reactions

144. Response to parasites in tissue

Questions 145 and 146

(A) Hageman factor
(B) adenosine diphosphate (ADP)
(C) platelet factor III
(D) histamine
(E) bradykinin

145. Pain of acute inflammation

146. Platelet aggregation

Questions 147 through 150

(A) granulation tissue
(B) fibrous tissue
(C) fibrin
(D) amyloid
(E) fat necrosis

147. Early acute inflammation

148. Early phase of wound healing

149. Abscess

150. Chronic inflammation

Questions 151 through 155

(A) fibrin deposition on serosal surfaces
(B) fibrin and mucus on epithelial surfaces
(C) PMN and localized necrosis of tissue
(D) protein-rich fluid in serous cavities
(E) diffuse PMN infiltration and fibrin throughout the tissue

151. Suppurative inflammation

152. Phlegmonous inflammation

153. Catarrhal inflammation

154. Fibrinous exudate

155. Serous exudate

Questions 156 through 159

(A) capillary buds and fibroblasts
(B) caseous necrosis and multinucleate giant cells
(C) central liquid necrotic debris mixed with neutrophils and bacteria
(D) collections of dense mature collagen
(E) coagulative necrosis and hemorrhage

156. Very early ischemic infarct

157. Abscess

158. Final stage of a healing wound

159. Response to tubercle bacilli

Questions 160 through 163

    (A) fluid from pericardium with low specific gravity and no inflammatory cells

    (B) fluid from pericardium with high specific gravity, many neutrophils, and bacteria

    (C) fluid from pericardium with high specific gravity, multinucleate giant cells, epithelioid cells, and lymphocytes

    (D) fluid from pericardium with mostly erythrocytes

    (E) fluid from pericardium with high specific gravity, abundant fibrin, but only rare inflammatory cells

160. Purulent exudate following pericardial wound infection

161. Transudate of congestive heart failure

162. Exudate of tuberculous pericarditis

163. Exudate of rheumatic pericarditis

Questions 164 through 166

    (A) ascorbic acid

    (B) interleukin II

    (C) chalones

    (D) histamine

    (E) fibronectin

164. Glycoprotein that is chemotactic for fibroblasts and stimulates capillary formation.

165. Product of mature cells that inhibits cell division by neighboring cells

166. Vitamin that promotes proper collagen formation

Questions 167 through 170

    (A) serotonin

    (B) epidermal growth factor

    (C) suppuration

    (D) sarcoidosis

    (E) eosinophilia

167. Promotes growth of surface epithelium in wounds

168. Delays proper wound healing

169. Associated with parasitic infections

170. Noncaseating granulomas

Questions 171 through 174

    (A) plasminogen activator and factor VIII

    (B) bradykinin

    (C) aspirin

    (D) myeloperoxidase

    (E) leukotrienes

171. Oxidant with antimicrobial activity found in neutrophils

172. Strongly chemotactic for inflammatory cells

173. Synthesized by endothelial cells

174. Production of local pain

Questions 175 through 178

    (A) C3a

    (B) myofibroblasts

    (C) prostacyclin

    (D) plasma cells

    (E) thromboxane A_2

175. Causes wound contraction

176. Anaphylatoxin

177. Inhibits platelet aggregation

178. Causes platelet aggregation

Questions 179 through 182

    (A) margination of leukocytes

    (B) fibrosis

    (C) granulation tissue

    (D) chronic foreign body inflammation

    (E) histamine

179. Tissue reaction to nonabsorbable suture material

180. Early event in the acute inflammatory response

181. Chemical mediator of fluid exudation in acute inflammatory reaction

182. Fibroblasts and capillary buds

Questions 183 through 186

    (A) collagen

    (B) procollagenase

    (C) laminin

    (D) fibroblast growth factors

    (E) elastin

183. Basement membrane glycoprotein

184. Major component of elastic tissue

185. Mitogenic and angiogenic

186. Cross-linking increases wound tensile strength

Questions 187 through 193

    (A) hyperacute inflammation

    (B) acute inflammation

    (C) chronic inflammation

    (D) noninflammatory fibrosis

    (E) noncaseating granulomatous
        inflammation

    (F) caseating granulomatous inflammation

    (G) eosinophilic inflammation

    (H) foreign body inflammation

187. A 38-year-old female is found to have bilateral hilar adenopathy on chest x-rays. She complains of a 2-month history of fever, fatigue, and increasing dyspnea. Lymphadenopathy is found on physical examination. A biopsy of one of her enlarged lymph nodes shows sarcoidosis. What pattern of inflammation did the lymph node demonstrate?

188. A 67-year-old male has been experiencing low grade fever, chest pains, cough, and bloody phlegm for about 6 weeks. A sputum sample is sent to the laboratory for examination. The sputum is found to contain numerous acid-fast bacilli. What pattern of inflammation is characteristic of this infectious disease?

189. A 45-year-old white female has noticed recent onset of symmetric swelling of the small joints of her hand, particularly in the morning. These joints are also painful and stiff. About 6 months later her knee joint also becomes swollen and painful. An arthroscopic examination of the joint finds abundant hypertrophic synovium with pannus formation. Shavings of the synovium examined pathologically display the typical histologic features of rheumatoid arthritis. What pattern of inflammation was present in the synovial tissue?

190. A 19-year-old male develops fever, right lower quadrant abdominal pain, and diarrhea. His peripheral leukocyte count is increased with many young band neutrophils and early toxic granulation. Surgery is performed to remove the appendix. At the time of surgery the appendix is tense, engorged with luminal purulent material, and has serosal fibrinous exudates. An obstructing fecalith is present at the appendiceal origin. What pattern of inflammation is the appendix most likely to display?

191. A 56-year-old female has a small 0.7-cm carcinoma of the left breast. She elects to have a lumpectomy excision followed by radiation therapy to the lumpectomy site. Five years later there is no evidence of recurrent or metastatic breast carcinoma. Her radiation site, however, is now sunken and hard. A biopsy of this tissue shows radiation damage and hypertrophic scar formation. What term best characterizes the radiation site changes?

192. A 14-year-old African boy has numerous lesions on his face. At first the skin lesions were only erythematous. But over the last 2 months he has noticed the center of these lesions to become hypopigmented and depressed. A biopsy of one of these skin lesions demonstrates tuberculoid leprosy. What pattern of inflammation was present on the biopsy?

193. At autopsy a 78-year-old male is found to have an impacted stone in his common bile duct and multiple hepatic abscesses. Pyogenic bacteria are cultured from the abscesses. What pattern of inflammation do the hepatic abscesses display?

DIRECTIONS (Questions 194 through 207): Each of the numbered items or incomplete statements in this section is followed by answers or by completions of the statement. Select the ONE lettered answer or completion that is BEST in each case.

Questions 194 through 196

A patient with a temperature of 101°F, headache, and stiff neck has the following laboratory findings: total leukocyte count of 18,000/mm³ (18×10^9/L) with 70% segmented neutrophils, 18% bands, 10% lymphocytes, and 2% monocytes; cerebrospinal fluid (CSF) turbid, glucose 35 mg/dL, protein 115 mg/dL, and 500 neutrophils/mm³ (75% segmented, 25% bands); blood glucose 110 mg/dL.

194. The most likely diagnosis is

   (A) chronic lymphocytic meningitis
   (B) granulomatous meningitis (tuberculous or cryptococcal)
   (C) subarachnoid hemorrhage
   (D) acute suppurative meningitis
   (E) pituitary gland carcinoma

195. Which is the most likely associated finding?

   (A) pulmonary tuberculosis
   (B) recent or current viral pneumonia
   (C) middle cerebral artery aneurysm
   (D) suppurative otitis media
   (E) diabetes insipidus

196. Which complication is most likely?

   (A) disseminated miliary tuberculosis
   (B) intracerebral hemorrhage
   (C) severe viremia
   (D) brain abscess
   (E) hyponatremia

197. The cause of erythema (redness) of an acute inflammatory process is secondary to

   (A) angiogenesis
   (B) vasodilatation of arterioles
   (C) the accumulation of interstitial fluid
   (D) the migration of neutrophils into the area of injury
   (E) vasoconstriction of arterioles

198. In an acute inflammatory process histamine produces

   (A) chemotaxis of neutrophils
   (B) secretion of immunoglobulins by plasma cells
   (C) contraction of endothelial cells in post-capillary venules
   (D) production of collagen by fibroblasts
   (E) phagocytosis by macrophages

199. What are selectins?

   (A) proteins produced by fibroblasts that regulate collagen synthesis
   (B) lysosomal components of macrophages involved in killing bacteria
   (C) not produced in chronic granulomatous disease
   (D) adhesion molecules
   (E) produced from membrane phospholipids by the action of phospholipases

200. Name a chemical mediator that in acute inflammation produces an important vasodilatation.

   (A) plasmin
   (B) histomine
   (C) bradykinin
   (D) leukotriene B4
   (E) prostacyclin

201. Edema is an acute inflammatory process that is secondary to

   (A) lymphatic obstruction
   (B) increased tissue osmotic pressure
   (C) necrosis of endothelial cells
   (D) intercellular endothelial junctions
   (E) increased intravascular hydrostatic pressure

202. The first intravascular event in the mobilization of leukocytes at the site of acute inflammation is

   (A) pavementing
   (B) margination
   (C) emigration
   (D) diapedesis
   (E) phagocytosis

203. In an acute inflammatory process, a localized accumulation of a protein exudate, degenerating cells, is characteristic of

(A) fibrinous pericarditis
(B) keloid
(C) an abscess
(D) cellulitis
(E) a blister

204. Peripheral eosinophilia is a common finding in

(A) bacterial infection
(B) congenital diseases
(C) parasitic infestation
(D) viral infection
(E) vitamin deficiency

205. Indicate the connective tissue cell that releases histamine in acute inflammatory process.

(A) mast cell
(B) plasma cell
(C) basophil
(D) eosinophil
(E) neutrophil

206. Indicate the most common type of collagen found in keloid.

(A) type III
(B) type II
(C) type I
(D) type V
(E) type IV

207. Select the most important product derived from fibroblasts in wound healing.

(A) elastic fibers
(B) collagen
(C) laminin
(D) fibronectin
(E) dermatan sulfate

Answers and Explanations

89. **(E)** This question is meant to establish the well-known basic cardinal signs of acute inflammation, which should be known by all students and is a fundamental question of factual knowledge. This is based on the writings of Celsus in the first century AD: "Rubor et tumor cum calore delore"—redness, swelling, heat, and pain being the manifestations of acute inflammation. See Figure 2–1 for the sequences of events and their relationships to other aspects of inflammation. *(Chandrasoma and Taylor, pp. 37–41)*

90. **(D)** The redness in the early phase of acute inflammation and in some of the later phases is basically a vascular phenomenon. In fact, acute inflammation is primarily a response of the small blood vessels to injury whatever the injury may be. (Figures 2–1, 2–10, and 2–11). Although edema of the tissue is also a manifestation of acute inflammation, it is not the cause of the redness, nor is margination of the white cells or fibrin deposition, which comes later in the event. Thrombosis of blood vessels, although it may cause a dusky discoloration of the skin, is a very late and severe complication of inflammation. *(Chandrasoma and Taylor, pp. 37–41)*

91. **(D)** The outpouring of protein-rich fluid into the tissue is the main cause of the swelling associated with acute inflammation. Although swelling is related to some of the other events described, it is the actual formation of the fluid that causes the swelling. In Figure 2–4, the relationship of this particular aspect to the other events in the manifestations of acute inflam-

mation can be seen. Although the proliferation of fibroblasts may, of course, produce some swelling, this is usually a much later complication of acute inflammation and more related to chronic inflammatory changes (Table 2–2). *(Cotran et al., pp. 52–55)*

92–93. **(92-E, 93-E)** All of the events in Question 92 describe the hydrostatic pressure related to the production of fluid with low specific gravity that does not clot on standing, because it has no fibrinogen. It is the characteristic description of a transiodate. In comparison, Question 93 describes the characteristic features of an exudate in which there is altered vascular permeability. The fluid has a high specific gravity and clots on standing, because it does contain fibrinogen. Table 2–1 summarizes the main features that distinguish transudates and exudates of different degrees of severity and summarizes the main features. *(Cotran et al., pp. 52–55)*

94. **(C)** This is another way of obtaining the information given in Questions 92 and 93; Table 2–1 summarizes the main distinguishing features, which are high protein, medium to high specific gravity, and coagulability because of the presence of fibrinogen, that characterize an exudate. Vascular changes have taken place rather than there being a transudate in which back pressure with no altered vascular permeability produces a different type of fluid. *(Chandrasoma and Taylor, pp. 37–40)*

95. **(E)** The sensation of pain associated with acute inflammation is a complex phenomenon and

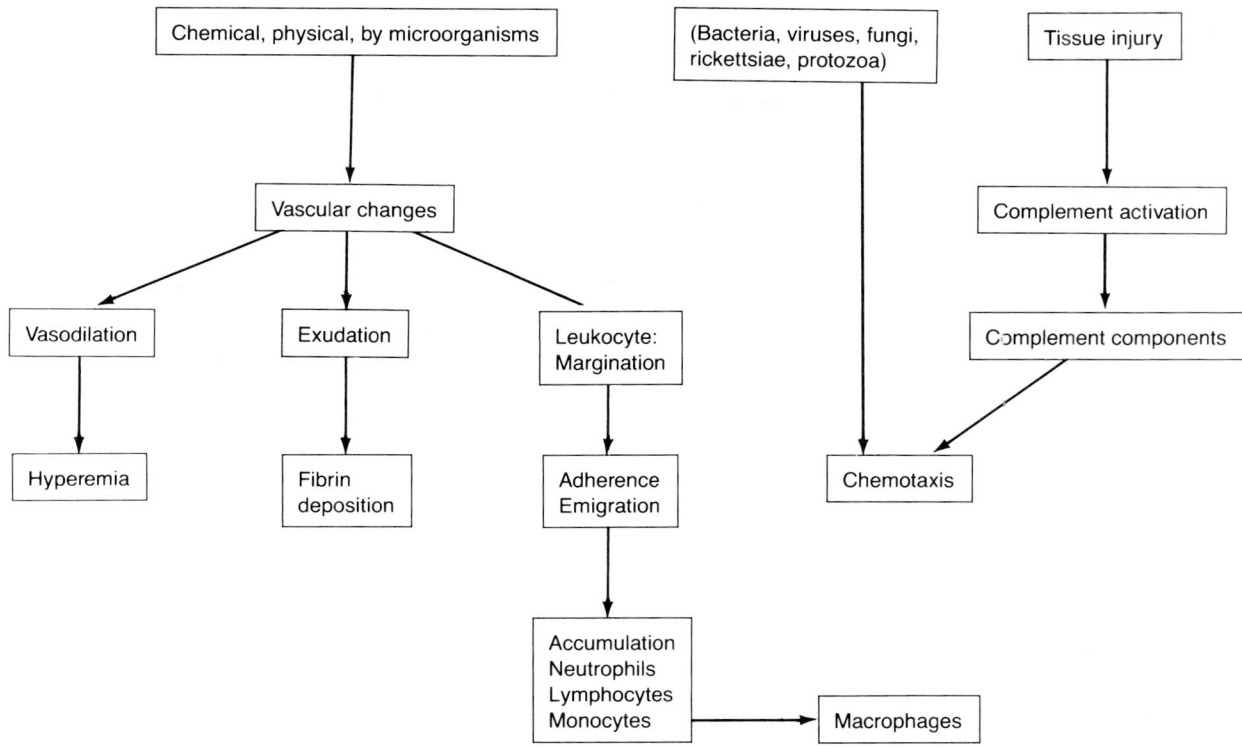

Figure 2–10. Schematic summary of events following injury.

can be produced in varying degrees by any of the mechanisms or substances mentioned. The combination of them, of course, makes the pain more severe, and the anatomic site also is of importance. For instance, a minor degree of inflammation in the subcutaneous tissue in the back of the neck will be more painful than a more extensive inflammation in the skin of the back of the hand, because the tissue tension in these two sites adds another element to the interaction. *(Cotran et al., pp. 50–55)*

96. **(E)** Histamines, serotonin, the kinins, and the prostaglandins are all considered to be chemical mediators of acute inflammation. Their relative importance in different stages and their effects on different components of the inflammatory response can be seen in Figure 2–12. Some of the mediators occur early in the vascular changes of acute inflammation, and others occur both early and late and act as an amplifying system to maintain the reaction in case the original stimulus is short lived. Some-

times, of course, this can be a disadvantage as well as an advantage. *(Cotran et al., pp. 65–79)*

97. **(D)** The accumulation of dead and dying polymorphs or neutrophils, dead and dying bacteria, and liquefaction necrosis of tissue is the characteristic description of suppurative inflammation. If found in a localized area, it is described as an abscess. Catarrhal inflammation may produce some of the features, including the neutrophils, and so can cellulitis, but the formation of an abscess requires all of these combined in a localized, encapsulated form. Granulomatous inflammation is considerably different and consists of a dry cellular proliferation of fibroblasts, epithelioid cells, and fibroblasts. The distinction between these two manifestations of acute and chronic inflammation can be seen in Table 2–2. *(Cotran et al., p. 78)*

98. **(B)** Although all of the events occur in acute inflammation, this particular sequence is an important distinction. It is the stasis of flow

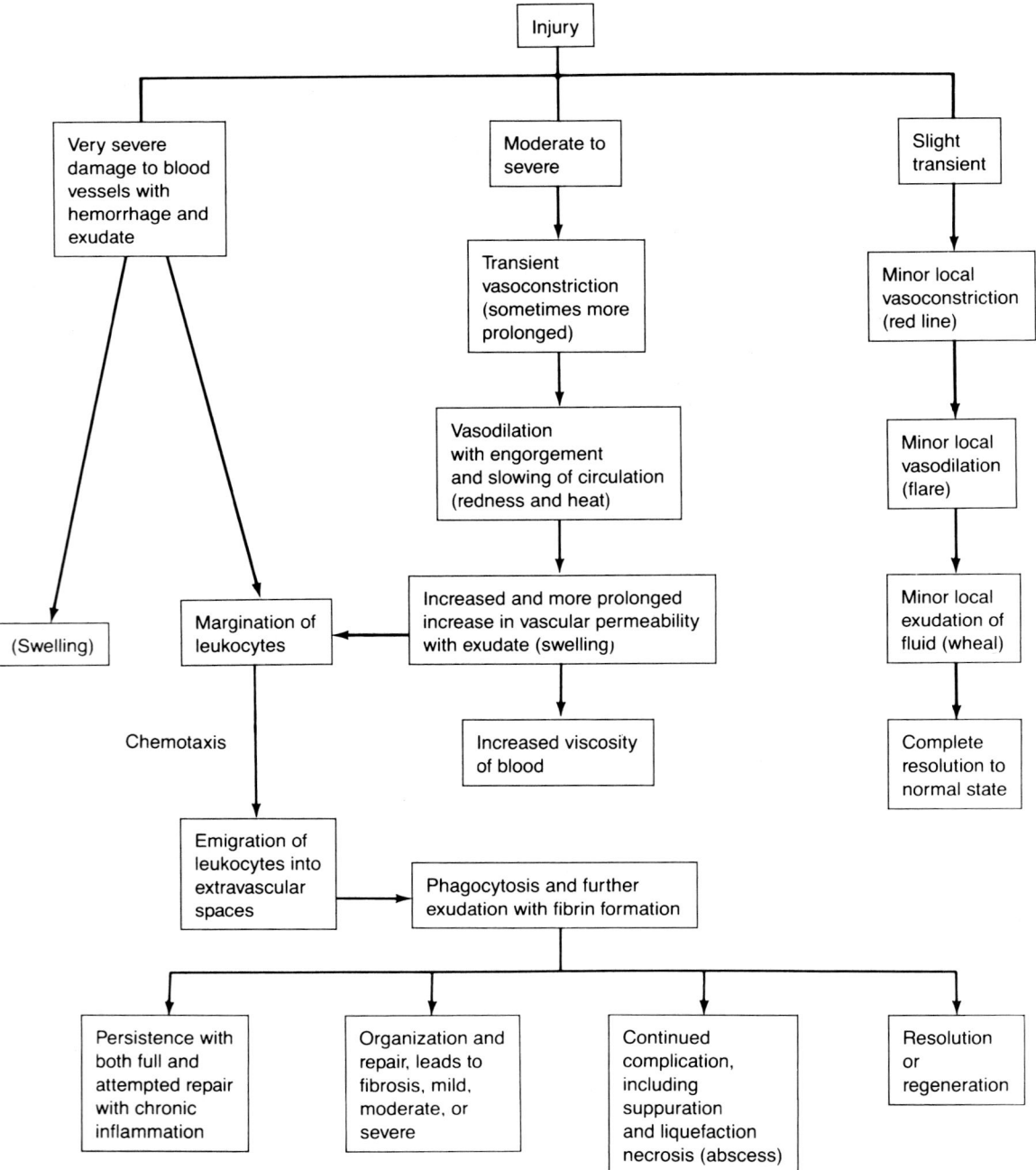

Figure 2–11. Possible sequences following tissue injury.

that leads to the margination of leukocytes, which leads to their emigration through the vessel wall, which results in phagocytosis. The term "lymphadenitis" is merely a description of inflammation in general in a lymph node and is in that sense an irrelevant component answer. The sequential events in acute inflam-mation are summarized in Figure 2–1 and out-lined in the introductory pages of this chapter. (*Cotran et al., pp. 53–55*)

99. (A) The best definition of inflammation is a reaction of the microcirculation in tissue to in-jury. Part of this, of course, consists of edema,

Mediators of Exudative Phase

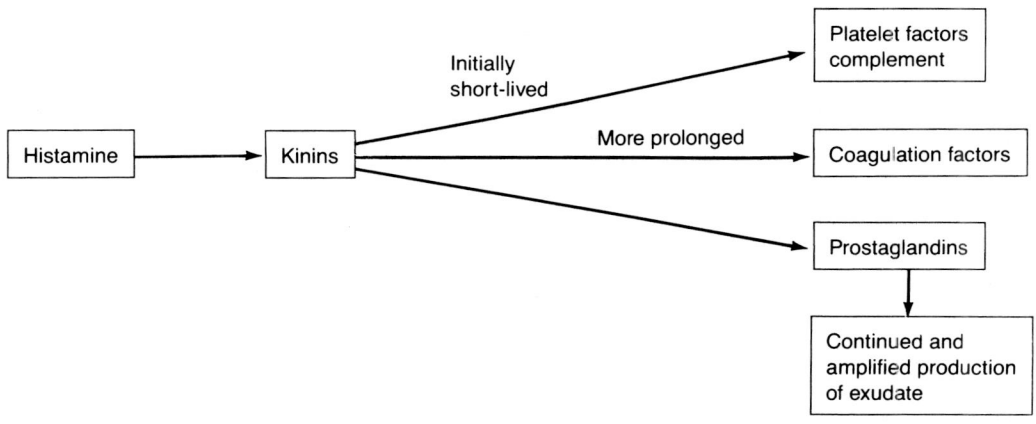

Mediators of Cellular Phase

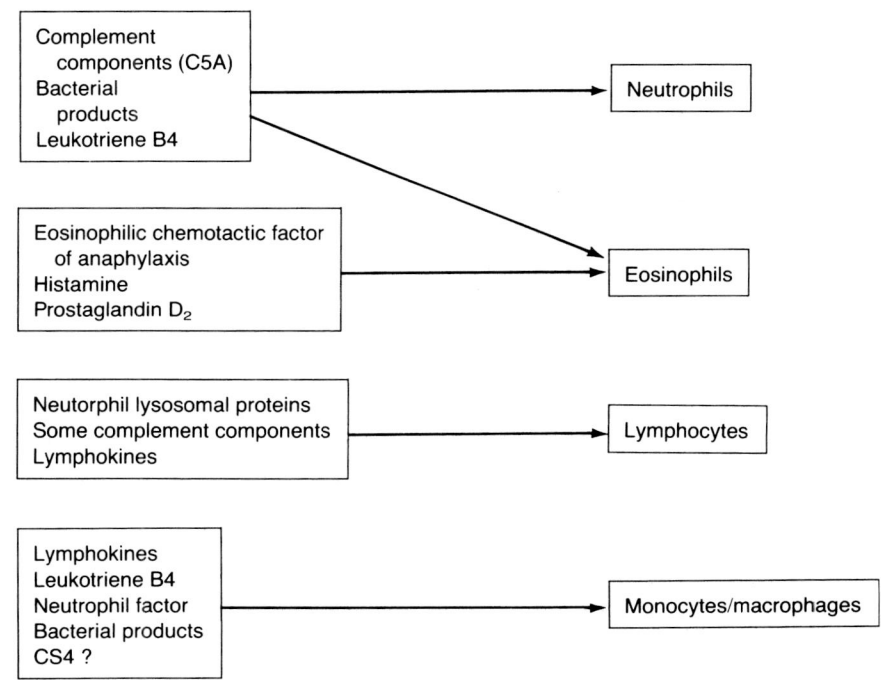

Figure 2–12. Chemical mediators of inflammation (sequential release).

chemotaxis, and some cellular changes resulting from injury. Abnormal cell growth usually is associated with neoplastic change, although some reaction may occur as a result of chronic inflammation. *(Chandrasoma and Taylor, p. 37)*

100. **(C)** The mediators of vascular permeability may act at different stages in the inflammatory response. They do not in and of themselves particularly increase intravascular hydrostatic pressure except by secondary events. The dissolution of the capillary basement membrane would be a very serious and irreparable injury and may occur as a complication but not as a fundamental mechanism. The binding of serum albumin into tissue is not a particularly important component. Contraction of endothelial cells, however, does open the otherwise potential spaces that have been shown to exist as gaps between endothelial cells, resulting in alterations in vascular permeability. *(Cotran et al., pp. 53–55)*

101. **(D)** Histamine is a very important substance in the transient aspects of early acute inflammation but may act at different stages. All of the others mentioned have some effect in vascular permeability but at different stages and by different mechanisms. Histamine is by far the most important in the transient, immediate phase. This is seen also in Figures 2–12 and 2–13, which show the sequential release of chemical mediators. *(Chandrasoma and Taylor, pp. 37–41)*

102. **(C)** Histamine is the most important early chemical mediator in the exudative or fluid phase of acute inflammation. The lymphokines, leukotriene B_4, the prostaglandins, and interleukin I occur at different stages of the inflammatory response. Many of them act in the more cellular phases, late in chronic inflammation (Figures 2–12 and 2–13). *(Chandrasoma and Taylor, pp. 37–41)*

103. **(A)** By definition regeneration is the renewal of lost tissue or part in which the lost cells are replaced by identical ones. Regeneration represents a compensatory mechanism, in reaction to the tissue loss. This has been studied most commonly in the skin, because the easy accessibility, and in particular study, on the regeneration on wound margins. The new cells, coming from reserved cells of the organ, and changing and adapting to the new circumstances in which mitoses occurs, until the process of growth and division stop. Later, it seems to be a process of maturation and differentiation with capillary resorption. The liver is one of the classic examples on which the cells regenerate to an estimate of 70% of the original mass. However, other organs did not respond as remarkably as the liver for regeneration, because of the quality of the tissue or the type of cells. *(Rubin and Farber, pp. 95, 96)*

104. **(D)** Aspirin is believed to have an effect via a number of complex interactions, including prostaglandins and their synthesis and action and other less well-understood pathways in acute inflammation. All of the other substances mentioned are, in fact, components of the chemical

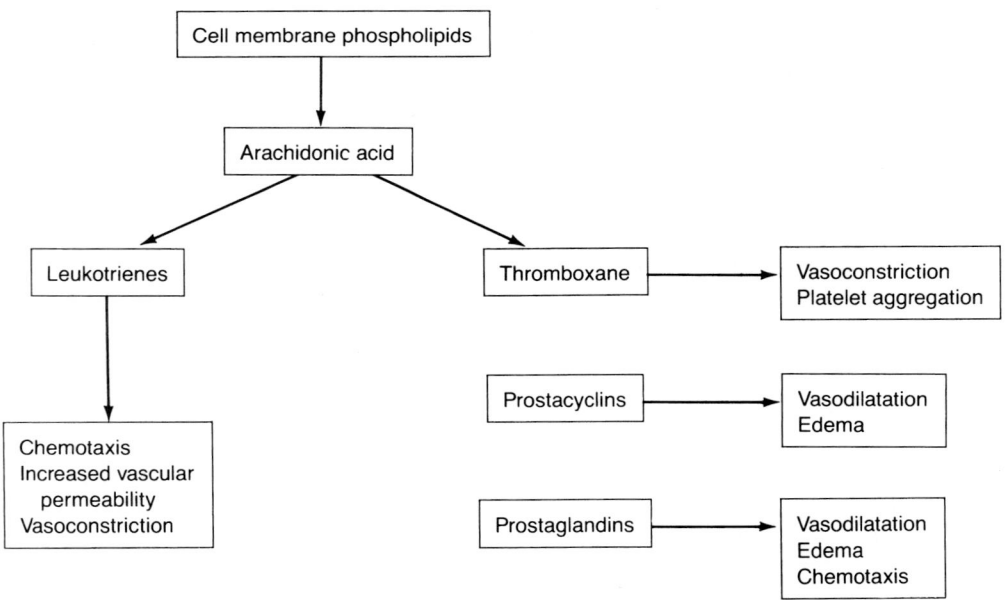

Figure 2–13. Simplified schema of role of phospholipids and their products as mediators of acute inflammation.

mediators of acute inflammation and, therefore, would hardly be used in the reduction of their effects. *(Cotran et al., pp. 70, 71)*

105. **(E)** The characteristic cell in acute inflammation is the polymorphonuclear leukocyte, which is seen in most forms of acute inflammation, although the amounts may be modified by either positive or negative chemotaxis later in the events. The plasma cell, foreign body giant cell, Langhans' giant cell, and lymphocytes are all characteristic of subacute and chronic inflammation (Table 2–2). *(Cotran et al., pp. 62–65)*

106. **(D)** The lymphocyte and monocyte series are the characteristic cells seen in more prolonged forms of inflammation, that is, chronic inflammation. The eosinophils and the polymorphonuclear leukocytes usually are associated with early or acute inflammatory responses. The mast cell is involved in liberating histamine in early inflammation. The platelets, although they may aggregate, are not characteristic of either. *(Cotran et al., p. 79)*

107. **(B)** Edema, fibrin, dilatation, and vascular engorgement are the characteristic manifestations of tissue responding to acute injury and are the underlying mechanisms for the cardinal signs of acute inflammation of redness, swelling, and heat. Chronic inflammation is a more cellular and much less vascular phenomenon (Table 2–2). Suppurative inflammation is characterized by destruction of tissue and an increase in polymorphonuclear leukocytes. Wound healing in the later stages would consist largely of a vascular connective tissue and granulation tissue. It is distinguished by its composition of newly formed blood vessels and fibroblasts. These characteristic differences are summarized in Figure 2–2 and in the introduction to this chapter. *(Cotran et al., pp. 52–54)*

108. **(D)** This is the reverse of Question 107. In this case, the features of monocytes, giant cells, fibroblasts, and lymphocytes are the highly cellular and relatively avascular components that occur late in response to injury and are characteristic of chronic inflammation (Table 2–2). *(Cotran et al., pp. 52–54)*

109. **(E)** Staphylococci are pyogenic bacteria; that is, they are pus producing. To produce pus, there must be some form of chemical attraction to the characteristic cell of acute suppurative inflammation that produces pus, namely, the PMN. Characteristic examples of such infections include boils, carbuncles, and abscesses. Although lymphocytes and monocytes may play a minor role in the outer limits and in the later stages of unresolved pyogenic infections of this type, and eosinophils occasionally may accompany PMNs; it is the PMNs that are the characteristic cell in this type of inflammation and its suppurative complication. *(Cotran et al., pp. 365–369)*

110. **(A)** Viral damage is usually at the cellular level, although in very early reactions to viral infections, an acute inflammatory response may occur. The more characteristic and prolonged viral infections usually result in a form of chronic inflammation, and because the lymphocyte is the characteristic cell of chronic inflammation, it is the one most likely to be seen. *(Cotran et al., p. 340)*

111. **(C)** Various types of protozoal proteins seem to stimulate chemotaxis of eosinophil leukocytes more than other cells. Although this is not universal, it is frequent enough to be of characteristic importance diagnostically. *(Chandrasoma and Taylor, pp. 195–201)*

112. **(C)** For reasons not entirely understood, species of *Salmonella,* particularly *Salmonella typhi,* produce a negative chemotaxis toward neutrophils or polymorphonuclear leukocytes (PMN) and eosinophils. Therefore, the predominant cell, despite acute inflammation, is the monocyte rather than the usual PMN. In many other respects, acute inflammation of typhoid is similar to that seen in other acute inflammatory situations, and only rarely do the lymphocyte and fibrosis become a characteristic response. The increase in monocytes in this form of inflammation is seen not only at the site of the lesion but also in the draining lymph nodes. *(Rubin and Farber, pp. 389–392)*

113. (A) Granulation tissue is the first phase of the healing process at the end of acute inflammation. New capillaries proliferate in the tissue, with fibroblasts and the first laying down of new collagen, which eventually will become largely avascular scar tissue. It is not to be confused with granulomatous inflammation or granuloma, which is the hallmark of a form of chronic inflammation in which healing and the stimulation for damage occur concurrently. Granulation tissue is a normal response in the normal healing process (Table 2–3). *(Cotran et al., pp. 102–104)*

114. (B) This is a corollary to Question 113. New capillaries, fibroblasts, and collagen describe granulation tissue occurring at the periphery of a hematoma or collection of blood. Although lysis of the blood clot may occur as a result, the actual formation of this response is known as organization and is an attempt to heal the area and fill the defect with collagen or scar tissue. If this occurs within a blood vessel, recanalization of the occluded lumen may take place subsequently and embolization may be an eventual complication. Infarction may be related to the formation of material in the lumen but has nothing to do with the process described. *(Cotran et al., pp. 102–104)*

115. (E) All these complications may occur following acute inflammation. The more obvious one of suppuration is an indication of breakdown of tissue, with bacterial lysosomal enzyme release, dead and dying neutrophils, and possibly the organisms that caused the inflammation. Abscess formation may occur as a subsequent complication of such suppuration. Dense scar tissue may complicate this or less complicated forms of acute inflammation, and a scar often may be the ultimate complication of acute inflammation that does not resolve. Organization with adhesions between these epithelial surfaces is merely a local anatomic setting in which such scar tissue may occur, binding fine delicate membranes together (Table 2–3 and Figure 2–11). *(Cotran et al., p. 78)*

116. (C) Vitamin C is particularly important in the formation of procollagen in the early form of wound healing. This was known in the days when scurvy was a prevalent disease and wounds did not heal correctly or in a timely fashion. *(Rubin and Farber, pp. 80, 81)*

117. (D) The term "callus" describes the modified and specialized form of granulation tissue that occurs in a healing bone. It is essentially the same phenomenon as granulation tissue, with the formation of new capillaries and fibroblasts and the laying down of collagen but with the rapid conversion of the ground substance and collagen to bone by osteoblasts. The remodeling by osteoblasts makes this particular form of granulation tissue so characteristic of bone. Involucrum is dead bone that is associated with inflammation that does not lead to correct resolution and healing. Laminated bone is a description of normal bone. Fibrocartilage is as stated. Periosteal new bone, although it may form as a result of a healing fracture, is a later remodeling manifestation and is not the callus described. *(Cotran et al., p. 1230)*

118. (B) Liver parenchymal cells are the best of the cells mentioned in regenerative capabilities. Although skeletal muscle may show some attempt at regeneration, in keeping with heart muscle and neurons, this is a very limited capacity. Neurons or the CNS have no such regenerative capacity. *(Rubin and Farber, p. 95)*

119. (C) The word "saponification" means the breakdown of fat, with soap formation in the tissues. Therefore, of all possible changes, the most likely one is fat necrosis. When this occurs, it inevitably produces an acute inflammatory response, and the combination of the two is best seen in enzymatic fat necrosis. A good example of this is acute pancreatitis, in which enzymes from the damaged pancreas destroy the fat in the surrounding tissue, causing saponification and resulting in an acute inflammatory response. *(Cotran et al., p. 905)*

120. (C) The combination of new capillary buds and fibroblasts is the hallmark of granulation tissue. The presence of collagen and giant cells is more in keeping with a prolonged response, as is seen in chronic inflammation. Similarly, fibroblasts and macrophages are seen in the later stages of chronic inflammation or in the stage before development of true healing. Capillary buds and lymphocytes would be seen when chronic inflammation was persisting and, therefore, healing was not adequate. Sometimes, this can be a mixed picture. Fibroblasts and giant cells are seen more typically in chronic granulomatous inflammation (Table 2–2 and Figure 2–12). *(Cotran et al., pp. 102–104)*

121. **(A)** The repair by connective tissue is produced by the regeneration of mesenchymal cells which serve the purpose of repairing the tissue damage. This occurs when the parenchymal cells fail to accomplish by themselves the regeneration of the organ. The connective tissue therefore grows and produces fibroblasts, accompanied by a process of angiogenesis, in which a vascular network is established to bring nutrients to the damaged area. Therefore, granulation tissue is characteristically formed in the surface of the wounds, and histologically it shows the formation of small capillaries and the proliferation of fibroblasts, that with maturation, and collagen deposition will lead to fibrosis and scarring. *(Cotran et al., pp. 102–103)*

122. **(A)** Vascular endothelial growth factor is produced by mesenchymal and stromal cells, and their receptors are restricted to the endothelial cells. The VEGF bind to one of its receptors on angioblasts and induce the formation of proliferation of endothelial cells. This is the initial step that triggers a cascade of events leading to the formation of new capillaries. VEGF is one of the most important growth factors in the formation of new capillaries. The VEGF expression is stimulated by certain cytokines and growth factors. *(Cotran et al., pp. 104–106)*

123. **(C)** Hemorrhagic inflammatory response usually results in a severe and more violent form of inflammation in which the small blood vessels are damaged in the inflammatory response (Figures 2–1 and 2–11). *(Cotran et al., p. 634)*

124. **(B)** It is the amount of collagen in a wound that determines the tensile strength. The contractility of the wound should not be confused with this, because it can occur at several stages and is not entirely dependent on collagen but on other factors. The ascorbic acid content of

the scar does not seem to be significant, because ascorbic acid availability in the body in general is adequate. The appearance of capillary sprouts merely indicates the early stages of the production of such a scar, and the level of substance that may produce keloid is not known and does not seem to have anything to do with the tensile strength of the developing scar tissue. *(Rubin and Farber, pp. 81–83)*

125. **(B)** The correct order of the events in acute inflammation are vascular dilatation, increased vascular permeability, local hemoconcentration and slowing of blood, margination of white cells, and emigration of white cells (Figures 2–1 and 2–11). *(Chandrasoma and Taylor, pp. 37–42)*

126. **(C)** When tissue necrosis has occurred in cells, the lack of enough regeneration power to cover the damaged areas a pathological excessive amount of fibrous tissue is formed, with scar formation. The granulation tissue that is formed by necessity becomes excessive, and there is an increased amount of synthesis of collagen, and also degradation. *(Cotran et al., p. 109)*

127. **(E)** One of the most important cells in the acute inflammatory process is the leukocytes (see Figure 2–14). The function of the polymorphonuclear cells is to phagocytize microorganisms, necrotic tissue, as well as killing bacteria and other microorganisms. They also release enzymes, chemical mediators, and toxic oxygen radicals. The extravasation of polymorphonuclear cells from the blood vessels in an acute inflammatory process follows a sequence of events that begins with the approach of the cells into the vessel wall (margination), rolling, and adherence. Then they are transported across the endothelium and wall of the capillaries (diapedesis). *(Cotran et al., pp. 55–57)*

128. **(C)** The cells have the multilobe structure and size of a PMN. This is the typical cell seen in acute inflammation. *(Chandrasoma and Taylor, pp. 41, 42)*

129. **(D)** The presence of polymorphonuclear leukocytes (PMN) in peritoneal fluid is typical of an acute inflammatory response of the suppurative

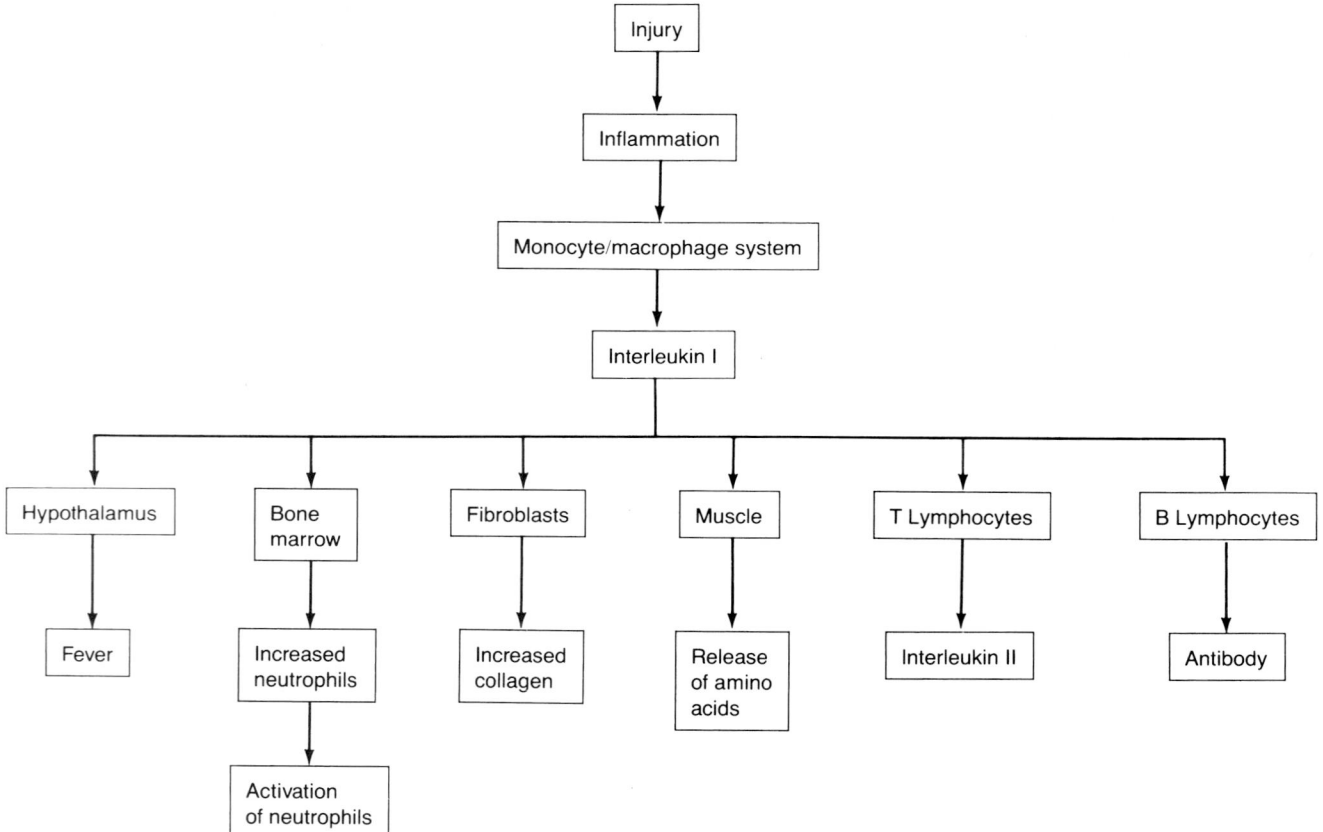

Figure 2–14. Diverse actions of interleukin I activation.

type, as seen in acute peritonitis. In ascites, although PMNs may be present, they are not necessarily characteristic. In chronic peritonitis, the lymphocytes are the predominant cell, with perhaps some monocytes. In tuberculous peritonitis, lymphocytes and monocytes are seen. In carcinomatous peritonitis, in some instances, PMNs may be present, but again, peritoneal macrophages also would be very strongly represented. *(Chandrasoma and Taylor, pp. 41, 42)*

130. **(D)** If one assumes that this is acute peritonitis and that these are polymorphonuclear leukocytes (PMN), rupture of the appendix would be by far the most common form of acute inflammation with suppuration occurring in the peritoneal cavity. *(Rubin and Farber, pp. 748–749)*

131. **(C)** The cells have eccentric nuclei of a cartwheel variety, and their shape and size are characteristic of plasma cells. The plasma cell is seen most frequently in subacute or in some early chronic inflammation but is not characteristic of acute suppurative inflammation. *(Cotran et al., p. 82)*

132. **(C)** A firm painless skin nodule consisting entirely of plasma cells is a highly characteristic response to a very few types of organisms, and the primary chancre of syphilis is the most common. Darkfield illumination for the presence of live spirochetes is more valuable than are gram stains, acid-fast stains, or stains for fungi or malignant cells. *(Rubin and Farber, pp. 408–413)*

133. **(E)** The only reasonable positive finding by darkfield illumination in a painless skin nodule containing plasma cells is spirochetes of syphilis and, therefore, the alternative are much less likely. *(Rubin and Farber, pp. 408–413)*

134. **(C)** Figure 2–7 shows a collection of cells in a background of lymphocytes. The cells form tubercles or granulomas in which giant cells can be seen. This is typical of a granulomatous form of chronic inflammation. *(Cotran et al., pp. 350–351)*

135. **(D)** Of the alternatives presented, a giant cell granulomatous lesion in a lymph node is not typical of a pyogenic infection produced by gram-positive cocci or gram-negative bacilli. *(Cotran et al., pp. 349–352)*

136. **(A)** Because the organisms are acid-fast bacilli, the only reasonable diagnosis is tuberculosis. *Trichinella spiralis* and the organisms causing syphilis, gonorrhea, and staphylococcal abscesses are not acid-fast bacilli. *(Cotran et al., pp. 349–352)*

137–138. **(137-C, 138-A)** Figures 2–8 and 2–9 depict sections through skin and subcutaneous tissue. **A** is epidermis, **B** is normal collagen bundles of the dermis, **C** is scar tissue that extends vertically from the surface into the dermis and is more amorphous in appearance than the surrounding epidermis. There is no evidence of acute or chronic inflammation cells or exudate and no evidence of necrosis or tumor. The appearance of bland, almost structureless collagen in this linear fashion is characteristic of scar tissue and is the end result of healing. *(Chandrasoma and Taylor, pp. 87–92)*

139–144. **(139-A, 140-D, 141-E, 142-A, 143-B, 144-B)** The PMN is the characteristic cell of acute inflammation (Table 2–2) and, therefore, would be expected in an abscess, which is a focal collection of such white cells in response to a number of stimuli in the presence of liquefaction necrosis. The PMNs also would be seen at the edge of a recent infarct, because the tissue damage elicits chemotaxis of PMNs early in the evolution of the process. Eosinophils are attracted to tissue by chemotactic substances in the walls of many protozoal and other forms of parasites. They would be seen in this condition and are seen classically in the bronchial wall in asthmatic reactions. Eosinophils are involved also in attraction to tissue in which certain types of allergic reactions have taken place presumably because of immune complexes and some complement pathways. They are seen in bronchial asthma in increased numbers both in the peripheral blood and in the tissue concerned.

Plasma cells are the main end production cells of the B lymphocyte series and produce immunoglobulins. The monocyte is the cell of origin of many of the cells of chronic inflammation, including the epithelioid cells of granulomas and the fused monocytes and epithelioid cells that produce the Langhans' giant cells in certain types of granulomatous inflammation and foreign body giant cells. *(Cotran et al., pp. 55–65)*

145–146. **(145-E, 146-B)** Although there are many factors that can be responsible for the pain of acute inflammation, the kinin group of chemical mediators is particularly known to be pain producing. Platelet aggregation can occur through a number of chemical mediators, some of which are summarized in Figures 2–12 and 2–13. However, ADP is both liberated by platelets and can cause further platelet aggregation and is, therefore, particularly important in this respect. *(Cotran et al., p. 52)*

147–150. **(147-B, 148-A, 149-E, 150-B)** Early acute inflammation produces an exudation of fluid rich in fibrinogen, and fibrin is precipitated on the surfaces of tissues. In the early phase of wound healing, granulation tissue is present, which eventually becomes fibrous tissue. Therefore, the early phase is associated with the production of granulation tissue. Chronic inflammation occurs after the early phase and is characterized by a number of events. Fibrous tissue is the hallmark, although it also could be the end result of a successful healing process (Figures 2–5 and 2–6). An abscess clearly is associated with pus and the presence of liquefaction necrosis and polymorphonuclear lymphocytes. *(Cotran et al., pp. 50–88)*

151–155. **(151-C, 152-E, 153-B, 154-A, 155-D)** These descriptions of the various manifestations of acute inflammation still are used extensively, although some of them are somewhat archaic. The deposition of fibrin on mucosal surfaces (fibrous exudate) is characteristic of the exudative phase of acute inflammation. Suppurative inflammation is characterized by the breakdown of tissue, with the presence of large numbers of leukocytes. In catarrhal inflammation, there is a mixture of fibrin on the surface of epithelium and mucus. A serous exudate is one in which fluid of high protein content accumulates in body cavities as a result of the inflammatory response. (Chandrasoma and Taylor, p. 45)

156–159. (156-E, 157-C, 158-D, 159-E) A very early ischemic infarct, such as a myocardial infarct due to coronary atherosclerosis, is characterized by coagulative necrosis and hemorrhage. Later there is neutrophilic and phagocytic resolution of the dead tissue. Granulation tissue ingrowth then occurs. The final stages of wound maturation are typified by collections of dense mature avascular collagen. Tissue reactions to pyogenic bacteria, such as staphylococci or streptococci, are typified by suppuration and abscess formation. The histology of an abscess includes liquid debris, neutrophils, and bacterial organisms. Tissue reactions to infections due to tubercle bacilli include granuloma formation, fibrosis, and lymphoplasmacytic inflammatory infiltrates. Capillary buds and fibroblasts are seen in the early healing stages of all wounds, regardless of etiology. (Cotran et al., pp. 59, 60; 83, 84)

160–163. (160-B, 161-A, 162-C, 163-E) Most abnormal collections of fluid (effusions) in a body cavity, such as a pericardial effusion, can be classified as either a transudate or as an exudate. Transudative fluid has a low specific gravity below 1.012, a total protein below 2 g/dL, and is essentially devoid of inflammatory cells. Transudates are an ultrafiltrate of blood and are usually caused by elevated hydrostatic pressure, such as during congestive heart failure. Exudates have a high specific gravity of 1.020 or more, a total protein of 2 g/dL or higher, and many inflammatory cells. Exudates usually occur with infectious or inflammatory processes. The type of inflammatory cell present in the exudate is determined by the etiology of the effusion. For example,

tubercle bacilli characteristically evoke a mixture of multinucleate giant cells, lymphocytes, epithelioid histiocytes, and fibroblasts. Pyogenic bacteria in an exudative effusion usually result in an abscess formation composed of many neutrophils and necrotic debris. Some immunologic disorders, such as rheumatic pericarditis, produce an exudate rich in fibrin with only a few lymphocytes. (Cotran et al., pp. 53, 54; 84, 85)

164–166. (164-E, 165-C, 166-A) A large number of chemical mediators are active in wound healing and repair. Growth-stimulating factors include fibronectin, platelet-derived growth factor, lymphokines, macrophage-derived growth factor, and fibrin. Fibronectin is a glycoprotein synthesized by fibroblasts that stimulates capillary formation and is chemotactic for fibroblasts. Platelet-derived growth factor is produced by platelets and stimulates capillary and fibroblast proliferation. Interleukin II is a lymphokine synthesized by T cell lymphocytes. Interleukin II stimulates T cell production. Macrophage-derived growth factor is mitogenic for fibroblasts. Chalones are growth-inhibiting chemical factors secreted by leukocytes and epidermal cells. Chalones inhibit cell division of neighboring cells (contact inhibition). Vitamin C, ascorbic acid, promotes proper collagen and matrix formation through hydroxylation of proline and lysine, and through the aggregation of tropocollagen fibrils. Histamine is present in mast cells and acts as a mediator of the acute inflammatory response through increasing vascular permeability. (Chandrasoma and Taylor, p. 88)

167. (B) A healing wound goes through several stages. The initial wound trauma engenders an acute inflammatory response with attendant leakage of plasma proteins, fibrin clot formation, and diapedesis of inflammatory cells. Next, granulation tissue composed of young collagen and capillary buds fill the wound defect. The surrounding epithelium and fibroblasts are stimulated by epidermal growth factor, a mitogenic polypeptide of about 6,000 daltons. Epidermal growth factor

stimulates cell division by binding to specific fibroblastic and epithelial tyrosine kinase receptors that trigger subsequent RNA synthesis, DNA synthesis, and mitosis. The final stages of wound healing are characterized by collagen deposition, collagen maturation, decreasing vascularity, and wound contraction. (Cotran et al., pp. 97–98; Chandrasoma and Taylor, pp. 86, 87)

168.   (C) A number of detrimental factors impede proper wound healing. Suppuration or pus formation is toxic to many cell types and delays the ingrowth of granulation tissue into a wound. If the suppurative process is unable to drain spontaneously, an abscess can develop, further complicating the resolution phase of wound healing. Abscesses may resolve spontaneously (pointing of an abscess) or through surgical drainage. Another adverse factor in wound healing is the presence of foreign material in the wound. Glass, wood splinters, and dirt in traumatic wounds mechanically obstruct orderly healing and provide a nidus for infection and suppuration. Additional factors that delay wound healing include vascular insufficiency, gapping wound defects, and a lack of collagen strengthening cofactors, such as ascorbic acid. Glucocorticoid therapy and diabetes also delay proper wound healing. (Chandrasoma and Taylor, pp. 89–91)

169.   (E) Eosinophils usually comprise less than 5% of peripheral blood leukocytes. A wide range of inflammatory, infectious, allergic, and neoplastic disorders produce increased circulating eosinophils (eosinophilia). Eosinophilia is a common manifestation of parasitic infections, especially with metazoan infestations. Allergic disorders that produce eosinophilia include allergic rhinitis, asthma, urticaria, drug allergies, and eczema. Immunologic diseases in which eosinophilia may occur include polyarteritis nodosa, pemphigus vulgaris, Loffler's syndrome, and eosinophilic gastroenteritis. Neoplasms associated with eosinophilia include Hodgkin's disease, mycosis fungoides, and eosinophilic leukemia. (Cotran et al., p. 648)

170.   (D) Sarcoidosis is a disease of unknown etiology characterized by noncaseating granulomas in multiple sites throughout the body. The presence of these distinctive granulomas suggests an immunologic or hypersensitivity reaction to an infectious agent. Clinically there may be peripheral lymphadenopathy, splenomegaly, hepatomegaly, fever, fatigue, cutaneous lesions, or eye involvement. Laboratory findings may identify hypercalcemia, elevated angiotensin-converting enzyme levels, and hyperglobulinemia. Radiographic studies usually demonstrate bilateral hilar adenopathy and lytic lesions of the phalangeal bones. There is no specific therapy, although some success is achieved with immunosuppression. The clinical course of the disorder is variable. Over half of affected individuals recover with minimal or no sequela. About 20% have permanent moderate pulmonary impairment. About 10% have progressive disease with terminal cor pulmonale, cerebral dysfunction, or cardiac insufficiency. (Cotran et al., pp. 350–351)

171.   (D) Myeloperoxidase is an enzyme present in the azurophilic granules of neutrophilic leukocytes. This enzyme actively converts peroxidase into a potent oxidative-free radical form which is bactericidal. The conversion reaction requires a halide cofactor, such as a chloride ion. The infrequent individuals who are born without normal myeloperoxidase activity suffer from a disorder termed "chronic granulomatous disease." With this genetic disease there is normal phagocytosis of bacteria. But the ingested organisms cannot be killed due to the hereditary impairment of myeloperoxidase. Thus, the organisms continue to multiply intracellularly. Histologically this sequence of events is observed as multifocal granulomas and microabscesses. The disease is usually inherited in an X-linked recessive mode, although a few individuals inherit the disorder in an autosomal recessive fashion. (Cotran et al., p. 76)

172.   (E) Arachidonic acid is found in the cell membranes of many inflammatory cells, such as neutrophils, macrophages, and mast cells. The enzymatic release of this twenty carbon unsaturated fatty acid by stimulated phos-

pholipases initiates a subsequent cascade of metabolites, including leukotrienes and prostaglandins, which serve as chemical mediators of the acute inflammatory response. Leukotrienes are strongly chemotactic for inflammatory cells. In addition, leukotrienes increase vascular permeability. The prostaglandins cause vasodilation, increase vascular permeability, and are chemotactic. Inhibitors of the acute inflammatory response act by either blocking the phospholipase release of free arachidonic acid (corticosteroids) or by blocking the cyclooxygenase pathway (aspirin). *(Cotran et al., pp. 70–72)*

173. **(A)** Endothelial cells line the interior wall of blood and lymphatic vessels providing a smooth nonclotting surface. Between the individual endothelial cells are small pores through which water and small molecules exchange with the interstitium. The widening of these pores by histamine results in edema formation during the acute phase of the inflammatory response. Endothelial cells, in addition, synthesize a diverse group of substances, including factor VIII, plasminogen activator, and prostaglandins. *(Cotran et al., pp. 119, 120)*

174. **(B)** Bradykinin is painful when injected into the skin. It also causes contraction of smooth muscles and dilation of blood vessels. Bradykinin is the end product of the kinin system. The kinin system is a series of plasma proteases that begins with activation of factor XII (Hageman factor) and ends with bradykinin production. Initial contact with collagen, basement membrane material, bacterial endotoxin, or other surface agents converts factor XII into factor XIIA (prekallikrein activator). The next step in the kinin system is the conversion of prekallikrein into kallikrein by factor XIIA. The kallikrein produced then cleaves high-molecular weight kininogen to produce bradykinin. The kinin system is only one of three plasma proteases whose components are useful in the acute inflammatory response. The other plasma proteases are the complement system and the blood clotting system. *(Cotran et al., pp. 68–69)*

175. **(B)** Myofibroblasts are mesenchymal-derived cells with features of both smooth muscle cells and fibroblasts. Like smooth muscle cells, the myofibroblasts contain the contractile protein bundles of actin and myosin. However, the myofibroblasts still retain the fibroblastic quality of collagen production. When a wound develops the myofibroblasts enter the defect on the 2nd or 3rd day concomitant with the ingrowth of granulation tissue. The contractile properties of the myofibroblast provide a mechanical reduction in the size of the wound defect to be repaired. In general, the smaller the defect to be repaired the more rapid the closure is completed. *(Rubin and Farber, pp. 87, 88)*

176. **(A)** Complement is a cascade of plasma proteases whose final goal is the lysis of cell membranes. In the classic pathway, complement is bound to the Fc portion of an antibody–antigen complex. In the alternative pathway, properdin initiates complement activation independent of an antibody–antigen complex. After initiation the complement cascade generates a wide number of fractions with diverse biologic activities. The C3a and C3b fractions are anaphylatoxic and opsonic, respectively. The C5a fraction is anaphylatoxic and chemotactic. The C1 and C5b67 fractions are chemotactic. These active products can modify the inflammatory response through the recruitment of additional inflammatory cells (chemotaxis) or through increasing vascular permeability (anaphylaxis). *(Rubin and Farber, pp. 53, 54)*

177. **(C)** Prostacyclin (prostaglandin PGI_2) is a potent inhibitor of platelet aggregation and is secreted principally by endothelial cells and macrophages. Prostacyclin is synthesized from free arachidonic acid via the cyclooxygenase pathway. A number of unstable prostaglandins (PGH_2 and PGG_2) are synthesized as intermediates prior to final synthesis of stable prostacyclin. Prostacyclin is a modifier of the inflammatory response through its vasodilatory action. The vasodilation increases the blood flow to an inflamed area, potentially increasing the plasma proteins and inflammatory cells available to mount an inflammatory response. Prostacyclin also reduces the functional activity of platelets and neutrophils by increasing their intracellular cyclic adenosine monophosphate levels. Prostacyclin synthesis,

like most of the other prostaglandins, is reduced by aspirin, indomethacin, and corticosteroids. *(Rubin and Farber, p. 483)*

178. **(E)** Thromboxane A_2 is a potent mediator of platelet aggregation. Thromboxane A_2 is synthesized from free arachidonic acid via the cyclooxygenase pathway. It is present in high concentrations within platelet granules. Its release plays a major role in the "second wave" of platelet aggregation. Thromboxane A_2 is also an active vasoconstrictor. Its dual ability to recruit platelets and constrict blood vessels is particularly useful in states of vascular disruption. *(Rubin and Farber, pp. 44–46)*

179. **(D)** Foreign body inflammation displays a constellation of histologic features: multinucleate giant cells, lymphocytes, nonepithelioid histiocytes, and fibrosis. The multinucleate giant cells seen in foreign body reactions demonstrate multiple nuclei randomly arranged throughout the cytoplasm, including nuclei present in the center of the cell. This is in contradistinction to the Langhans' giant cell seen with granulomatous inflammation. The Langhans' cells has its multiple nuclei arranged at the periphery of the cytoplasm, usually without any nuclei in the center of the cell. The mononuclear epithelioid histiocytes from which the Langhans' cell is derived are also seen in granulomatous inflammation. With foreign body inflammation only normal, nonepithelioid histiocytes are usually seen. Fibrosis may be a very prominent feature of foreign body inflammation, such as that seen with inhaled silicon particles (silicosis). Fibrosis plays only a minor role in granulomatous inflammation until the final healing stages. Nonabsorbable sutures, such as those made of silk or plastic, would evoke a foreign body inflammatory response. The use of adsorbable suture material, such as chromic-treated cat gut, would evoke a foreign body response until the suture material was completely metabolized. *(Rubin and Farber, pp. 73, 74)*

180. **(A)** In the acute inflammatory response, there is immediate transient vasoconstriction (blanch), followed by vasodilation (flare), and fluid exudation (wheal). Margination of leukocytes occurs early in the acute inflammatory response. A number of chemical mediators, including epinephrine, are able to marginate leukocytes. The presence of leukocytes on the inner wall of blood vessels ensures that sufficient leukocytes will be available for recruitment into the adjacent damaged tissue. As the inflammatory process progresses, the marginated leukocytes will exit through the newly expanded holes in the blood vessel walls (diapedsis) in response to chemotactic products liberated by tissue damage. *(Rubin and Farber, pp. 55, 56)*

181. **(E)** Histamine is a chemical mediator of fluid exudation in the acute inflammatory response through its ability to produce endothelial cell contraction. Histamine is found mainly in mast cells and basophils, and to a lesser extent in platelets. Histamine acts on the vasculature by binding to specific H_1-receptor sites on endothelial cells. Once bound, histamine initiates a reversible contraction of the endothelial cell cytoplasm. This cytoplasmic contraction widens the miniscule gaps already present between endothelial cell membranes and allows the exudation of fluid and larger molecules out into the interstitium. *(Rubin and Farber, pp. 47, 48)*

182. **(C)** Granulation tissue is composed of fibroblasts and capillary buds. Histologically, there is usually accompanying mild edema, a few inflammatory cells, and a rare extravisated erythrocyte. In a clean, nonsuppurative wound granulation tissue appears during the 2nd through 5th day. Beginning at the periphery of the defect it advances centrally. As the wound matures the granulation tissue becomes less vascularized and more collagenized. There is contraction of the wound site from myofibroblasts and the cross-linking of the young collagen imparts increased tensile strength to the healing tissue. The final stages of a healed wound result in fibrosis. *(Rubin and Farber, pp. 88, 89)*

183. **(C)** Basement membranes separate the epithelial and mesenchymal compartments. The basement membrane is composed of type IV collagen, laminin, and heparin sulfate proteo-

glycan. The glycoprotein laminin is the major component of the basement membrane and serves a glue-like function simultaneously attaching to collagen, epithelial cells, and proteoglycans. The large laminin molecule has three short arms, a central core, and a single long arm. Type IV collagen can bind to each of the laminin molecule's three short arms. The central core of the laminin molecule attaches to specific receptors present on the external surface of epithelial cells. The long arm of laminin binds to heparin. The laminin molecule is an important structural barrier that malignant cells must overcome before they can invade into the interstitium. *(Rubin and Farber, pp. 56, 57)*

184. **(E)** Elastic connective tissue is found at many sites throughout the body, such as the ears, the spinal column, skin, lungs, the epiglottis, and in blood vessels. The major component fiber of elastic connective tissue is elastin. The precursor fiber, tropoelastin, measures about 70,000 daltons and matures into elastin by covalent desmosine and isodesmosine cross-linkages. The half-life of elastin is longer than the normal human life span. However, actinic damage, trauma, and certain bacterial elastases can all retard the longevity of elastin. *(Cotran et al., pp. 99, 100)*

185. **(D)** In the repair phase of a healing wound, a number of growth factors are active. These growth factors include fibroblast growth factor, epidermal growth factor, transforming growth factors, interleukin I, and tissue necrosis factor. The fibroblast growth factor is synthesized by a wide variety of epithelial and mesenchymal tissues. It is mitogenic for fibroblasts. In addition, it has the ability to stimulate the production and growth of new blood vessels (angiogenesis). *(Cotran et al., pp. 97, 98)*

186. **(A)** Collagen cross-linking increases wound tensile strength. This cross-linkage takes place between tropocollagen fibers at the site of previously oxidized lysine and hydroxylated proline residues. The oxidation and hydroxylation steps require the presence of ascorbic acid (vitamin C) and specific enzymes. *(Rubin and Farber, pp. 76–80)*

187. **(E)** Sarcoidosis produces a noncaseating pattern of granulomatous inflammation. Although the exact cause is unknown, an infectious or disordered immune etiology is suspected. Sarcoidosis occurs more frequently in North American blacks than in whites, and is common in Scandinavia. The clinical symptoms include fever, fatigue, malaise, weight loss, dyspnea, skin lesions, splenomegaly, eye lesions, and lymphadenopathy. Affected sites demonstrate the characteristic noncaseating granulomas on histologic examination. The majority of individuals with sarcoidosis recover uneventfully or suffer only minor pulmonary impairment. Only about 10% of patients suffer end-stage lung disease or succumb to cardiac complications. *(Rubin and Farber, p. 1273)*

188. **(E)** Tuberculosis produces a caseating pattern of granulomatous inflammation. Tuberculosis is divided into primary and secondary forms. An individual's first infection with tubercle bacilli is termed "primary tuberculosis." The inhaled bacilli lodge in the distal airways of the lung where they multiply freely until cell-mediated immunity develops. The typical caseating granulomatous pattern of inflammation coincides with the development of cellular immunity. Secondary tuberculosis occurs with reinfection of an individual from a dormant primary focus. If there is adequate cellular immunity, a caseating granulomatous reaction occurs. Histologically, there is central cheesy necrosis and a peripheral wall formed by lymphocytes, epithelioid histiocytes, Langhans' giant cells, and early fibrous tissue. The waxy cell walls of the tubercle bacilli retain carbolfuchsin dyes after acid rinsing. This "acid-fast" property is useful in the laboratory identification of mycobacterial infections. *(Rubin and Farber, pp. 426, 427)*

189. **(C)** The pattern of inflammation seen in rheumatoid arthritis is chronic inflammation. The synovium displays villiform hypertrophy, a mixed lymphocytic and plasmacytic infiltrate, germinal follicle formation, and fibrin deposition. Most affected individuals possess a rheumatoid factor in their serum which can be

detected by laboratory testing. This factor is an IgM molecule that reacts against IgG. The disease is most commonly observed to occur in middle-aged females. Symmetric swelling of the small joints of the hands is the usual presenting feature. *(Cotran et al., pp. 1251–1253)*

190. **(B)** The basic fact that the narrow lumen of the appendix is continuous with that of the bowel predisposes to its obstruction by an impacted fecalith. Continued secretion of mucinous fluid distal to the obstruction causes increased intraluminal pressure, which impedes venous drainage and causes ischemic damage and transudation of fluid into the wall, and possibly venous thrombosis, as well. The mucosa, especially if ischemically injured, is subject to damage by the fecalith, leading to invasion by the normal mixed bacterial flora of the bowel, with consequent exudation of fluid and neutrophils into the wall and onto the serosa. The vicious cycle of ischemia, bacterial infection, and swelling due to acute inflammation often increases tension in the tissue enough to impede blood flow, causing more ischemia and even gangrene, with rupture and peritonitis. This sequence of events is a particular problem in this location because the venous return and end-arterial supply are easily compromised, and adequate collateral circulation is not present. Thus, resolution is not likely to follow significant acute inflammation in this anatomic site. The appendix may also be occluded by calculus, tumor, *Enterobius vermicularis* infestation, and possibly lymphoid hyperplasia associated with viral or bacterial infection. Some cases of acute appendicitis apparently are not associated with luminal obstruction and may result from sharp angulation of the appendix caused by adhesions, fibrous bands, or retrocecal location. The pathogenesis of similar situations can be predicted, such as a loop of bowel incarcerated within a hernia and possibly strangulated, twisted around its mesentery (volvulus), or telescoped into itself (intussusception), or a colonic diverticulum can become obstructed and inflamed. *(Lewis and Raudin, pp. 10–19)*

191. **(D)** Noninflammatory fibrosis commonly follows in sites of radiation therapy. Chronic radiodermatitis is characterized by loss of adnexal structures, poor vascularity with perivascular fibrosis, increased collagen deposition in the dermis, and a thinning of the epidermis. These histologic changes are accompanied by the clinical observations of a shrunken, hard, thin-skinned surface that heals poorly, or not at all, if injured. *(Cotran et al., p. 429)*

192. **(F)** Tuberculoid leprosy displays a caseating granulomatous pattern of inflammation. In tuberculoid leprosy there is a type IV delayed hypersensitivity reaction to leprosy bacilli antigens producing caseating granulomas. Clinically, these lesions are hypopigmented and are depressed centrally. Leprosy bacilli characteristically involve nerves producing the additional later clinical findings of wristdrop, footdrop, and other palsies. Leprosy is seen in tropical countries, including portions of the southern United States, California, and Hawaii. *(Chandrasoma and Taylor, pp. 2, 385, 386)*

193. **(B)** Hepatic abscesses have an acute inflammatory reaction pattern. Bacterial hepatic abscesses usually result from either biliary obstruction or septicemia. The pyogenic and coliform bacteria are the most frequent pathogens. The mortality rate for hepatic abscesses is about 60%. Histologically, there is central necrotic debris, fibrin precipitates, abundant neutrophils, and scattered bacteria. *(Chandrasoma and Taylor, pp. 867, 868)*

194–196. **(194-D, 195-D, 196-D)** The presence of fever, headache, and stiff neck may be seen in all of the conditions and simply results from irritation of the meninges. However, the blood and CSF neutrophilic leukocytosis with an increased proportion of immature forms (left shift) is strong evidence of acute suppurative inflammation, most probably due to bacterial infection likely associated with bacterial otitis media. Chronic lymphocytic meningitis, tuberculous and fungal meningitis, and allergic encephalomyelitis classically produce a lymphocytic or monocytic cellular response. The most likely complication is brain abscess. *(Cotran et al., pp. 1315, 1316)*

197. **(B)** Vasodilatation of small arterioles, and stasis follows an initial very short period of vasoconstriction. The vasodilatation of the arterioles, capillary, and venules (hyperemia) causes a marked increase in the blood flow to the acute inflamed area. This increase in the blood flow to the area, will be translated as redness of the injured tissue. The accumulation of interstitial fluid, the migration of neutrophils or the vasoconstriction of the arterioles will not produce this phenomenon. Angiogenesis is a late development in the inflammatory process (chronic inflammation). *(Chandrasoma and Taylor, pp. 37, 38)*

198. **(C)** Histamine, also called vasoactive amine, are released from the mast cells and platelets and is also present in the early stages of acute inflammation. Histamine is responsive for the vessel dilatation and increased permeability that acts in the immediate acute inflammatory response. Histamine levels decrease rapidly within an hour after the onset of inflammation. The histamine acts by contraction of endothelial cells in the post capillary venules. *(Chandrasoma and Taylor, pp. 42–45)*

199. **(D)** The migration of polymorphonuclear cells through the wall of the capillaries is proven to be mediated by binding of different type of adhesion and transmigration molecules. One type of these molecules is called selectins, which is secreted by the endothelial cells, and act on the surface of the polymorphonuclear cells, with the interaction of another adhesion molecule. *(Cotran et al., pp. 55–57)*

200. **(C)** Bradykinin is the final product of the kinin system and is formed by the action of kallikrein on a precursor plasma protein. Bradykinin causes increased vascular permeability and also stimulates the pain receptors. The other elements cited in this question do not accomplish this function. *(Chandrasoma and Taylor, p. 44)*

201. **(D)** The increase in vascular permeability of the capillary and venules of the acute inflamed area is produced as a function of the intercellular junction between vascular endothelial cells. The pores that exist in between these endothelial cells permit the filtration of small molecules. In acute inflammation, there is an immediate marked increase in the permeability in the venules and capillaries because of the active contraction of acting filaments in endothelial cells. The effect is separation of intercellular junctions from one to another, which leads to accumulations of large amounts of fluid capable of passing through these abnormally permeable vessels, producing the swelling (of the soft tissues) and edema. *(Chandrasoma and Taylor, pp. 38–40)*

202. **(B)** Margination is the phenomenon in which the polymorphonuclear cells that usually travel in the center of the bloodstream in the capillary and venules, approach the periphery of the vessel, and get close to the endothelial cells. In normal circumstances, these endothelial cells are, for the most part, covered by plasma. The stasis, as well as the damage of the tissue allow the cells to marginate on the periphery of the capillary walls. *(Rubin and Farber, p. 55)*

203. **(C)** An abscess is a collection of inflammatory cells, with aggregate of tissue cell destruction, proteins, and a wall composed of fibroblasts, as well as acute and chronic inflammatory cells. Keloid formation is hypertrophic scar. Cellulitis is an acute inflammatory process with no collection of pus. A blister is composed mostly of proteinaceous material as is fibrinous pericarditis. *(Rubin and Farber, pp. 41, 42)*

204. **(C)** Eosinophilia is a condition that could be seen in many different types of diseases, or reactions. In general, bacterial, viral infections are not characterized by a high eosinophilic count. Vitamin deficiency and congenital diseases are not known to have a high eosinophil count. Other disorders that can produce eosinophilia are asthma, high fever, and allergic skin reactions. Such malignancies as Hodgkin's and non-Hodgkin's lymphomas are known to have occasional eosinophilia. Collagen vascular disorders, vasculitis can produce an increased amount of eosinophils in the peripheral blood. *(Cotran et al., p. 648)*

205. **(A)** Mast cells are the major and richest source of histamine, and they are normally present in the connective tissue adjacent to the blood vessels. Also, to a lesser degree, histamine can be produced by basophils and platelets. The histamine is present in the mast cell granules and is released by a variety of stimuli. *(Cotran et al., p. 66)*

206. **(C)** Type I collagen is the major collagen of the mature scars and also is seen on normal tissues in the bone, skin, and tendons. Collagen type II is the major collagen in cartilage, vitreous humor, and nucleus pulposus. Collagen type III is abundant in embryonic tissue, and in adults predominant in the pliable organs, such as blood vessels, uterus, and gastrointestinal tract. Collagen type IV is found exclusively in basement membrane. Collagen type V is widely distributed in most of the tissues but never as a major component. *(Rubin and Farber, pp. 79–81)*

207. **(B)** Wound healing that is the accumulation of mostly collagen type I is produced by activated and proliferation of fibroblasts. Fibroblasts originate in the mesenchymal stem cells, which are detected 2 or 3 days after the injury. After 4 or 5 days, the activated fibroblasts show abundant rough endoplasmic reticulum and prominent Golgi complex. They secrete extracellular matrix components, including the collagen types I and III. *(Rubin and Farber, p. 94)*

REFERENCES

Chandrasoma P, Taylor CR. *Concise Pathology*, 3rd ed. Norwalk, CT: Appleton & Lange, 1998.

Cotran RS, Kumar V, Robbins SL. *Robbins Pathologic Basis of Disease*, 6th ed. Philadelphia: Saunders, 1999.

Lewis MG, Rowden G. *Histopathology: A Step by Step Approach*. Boston: Little, Brown, 1987.

Rubin E, Farber JL. *Pathology*. Philadelphia: Lippincott, 1999.

CHAPTER 3

Alterations of Fluid Balance, Hemodynamics, Coagulation, and Acid–Base

The constant cellular demand for oxygen, metabolites, electrolytes, and waste removal requires precisely tuned homeostatic mechanisms for fluid balance and hemodynamics. Perturbations in fluid balance, acid–base, hemodynamics, and coagulation are commonly encountered in medicine and can result in a wide range of pathologic entities such as dehydration, edema, shock, thrombosis, embolization, infarction, and hemorrhage.

BASIC FACTS AND CONCEPTS

The human body is mostly (60%) water, and total body water is divided between intracellular and extracellular compartments. The relative volume of intracellular water is about twice that of extracellular water. In the normal physiologic state, the interstitium is free of excess water (nonedematous) because of the draining action of terminal lymphatics.

	DIRECTION OF FLUID FLOW (MM HG)		
CAPILLARY			**INTERSTITIUM**
Oncotic pressure	← (28)	→ (5)	Oncotic pressure
Hydrostatic pressure	→ (17)	→ (−6.5)	Hydrostatic pressure
	net 0.5 → drawn off by lymphatics		

When the ability of the terminal lymphatics to absorb excess fluid is impaired or the quantity of fluid is excessive, edema can occur. Depending on the site and disease process considered, the resultant edema may be either localized (e.g., urticaria) or diffuse (e.g., anasarca). The usual pathologic mechanisms of edema formation are:

1. Decreased plasma oncotic pressure: hypoalbuminemia secondary to cirrhosis, severe starvation, or nephrotic syndrome;
2. Increased hydrostatic capillary pressure: congestive heart failure;
3. Lymphatic obstruction: filariasis or metastatic cancer;
4. Increased endothelial permeability: urticaria or thermal burns; and/or
5. Increased sodium retention: excessive salt intake.

Decreased total fluid volume is termed "dehydration" and may be seen with insufficient fluid intake and/or with excessive loss of bodily fluids. Excessive loss of selective bodily fluids, such as loss of gastric acid by repeated vomiting, may result not only in dehydration, but may additionally cause abnormalities in electrolyte and acid–base balance.

Decreased vascular perfusion of tissues is termed "shock" and may be caused by:

1. Hypovolemic shock: hemorrhage, dehydration, or diarrhea;
2. Vasodilatory shock: sepsis or anaphylaxis; and/or
3. Cardiogenic shock: myocardial infarct, myocarditis, or tamponade.

Normal hemodynamics is defined as nonturbulent laminar flow of liquefied blood within blood vessels. Abnormal hemodynamics usually occurs with damaged endothelium, vascular stasis, or increased blood coagulability. Pathologic hemodynamics predisposes to intravascular clotting and thrombogenesis that may further engender embolization, hemorrhage, and infarction. Occlusive thrombi or emboli in distal-end arteries of the heart, spleen, or kidney produce wedge-shaped pale infarcts with coagulative necrosis. Thromboses in a dual blood supply organ, such as lung and intestine, characteristically produce a hemorrhagic infarct. Brain infarcts display a unique pattern of liquefaction necrosis.

Bleeding, coagulation, and hemorrhage are intimately related to abnormal hemodynamics, usually as a contributor to the disordered process, a result of the process, or both. The normal coagulation system is a complex cascade of interactive proteins with varying activator, inhibitor, and modifying properties. The task of the coagulation system alternates between the maintenance of blood in the native liquid state and the prompt formation of a stable fibrin clot when activated. The two initiating arms of the coagulation system are divided into the extrinsic and intrinsic systems. The intrinsic system is usually activated by intravascular damage, such as collagen exposed at an ulcerated atheromatous plaque. The extrinsic system is activated by tissue damage, such as a surgeon's incision with liberation of lipoprotein tissue factors. In many instances, the dual systems are coactive. Both pathways share a terminal goal of thrombin–fibrin production. "Fibrinolysis" is the term used to describe the physiologic dissolution of the fibrin clot. Hyperactive fibrinolysis is operative in a number of disease states, such as disseminated intravascular coagulation, carcinomatosis, and multiple recurrent deep vein thromboses.

Alterations of pH deleteriously affect a myriad of intracellular enzymatic processes that sustain life. Disturbances of acid–base in their pure form are pathologically sorted into four categories: respiratory acidosis, respiratory alkalosis, metabolic acidosis, and metabolic alkalosis.

FORM	pH	P_{CO_2}	H_{CO_3}	EXAMPLE
Respiratory acidosis	↓	↑	↑	Hypoventilation
Respiratory alkalosis	↑	↓	↓	Hyperventilation
Metabolic acidosis	↓	Normal	↓	Diabetic ketoacidosis
Metabolic alkalosis	↑	Normal	↑	Gastric suction

Questions

DIRECTIONS (Questions 208 through 250): Each of the numbered items or incomplete statements in this section is followed by answers or by completions of the statement. Selection the ONE lettered answer or completion that is BEST in each case.

208. The single largest constituent of the body by weight is

    (A) lysosomes
    (B) ribosomes
    (C) nucleic acid
    (D) water
    (E) blood

209. The tissue that has the lowest percentage of water is

    (A) spleen
    (B) heart
    (C) liver
    (D) adipose tissue
    (E) skeletal muscle

210. Which of the following factor(s) is/are involved in thrombus formation?

    (A) endothelial injury
    (B) turbulence of blood flow
    (C) stasis of blood
    (D) blood hypercoagulability
    (E) all of the above

211. Identify the factor or factors in which vitamin K is required for synthesis.

    (A) factor II (Prothrombin)
    (B) clotting factor VII

    (C) clotting factor IX
    (D) clotting factor X
    (E) all of the above

212. The purpose of the lymphatic valves is

    (A) to allow lymph because flow in only one direction
    (B) nonexistent, because lymphatics do not have valves
    (C) to reduce lymphatic oncotic pressure
    (D) to reduce lymphatic hydrostatic pressure
    (E) to increase lymphatic oncotic pressure

213. Predisposing conditions for vascular thrombosis include

    (A) turbulent blood flow
    (B) increased blood viscosity
    (C) stasis of blood
    (D) injury to the endothelial barrier
    (E) all of the above

214. Identify the factor that inhibits platelet aggregation.

    (A) prostacyclin (PG12)
    (B) epinephrine
    (C) adenosine diphosphate
    (D) 5-hydroxytryptamine
    (E) thrombin

215. Hypostatic pneumonia is

(A) usually caused by a virus
(B) secondary infection of chronic pulmonary edema
(C) associated with low blood pressure
(D) associated with low electrical charges
(E) infections of the legs with pulmonary complications

216. Which are likely causes of edema?

(A) increased vascular hydrostatic pressure
(B) lymphatic obstruction
(C) increased vascular oncotic pressure
(D) increased vascular permeability
(E) all of the above

217. Clinical states associated with generalized edema may include

(A) congestive heart failure
(B) nephrotic syndrome
(C) protein malnutrition
(D) cirrhosis
(E) all of the above

218. Identify the bleeding disorder that showed elevated prothrombin time (PT).

(A) vascular defects
(B) platelet defects
(C) hemophilia A
(D) deficiency of vitamin K
(E) thrombocytopenia

219. When viewed under the microscope with routine hematoxylin and eosin (H & E) stains, edema fluid appears as

(A) pink acellular precipitates
(B) blue nuclei, pink cytoplasm
(C) depends on cell type
(D) bile-stained gelatinous plugs
(E) lines of Zahn

220. Chronic passive congestion of the lung might include which of the following?

(A) brown induration

(B) hemosiderin macrophages
(C) congested alveolar capillaries
(D) pulmonary edema
(E) all of the above

221. What is the most common effect of pulmonary thromboemboli?

(A) results in pulmonary edema
(B) produces infarction by occluding the bronchial artery
(C) can produce right-sided heart failure
(D) usually produces pulmonary fibrosis
(E) causes hyaline membrane disease

222. Hydrogen ion concentration is expressed as

(A) mg/dL
(B) mg%
(C) pH
(D) P_{CO_2}
(E) mEq/L

223. An anxious man is brought to the emergency department feeling light-headed. His arterial blood gas is pH 7.52, HCO_3 is 21 mmol/L, and P_{CO_2} is 20 mm Hg. The most likely diagnosis is

(A) metabolic acidosis
(B) respiratory alkalosis
(C) inappropriate anion gap
(D) respiratory acidosis
(E) metabolic alkalosis

224. A 63-year-old female has been vomiting for several hours. Her blood gases are pH 7.51, HCO_3 32 mmol/L, and P_{CO_2} 40 mm Hg. The most likely diagnosis is

(A) anion gap metabolic acidosis
(B) nonanion gap metabolic acidosis
(C) metabolic alkalosis
(D) respiratory acidosis
(E) respiratory alkalosis

225. Which would be an UNEXPECTED finding with an elevated serum hydrogen ion concentration?

(A) acidosis

(B) renal compensation by increased urinary H^+

(C) pulmonary compensation by hypoventilation

(D) pH 7.20

(E) elevated serum K^+

226. Which item is important in determining if a vascular occlusion will cause infarction?

(A) rate at which the occlusion develops

(B) anatomic pattern of blood supply

(C) vulnerability of the tissue to ischemia

(D) presence of a collateral blood supply

(E) all of the above

227. Indicate the factor(s) that may cause hyperkalemia.

(A) triamterene

(B) acidosis

(C) juvenile diabetes mellitus

(D) adrenal insufficiency

(E) all of the above

228. In a failing cirrhotic liver, the edema is secondary to

(A) anemia

(B) hypocalcemia

(C) hypertension

(D) hypoproteinemia

(E) hyponatremia

229. An organized thrombus that begins to be recanalized, the cells involved in the process are

(A) the fibrinolytic system

(B) monocytes and macrophages neutrophils and fibroblasts

(C) neutrophils and fibroblasts

(D) platelets and fibroblasts

(E) fibroblasts and endothelium

230. The enzyme responsible for the conversion of bicarbonate and carbon dioxide into carbonic acid is

(A) adenosine triphosphatase (ATPase) sodium pump

(B) chloride anhydrase

(C) carbonic acid transferase

(D) carbonic anhydrase

(E) acetazolamide

231. Normal serum osmolality is about

(A) 210 mmol/kg

(B) 250 mmol/kg

(C) 290 mmol/kg

(D) 325 mmol/kg

(E) 350 mmol/kg

232. When a mural thrombus is examined grossly, the Lines of Zahn are more easily demonstrated in

(A) intra-abdominal blood clots

(B) intra-arterial thrombi

(C) right ventricular thrombi

(D) fresh gastrointestinal hemorrhage

(E) deep venous thrombi

233. The development of new blood channels through an occlusive thrombus is called

(A) infarction

(B) fibrinolysis

(C) recanalization

(D) propagation

(E) embolization

234. Chronic passive congestion of the spleen would be expected to include

(A) increase in splenic weight

(B) sinusoids filled with erythrocytes

(C) cyanosis

(D) hemosiderin deposition

(E) all of the above

235. Indicate a factor that promotes thrombosis.

(A) protein C

(B) prostacyclin

(C) nitric oxide

(D) tissue plasminogen activator

(E) von Willebrand factor

236. Identify the solution with the highest osmolality

    (A) 2 mol of NaCl dissolved in 1 L of H_2O
    (B) 1 mol of $MgSO_4$ dissolved in 1 L of H_2O
    (C) 1 mol of KCl dissolved in 1 L of H_2O
    (D) 1 mol of KCl dissolved in 2 L of H_2O
    (E) 1 mol of NaCl dissolved in 2 L of H_2O

237. Which tissue undergoes liquefaction when infarcted?

    (A) kidney
    (B) small bowel
    (C) heart
    (D) spleen
    (E) brain

238. The single necessary criterion to define shock is

    (A) rapid bleeding
    (B) inadequate tissue perfusion
    (C) loss of plasma proteins
    (D) severe burns
    (E) massive internal injuries

239. The earliest step in arterial thrombosis is

    (A) activation of common pathway
    (B) adherence of platelets to vessel walls
    (C) activation of intrinsic pathway
    (D) activation of plasminogen
    (E) activation of Hageman factor

240. The factor least likely to cause thrombosis is

    (A) damaged vascular wall
    (B) turbulent blood flow
    (C) decreased factor VIII
    (D) venous stasis
    (E) increased platelet count

241. Which cell secretes von Willebrand factor?

    (A) hepatocyte
    (B) neutrophil
    (C) lymphocyte
    (D) endothelial cell
    (E) platelet

242. A mural thrombus is most likely found in the

    (A) heart
    (B) coronary artery
    (C) right middle cerebral artery
    (D) right anterior cerebral artery
    (E) spleen

243. Which would be an unexpected finding in occlusive coronary thrombosis?

    (A) thrombus at site of abnormal blood vessel wall
    (B) ischemic necrosis
    (C) myocardial infarct
    (D) coronary atherosclerosis
    (E) thrombocytopenia

244. Which factor is part of the extrinsic clotting system?

    (A) factor VII
    (B) factor XII
    (C) factor XI
    (D) factor IX
    (E) factor VIII

245. Thrombi would not be likely to form with

    (A) deficiency of antithrombin III (AT III)
    (B) venous stasis
    (C) endothelial damage
    (D) turbulent blood flow
    (E) decreased clotting factors

246. A hemorrhagic infarct is most likely in which site?

    (A) spleen
    (B) kidney
    (C) anterior left cardiac ventricle
    (D) posterior left cardiac ventricle
    (E) lung

247. Which statement is true concerning occlusive arterial thrombi?

    (A) encountered frequently in coronary arteries
    (B) may be associated with atherosclerotic lesion

(C) arteritis may be the initiating event

(D) may be seen in arterial trauma

(E) all of the above

248. The term "paradoxical embolism" is best defined as

(A) death in a healthy person from a saddle-type pulmonary embolism

(B) an embolism that does not cause an infarct

(C) an organized embolus

(D) a venous embolus that gains access to the arterial side through a heart wall defect

(E) emboli from deep venous thrombosis

249. Gas embolism can be seen in which of the following?

(A) uterine delivery or abortion

(B) caisson disease

(C) traumatic injury to chest wall or lung

(D) decompression sickness

(E) all of the above

250. Shock can be seen commonly in which of the following events?

(A) massive hemorrhage

(B) septicemia

(C) myocardial infarct

(D) anaphylaxis

(E) all of the above

DIRECTIONS (Questions 251 through 297): Each group of items in this section consists of a list of lettered options followed by a set of numbered words or phrases. For each numbered word or phrase, select the ONE lettered option that is most closely associated with it. Each lettered option may be selected once, more than once, or not at all.

Questions 251 through 254

(A) alpha-1 antitrypsin

(B) streptokinase

(C) Stuart–Prower factor

(D) adenosine diphosphate (ADP)

(E) thrombin

251. Exogenous plasmin

252. Common name for factor II

253. Plasmin inhibitor

254. Platelet adherence factor

Questions 255 through 258

(A) aldosterone

(B) lactic acid

(C) methotrexate

(D) acetazolamide

(E) bicarbonate

255. Important extracellular buffer

256. Markedly elevated with tissue anoxia

257. Hormone involved in sodium regulation

258. Carbonic anhydrase inhibitor

Questions 259 through 262

(A) total body water

(B) intracellular water

(C) extracellular water

(D) plasma

(E) fibrin

259. 40% of lean body weight

260. 60% of lean body weight

261. 5% of lean body weight

262. 20% of lean body weight

Questions 263 through 266

(A) hydropericardium

(B) hydroperitoneum

(C) hydrosalpinx

(D) hemothorax

(E) pyarthrosis

263. Collection of blood in a pleural cavity

264. Collection of pus in a joint space

265. Collection of fluid in the peritoneal cavity

266. Collection of fluid in a fallopian tube

Questions 267 through 270

- (A) bleeding time
- (B) prothrombin time
- (C) partial thromboplastin time
- (D) clot retraction test
- (E) clot lysis test

267. In vitro test that evaluates the extrinsic clotting system

268. In vitro test that evaluates the intrinsic clotting system

269. In vivo test that evaluates platelet and capillary function

270 In vitro test that evaluates platelet actomyosin contraction

Questions 271 through 274

- (A) filariasis
- (B) urticaria
- (C) psoriasis
- (D) congestive heart failure
- (E) hypoalbuminemia

271. Edema due to decreased vascular oncotic pressure

272. Edema due to increased endothelial permeability

273. Edema due to lymphatic obstruction

274. Edema due to increased capillary hydrostatic pressure

Questions 275 through 278

- (A) air embolism
- (B) fat embolism
- (C) amniotic fluid embolism
- (D) nitrogen embolism
- (E) serosal embolism

275. Usually associated with DIC and caused by childbirth

276. Usually seen with multiple fractures of large bones

277. Usually seen as decompression sickness in scuba divers

278. Usually seen with thoracic puncture wounds and pneumothorax

Questions 279 through 282

- (A) renal infarct
- (B) angina pectoris
- (C) intermittent claudication
- (D) stroke
- (E) amaurosis fugax

279. Emboli to ophthalmic artery

280. Emboli to middle cerebral artery

281. Thrombosis of a coronary artery

282. Emboli to branches of the renal artery

Questions 283 through 286

- (A) calcium
- (B) chloride
- (C) potassium
- (D) bicarbonate
- (E) sodium

283. Major intracellular cation

284. Major extracellular cation

285. Anionic form of a major body buffer

286. Cation active in coagulation and muscle contraction

Questions 287 through 289

- (A) acute metabolic acidosis
- (B) acute metabolic alkalosis
- (C) acute respiratory acidosis
- (D) acute respiratory alkalosis
- (E) chronic metabolic acidosis
- (F) chronic metabolic alkalosis
- (G) chronic respiratory acidosis
- (H) chronic respiratory alkalosis

287. A medical student is taking part in an experiment and volunteers to breathe air to which 10% carbon dioxide has been added. After 10 minutes, the student's blood gases are pH 7.28, P_{CO_2} 51 mm Hg, and HCO_3 32 mmol/L.

288. A young child is about to have an arterial blood gas study and begins hyperventilating. The laboratory reports the blood gases as pH 7.51, P_{CO_2} 26 mm Hg, and HCO_3 18 mmol/L.

289. A depressed man drinks ethylene glycol in an attempted suicide. In the emergency department his blood gases are pH 7.19, P_{CO_2} 40 mm Hg, HCO_3 19 mmol/L.

Questions 290 through 292

 (A) air emboli
 (B) amniotic fluid emboli
 (C) fat emboli
 (D) nitrogen emboli
 (E) mesenteric venous thromboses
 (F) candidiasis
 (G) hydropericardium
 (H) hemopericardium

290. A 32-year-old female with a family history of antithrombin III deficiency dies suddenly after complaining of abdominal pain for 7 days. At autopsy, there is a segment of gangrenous bowel which anatomically is drained by the superior mesenteric vein. What is most likely to be found in this vein?

291. A 21-year-old pregnant female is having a very difficult and prolonged labor. She begins to develop disseminated intravascular coagulation. What is likely to be found in her lungs?

292. A 47-year-old man with Marfan's syndrome complains of chest pain and dies suddenly. At autopsy there is a dissecting aneurysm of the thoracic aorta due to cystic medial necrosis. Proximally, the dissection extends through the root of the aorta into the pericardial sac. What is likely to be found in the pericardial space?

Questions 293 through 297

 (A) fat embolism
 (B) pulmonary embolism
 (C) nitrogen embolism
 (D) amniotic fluid embolism
 (E) anasarca
 (F) hydrosalpinx
 (G) exudate
 (H) transudate

293. An inexperienced scuba diver ascends from a depth of 60 meters to the surface in about 4 minutes. Shortly after surfacing the diver complains of severe muscle contractions and intense abdominal pain.

294. A 26-year-old male fractures his pelvis and femur in a motor vehicle accident. On the third hospital day he dies after developing a hemorrhagic rash, respiratory distress, and cerebral dysfunction. At autopsy, fat globules are found scattered in the cerebral cortex, kidney, and lung.

295. A 43-year-old obese female is admitted to the hospital for treatment of deep vein thromboses. On the night of admission she suddenly dies. At autopsy, a large plug of laminated blood clot is found to occlude the main pulmonary artery.

296. A 63-year-old man in congestive heart failure has a fluid accumulation withdrawn from his right pleural space. The laboratory analysis of the fluid is: specific gravity 1.008, albumin 0.2 g/dL, white blood cells 2/μL, and red blood cells O/μL.

297. A 59-year-old female with widely metastatic breast carcinoma has a fluid accumulation withdrawn from her left pleural space. The laboratory analysis of the fluid is: specific gravity 1.028, albumin 3.1 g/dL, white blood cells 32, 200/μL, and red blood cells 2,900/μL.

Answers and Explanations

208. (D) Approximately 60% of the lean body weight is water, two-thirds of which is intracellular, and the remaining will be in the extracellular components mostly as interstitial fluid. (*Cotran et al., pp. 113–114*)

209. (D) Adipose tissue is 10% water. The other tissues are about 60% water. Because adipose tissue contributes 100% of its mass to total body weight but only 10% of its mass to total body water, all discussions of total body water use an idealized lean body, without any significant adipose tissue. In this way, water compartments can be discussed regardless of the body's nutritional status or habitus. (*Cotran et al., pp. 113–114*)

210. (E) The so-called Virchow's Triad are the primary causes that influence thrombous formation which are: endothelial injury, stasis and turbulence of the blood and hypercoagulability of the blood. (*Cotran et al., p. 124*)

211. (E) Vitamin K deficiency will lead to an impairment of the synthesis of coagulation factors such as VII, IX, X, and II (prothrombin). In vitamin K deficiency the PT is typically prolonged and PTT may also be prolonged. Because fibrinogen synthesis is not vitamin K dependent, the TT remains normal. (*Henry, p. 740*)

212. (A) The lymphatic valves are important in maintaining unidirectional flow. Both lymphatics and capillaries possess valves. The oncotic pressure is a function of the number of particles in solution, and valves do not affect it. Lymph trying to flow backward tends to build up next to valves, raising the lymphatic hydrostatic pressure, not lowering it. (*Cotran et al., p. 115*)

213. (E) Vascular thrombosis is usually seen in association with alterations in blood flow, damage to the endothelial barrier, and in hypercoagulable states. Normal blood flow is laminar and nonturbulent. Abnormalities of blood flow that predispose to thrombus formation include sluggish flow, stasis, increased viscosity, and turbulence. Damage to the endothelial barrier may expose collagen or lipid fractions that are potent initiators of thrombogenesis. Hypercoagulable blood has an increased potential for thrombosis. Hypercoagulable states include those with increased platelets (thrombocytosis), acquired or hereditary absence of coagulation cascade inhibitors (antithrombin III deficiency), and premature activation of protein clotting factors (disseminated intravascular coagulation). (*Cotran et al., pp. 124–129*)

214. (A) Autacoids is a potent bioactive compounds that are released locally and act in short distances, and they are rapidly inactivated. Endothelial cells release autacoids and, thereby, exert effect on vascular tone and platelet activity. For example, prostacyclin is the first autacoid observed relaxes smooth muscle and inhibits the aggregation of platelets. (*Rubin and Farber, p. 483*)

215. (B) Secondary infection of chronic pulmonary edema is termed "hypostatic pneumonia." It is almost always a bacterial not a viral infection. It has no specific relationship to low blood pressure, low electrical charges, or leg infections. (*Cotran et al., pp. 116–117*)

216. (E) Edema, the fluid expansion of the interstitial space, has numerous causes, including increased vascular hydrostatic pressure (congestive heart failure), decreased vascular oncotic pressure (hypoalbuminemia), lymphatic obstruction (lymphedema), increased capillary permeability (burns), and increased interstitial osmotic pressure (poor renal perfusion). *(Cotran et al., pp. 113–116)*

217. (E) Congestive heart failure increases the venous hydrostatic pressure, favoring edema formation. Protein malnutrition and nephrotic syndrome both lower vascular oncotic pressure, and cirrhosis increases venous hydrostatic pressure and, by hypoalbuminemia, lowers vascular oncotic pressure. Both of these factors promote edema. *(Cotran et al., pp. 113–116)*

218. (D) Please refer to Answer 211. *(Guyton, p. 431)*

219. (A) Edema fluid is acellular proteinaceous material that appears as a pink precipitate with H & E stain. Because edema fluid is acellular, it is not dependent on cell type, nor does it have nuclei or cytoplasm. Lines of Zahn describe alternating strata of fibrin and red blood cells in thrombi. Bile-stained gelatinous plugs bear no relationship to the microscopic appearance of edema fluid. *(Cotran et al., p. 116)*

220. (E) Chronic passive congestion must, by definition, have congested alveolar capillaries. In more severe or long-standing cases, fluid and red blood cells leak out into the alveolar spaces. This transudate fluid in the alveolar space is termed "pulmonary edema." The red blood cells are broken down to form hemosiderin (brown pigment) inside macrophages. Occasionally, a fibrotic process will occur grossly that is called "brown induration." Erythema, a reddish hue, is seen in states of active hyperemia not the passive hyperemia of pulmonary passive congestion. *(Cotran et al., p. 116)*

221. (C) Occlusions of the pulmonary arteries by blood clots are almost always embolic in origin. These complications in patients who are already suffering from such underlying disorders as hypercoagulable states, malignancies, or long periods of embolization may lead to infarct. In general, the clinical significance of pulmonary embolism depend on the extent to which the pulmonary artery blood flow is obstructed. It could be a hemodynamic compromise with pulmonary hypertension and acute right-sided failure. A large pulmonary emboli could produce sudden death, without leading to an infarct. *(Cotran et al., pp. 703, 704)*

222. (C) Hydrogen ion concentration is expressed as pH units, representing the antilog of hydrogen ion concentration. This logarithmic expression is useful to cover the wide range of hydrogen ion concentration found in nature. *(Henry, pp. 134–135)*

223. (B) When evaluating acid–base problems, look first at the pH and P_{CO_2}. The man's pH is more than 7.4, so he is alkalotic (acidotic choices then cannot be correct). The P_{CO_2} is not 40 mm Hg, so there is a respiratory component. Changes in P_{CO_2} are only respiratory, not metabolic. With these two datapoints, only one choice remains, respiratory alkalosis. The presentation, one of nervous hyperventilation, is the classic example. The anion gap is useful in separating forms of metabolic acidosis but provides no useful information in this instance. *(Guyton, pp. 340–342)*

224. (C) The pH is elevated (alkalotic), so there is no acidosis. The P_{CO_2} is normal at 40 mm Hg, indicating that there is no respiratory component. This clinical presentation is classic for metabolic alkalosis. Prolonged vomiting loses HCl from the stomach and allows a metabolic alkalosis to develop. In a real clinical setting, there usually would be compensatory hypoventilation (respiratory acidosis) to attempt to correct the pH to 7.4. *(Guyton, pp. 340–342)*

225. (C) An increased serum hydrogen ion concentration is an acidotic state with a pH less than 7.4. Common bodily compensatory mechanisms include movement of K^+ out of cells into the serum in exchange for H^+, increased renal secretion of H^+, and hyperventilation. Hypoventilation would exacerbate the acidosis by alveolar retention of P_{CO_2}. *(Guyton, pp. 330–342)*

226. (E) The rate at which the occlusion develops is important, because an acute rapid obstruction can lead to infarction, whereas, a slow occlusion of an artery may give time for the formation of collateral circulation and preventing, in this way, the injury. The organs that have an alternative blood supply (lungs, liver) are more resistant to develop infarcts. The tissues that are highly dependent on oxygen (brain) can have a irreversible damage in minutes. (*Cotran et al., p. 133*)

227. (E) Hyperkalemia is an increase in blood potassium concentration. Increases are associated with acidosis, such as in diabetes, with K+ moving out of the cell into plasma in exchange for H+. Triamterene is a potassium-sparing diuretic and, unlike most of the other diuretics, can cause hyperkalemia by renal potassium retention. Aldosterone saves renal sodium at the expense of K+. In states of low aldosterone (such as adrenal insufficiency), there is hyperkalemia. In states of high aldosterone (such as aldosterone-secreting tumors), there is hypernatremia with hypokalemia. (*Henry, pp. 130–131*)

228. (D) Reduced plasma osmotic pressure can result from excessive loss, or reduced synthesis of albumin, in a condition such as liver failure. The serum albumin and proteins are most responsible for maintaining the colloid osmotic pressure. Reduced albumin synthesis that is a consequence of the liver failure or protein malnutrition can lead to extravasation of fluids with the typical clinical picture of edema. (*Cotran et al., p. 115*)

229. (E) Following thrombotic vascular occlusion the thrombi undergo different events that could include propagation, embolization, dissolution, and organization with recanalization. On the latter, the thrombi may undergo fibrosis, with organization that eventually may become recanalized with re-establishment of the vascular flow. The thrombi may end up incorporated into the vessel wall. On the recanalization, the most important cells that play a role are the fibroblasts and endothelium. (*Cotran et al., p. 127*)

230. (D) The enzyme responsible for the conversion of carbon dioxide and bicarbonate into carbonic acid is carbonic anhydrase. Acetazolamide is a potent inhibitor of carbonic anhydrase and a diuretic. (*Guyton, pp. 331–334*)

231. (C) Normal serum osmolality is about 290 mmol/L. A quick approximation is given by the formula

$$osmolality = 2(sodium) + (glucose/20) + (BUN/3)$$

where osmolality is calculated as mmol/L, the sodium is in mmol/L, the glucose is in mg/dL, and the BUN (blood urea nitrogen) is in mg/dL. The factors of 20 and 3 convert the mg/dL units of glucose and BUN, respectively, into mmol/L. Serum osmolality is controlled principally by antidiuretic hormone (ADH) which is synthesized by the hypothalamus and then stored in the posterior pituitary. States of high serum osmolality (dehydration) result in increased ADH release. Circulating ADH acts on the kidney to elevate urinary osmolality. The free water generated in the kidney is used to dilute the blood back to its normal osmolality of about 290 mmol/L. (*Henry, pp. 143–146*)

232. (B) In the major arteries, particularly in the aorta, as well as in the heart, the thrombi may exhibit on cross section apparent laminations. These are called Lines of Zahn. They are produced by alternating pale layers of platelets admixed with some fibrin and darker layers containing red cells. Lines of Zahn are significant only in that they imply thrombosis at a site of blood flow. In vein or smaller arteries, the laminations are typically not as apparent, and, in fact, thrombi formed in the sluggish venous flow usually resemble statically coagulated blood. (*Cotran et al., p. 126*)

233. (C) Recanalization is the development of new channels in an occlusive thrombus. Infarction is tissue death from inadequate blood supply, a common result of arterial occlusive thrombi. Fibrinolysis is the dissolving of thrombus clot by plasma proteins, particularly plasmin. Propagation is the continued enlargement of a thrombus and predisposes to embolization, which is the breaking off of parts of a thrombus that are then carried in the bloodstream to a different site. *(Cotran et al., pp. 127–129)*

234. (E) Passive splenic congestion produces a heavy, cyanotic spleen. The cut surface freely exudes blood. The sinusoids are dilated and filled by erythrocytes. The splenic capsule is expanded and tense. *(Cotran et al., pp. 750–751)*

235. (E) Hemophilia A and von Willebrand disease, two of the most commonly inherited disorders of bleeding, are caused by qualitative or quantitative defects involving the factor VIII, von Willebrand factor complex. The plasma factor VIII–vWF is a complex made up of two separate proteins (factor VIII and vWF) that can be distinguished by functional, biochemical, and immunologic criteria. One component, which is required for the activation of factor X in the intrinsic coagulation pathway, is called factor VIII procoagulant protein. The most important function of vWF in vivo is to facilitate the adhesion of platelets to subendothelial collagen. vWF is crucial to the normal process of hemostasis and its absence in von Willebrand disease leads to bleeding diathesis. *(Cotran et al., p. 638)*

236. (A) Osmolality depends on the number of particles per unit volume, irrespective of charge. The term used to describe electrical charges per unit volume is "equivalents." In the choices listed, each chemical rapidly separates into ions in H_2O. To find the choice with the highest osmolality, find the one with the most particles per unit volume.

RELATIVE OSMOLALITY

A	2
B	1
C	1
D	½
E	½

To find the solution with the highest equivalence, find the one with the most electrical charges per concentration. *(Henry, pp. 42–43, 125–126)*

237. (E) Infarcts cause coagulative necrosis in most organs (including kidney, small bowel, heart,

and spleen) whether caused by a white or a red infarct. Coagulative necrosis microscopically appears as an acellular, nuclei-depleted ghost image of the normal tissue architecture. The brain is an exception and undergoes liquefaction with infarcts. The infarcted brain tissue is rapidly liquefied, losing its usual architecture, and phagocytized by microglia. *(Rubin and Farber, pp. 294–299)*

238. (B) Shock is defined succinctly as inadequate tissue perfusion. All the other answers are common causes of inadequate tissue perfusion but do not define the single necessary criterion for shock. *(Rubin and Farber, pp. 300–304)*

239. (B) Adherence of platelets to the vessel wall is the earliest event in arterial thrombosis. This is followed by activation of Hageman factor of the intrinsic system and a cascade effect with subsequent activation of the rest of the intrinsic system components. The end result of intrinsic system activation is activation of the common pathway. Plasminogen activation is part of the fibrinolysis system and would dissolve clots, not form them. *(Cotran et al., pp. 117–119)*

240. (C) A system of checks and balances in the body maintains the fine line between bleeding and thrombosis. *(Cotran et al., pp. 638–639)*

241. (D) von Willebrand factor, a component of coagulation factor VIII, is made by endothelial cells and is a necessary cofactor for the adherence of platelets to subendothelial tissue. Although hepatocytes take many of the circulating protein coagulant factors, they do not produce von Willebrand factor. Platelets are crucial for coagulation but do not synthesize von Willebrand factor. Neutrophils and lymphocytes are not significantly involved in hemostasis. *(Cotran et al., pp. 638–639)*

242. (A) A mural thrombus is a nonocclusive blood clot that forms on the wall of a large volume blood-filled organ, such as the heart or aorta. Small arteries, such as the cerebral and coronaries, form occlusive thrombi. Since the spleen is a solid organ, mural thrombi could not form. *(Cotran et al., pp. 119–120)*

243. **(E)** An occlusive arterial thrombus, such as coronary thrombosis, is almost always at the site of a vessel abnormality. The most common abnormality is atherosclerosis. Rarer abnormalities include arteritis and trauma. An expected finding in coronary thrombosis is infarction of the myocardium, with ischemic (coagulative) necrosis. Thrombocytopenia is not expected in coronary thrombosis, since platelets must be present in adequate numbers and function to initiate a thrombus. A low platelet count would make thrombus formation unlikely. *(Rubin and Farber, pp. 292–293)*

244. **(A)** Factor VII is part of the extrinsic pathway. All the other choices are part of the intrinsic clotting mechanism. *(Cotran et al., pp. 122–124)*

245. **(E)** The three major influences in thrombogenesis are injury to endothelium, alterations in normal blood flow (turbulent flow or stasis), and hypercoagulability (as in rare AT III-deficient people). A decrease in the clotting factors would make the blood potentially hypocoagulable, with subsequent thrombus formation unlikely. *(Cotran et al., pp. 119–121)*

246. **(E)** Hemorrhagic infarcts, also called "red infarcts," are encountered usually with venous occlusions, in loose tissues, in tissues with a double circulation, and in tissues previously congested. The other type of infarct, white or anemic infarcts, is usually seen with arterial occlusion, single end-artery blood supply, and in solid tissues. The lungs characteristically have hemorrhagic infarcts. *(Rubin and Farber, p. 293)*

247. **(E)** Occlusive arterial thrombi occur frequently in the coronary arteries, usually at the site of an atherosclerotic lesion. Other affected vessels include cerebral, iliac, and femoral arteries. Rarely, occlusive thrombi occur at sites of trauma or arteritis. Emboli almost never occur with occlusive arterial thrombi, since the artery's diameter decreases distally. *(Cotran et al., pp. 124–129)*

248. **(D)** Paradoxical emboli are those from the venous system that gain access to the arterial circulation through a heart wall defect. Sudden death from a pulmonary embolus in healthy people is not common. These pulmonary emboli usually originate in the deep veins of the leg (deep venous thrombosis). Not all emboli cause infarcts. An organized embolism is one that has an ingrowth of young blood vessels and fibrous tissue. *(Cotran et al., p. 289)*

249. **(E)** Gas embolism is the abnormal occurrence of gas bubbles in the circulation. They gain entrance to the circulation by trauma (lung, chest wall, ruptured uterine veins) or by coming out of solution from fatty tissues (decompression sickness, or Caisson disease). *(Rubin and Farber, pp. 290–292)*

250. **(E)** Shock, or inadequate tissue perfusion, commonly is associated with cardiogenic failure, hypovolemia, pooling of blood in periphery, anaphylaxis, disseminated intravascular coagulation and septicemia. *(Rubin and Farber, pp. 300–306)*

251–254. **(251-B, 252-E, 253-A, 254-D)** All of the listed choices are effectors of coagulation or fibrinolysis. The fibrinolytic system dissolves clots mainly through activation of plasmin. A potent inhibitor of plasmin activation is alpha$_1$-antitrypsin. A nonhuman source (exogenous) of plasmin activity is streptokinase, which is used therapeutically to dissolve thrombi, particularly those in the coronary circulation. Thrombin is the common name for factor II, an element of the common pathway. ADP is a platelet-aggregating factor. *(Cotran et al., pp. 122–124)*

255–258. **(255-E, 256-B, 257-A, 258-D)** The major extracellular buffer is bicarbonate. It is the buffering salt of carbonic acid (H_2CO_3). Lactic acid is produced by anaerobic glycolysis in states of tissue anoxia. Aldosterone, a hormone, and antidiuretic hormone regulate sodium concentration in the body. Acetazolamide is an inhibitor of carbonic anhydrase, which is an enzyme present in lung and kidney and is involved in acid–base regulation. *(Guyton, pp. 331–334)*

259–262. **(259-B, 260-A, 261-D, 262-C)** Total body water is about 60% of lean body weight (LBW).

The total body water is two-thirds (40% LBW) intracellular and one-third (20% LBW) extracellular. Plasma, part of the extracellular component, makes up about 5% LBW. *(Guyton, pp. 273–279)*

263–266. (263-D, 264-E, 265-B, 266-C) Abnormal collections of fluid in the body are named by both the site of occurrence and the character of fluid that accumulates. The most common sites include peritoneum, pericardium, thorax, joints, and fallopian tube. If the fluid that accumulates is watery or serous, the prefix "hydro" is used. If the fluid is bloody, the prefix "hemo" is used. Purulent collections are characterized by the prefix "py." For example, a collection of bloody fluid in the pericardium is termed "hemopericardium." Watery fluid accumulations in the pleural cavity of the chest are called "hydrothorax." Purulent expansions of the joint space are called "pyarthroses." *(Rubin and Farber, pp. 299–302)*

267–270. (267-B, 268-C, 269-A, 270-D) Laboratory tests are commonly used to evaluate the hemostatic status of patients. The prothrombin time (PT) and partial thromboplastin time (PTT) are in vitro tests of the extrinsic and intrinsic clotting systems, respectively. Both employ activators (PT = thromboplastin, PTT = kaolin–cephalin) in the presence of added calcium to stimulate the patient's calcium-depleted plasma to produce a fibrin clot. The clot normally forms in about 12 seconds for the PT and about 25 seconds for the PTT. Decreased protein clotting factors or circulating anticoagulants will prolong these tests. The bleeding time is an in vivo test used to evaluate platelet and capillary function. After placing a blood pressure cuff at 40 mm Hg on the upper arm, a small incision is made on the forearm. Every 30 seconds thereafter, the wound is gently touched with blotter paper to see if it is still bleeding. The time it takes the incision to stop bleeding is termed the "bleeding time." Normal values are usually under than 8 minutes. Abnormal platelet function, thrombocytopenia, or capillary abnormalities all can prolong the bleeding time. The clot retraction test is an in vitro test of platelet contraction. Normally, a clot will retract from 40–60% of its initial volume during 4 hours when incubated at 37°C. The clot lysis test is an in vitro test for fibrinolysis. If the fibrinolytic system is hyperactive (DIC, carcinomatosis), the clot will lyse in only a few hours, instead of the normal 18–24 hours. *(Cotran et al., pp. 633–634)*

271–274. (271-E, 272-B, 273-A, 274-D) The draining suction of the terminal lymphatics and vascular oncotic pressure work together to maintain the interstitium in a dry, nonedematous state. Decreased oncotic pressure due to hypoalbuminemia can result in edema. Obstruction of the lymphatic channels occurs in filariasis and can produce edema. Urticaria is localized edema caused by histamine release, with increased endothelial permeability, and subsequent leakage of fluid into the interstitium. Congestive heart failure may produce edema via increased capillary hydrostatic pressure. *(Cotran et al., pp. 113–116)*

275–278. (275-C, 276-B, 277-D, 278-A) The partial or complete obstruction of vascular channels from a traveling fragment of blood clot or other substance is termed "embolism." Amniotic embolism usually occurs during prolonged, strenuous labor because of the forceful introduction of amniotic fluid contents into the uterine venous sinuses. The pernicious nature of amniotic embolism results from DIC which amniotic fluid's potent thromboplastin activity initiates. Major boney fractures almost always release particles of fat into the venous circulation to embolize in brain, lung, and kidney. In certain instances adult respiratory distress syndrome and cerebral confusion may result. Decompression sickness is seen in divers who surface too rapidly after being submerged for long periods. As they ascend, nitrogen gas comes out of solution as bubbles that act as emboli. Air embolism occurs when air enters the vascular system, usually due to thoracic trauma. Only about 150 mL of embolic air is fatal. *(Cotran et al., pp. 129–132)*

279–282. (279-E, 280-D, 281-B, 282-A) As emboli travel through the vascular system, they may totally or partially occlude the vessel lumen. Ischemia, functional impairment, or infarction of the tissue may result from this luminal stenosis. For example, an embolic stenosis of the ophthalmic artery may produce transient monocular blindness (amaurosis fugax). Emboli to the middle cerebral artery often cause cerebral infarcts (strokes). Emboli to branches of the renal artery may result in a typical fan-shaped pale renal infarct of the end-artery type. "Angina pectoris" is the term used for chest pain due to myocardial ischemia. The usual etiology of angina pectoris is atherosclerosis with subsequent coronary artery stenosis. Ischemic leg pains that develop with exercise are called "intermittent claudication." Atherosclerotic stenosis of the femoral or popliteal artery is the usual cause of intermittent claudication. *(Cotran et al., pp. 132–134)*

283–286. (283-C, 284-E, 285-D, 286-A) Cations are positively charged ions. Anions are negatively charged ions. The major intracellular and extracellular cations are potassium and sodium, respectively. The bicarbonate anion is the ionic component of the body's most important buffering mechanism. Calcium is a cation which is active in coagulation and muscle contraction. Chloride is an important extracellular anion. *(Henry, pp. 128–132; Guyton, p. 333)*

287–289. (287-C, 288-D, 289-A) In solving acid–base problems, first look at the pH. If the pH is less than 7.4, there is acidosis. If the pH is more than 7.4, there is alkalosis. Next look at the P_{CO_2} to see if there is a respiratory component. Pure acute metabolic processes will lack any contributing respiratory component and should demonstrate a normal P_{CO_2} of about 40 mm Hg. If there is a respiratory component present, the uncompensated acid–base disturbance should have an abnormal P_{CO_2}.

Question 287 has a pH of 7.28 so the student is acidotic. The P_{CO_2} is abnormal so there is a respiratory component. Thus, the student has respiratory acidosis. It is acute because the experiment has had only a 10-minute duration and because there has not been sufficient time for compensatory renal actions to occur. Breathing air with an increased carbon dioxide concentration (respiratory failure, chronic lung disease, breath holding) will produce respiratory acidosis.

Question 288 has a pH of 7.51 so the child is alkalotic. The P_{CO_2} is abnormal so there is a respiratory component. Thus, the child has respiratory alkalosis. It is acute because of the immediate time frame of the hyperventilation and because there has not been sufficient time for compensatory renal actions to occur. Hyperventilation characteristically produces respiratory alkalosis.

Question 289 has a pH of 7.19 so there is acidosis. The P_{CO_2} is normal so there is no respiratory component. Thus, the man is in metabolic acidosis. The acidosis is acute because there is no evidence of compensatory respiratory actions. The ingestion of ethylene glycol will produce a marked metabolic acidosis with a large anion gap. Ingestion of sufficient ethylene glycol can be fatal. *(Guyton, pp. 340–342)*

290–292. (290-E, 291-B, 292-H) The first scenario depicts a young woman with a hypercoagulable state (antithrombin III deficiency). At autopsy the bowel is gangrenous in a segment drained anatomically by the superior mesenteric vein. A thrombosis of the vein is likely. Factors that predispose to thrombus formation include nonlaminal flow, hypercoagulable states, or damage to the endothelium. Mesenteric vein thrombosis is a common occurrence in antithrombin III deficient individuals. The second scenario describes diffuse intravascular coagulation resulting from amniotic fluid emboli. During prolonged labor, amniotic fluid material may enter the uterine venous sinuses and subsequently embolize to the lungs. Amniotic material is a potent thromboplastin that can initiate intravascular coagulation. The third scenario describes a man with Marfan's syndrome. Cystic medial necrosis and dissecting thoracic aneurysms are common complications seen in aged individuals with Marfan's syndrome. Proximal dissection into the pericardium invariably produces hemopericardium and cardiac tamponade. *(Cotran et al., pp. 129–134)*

293. (C) Nitrogen embolism (acute decompression sickness) is seen in scuba divers who ascend too rapidly after a deep dive. While deeply submerged, inhaled compressed air becomes partially dissolved in the blood, tissue fluids, and fat. As the diver rapidly ascends, the dissolved air comes back out of solution as bubbles. The oxygen component of the bubbles is rapidly redissolved or metabolized. The nitrogen component, however, persists as minute bubbles that mechanically obstruct the minor vasculature with subsequent multifocal ischemia. Ischemia in the skeletal muscles produces severe pain (the bends). Mechanical blockage of pulmonary vessels impedes efficient respiratory exchange with resultant respiratory distress (the chokes). In the most serious cases, mechanical obstruction of cerebral vessels by nitrogen emboli may lead to obtundation, coma, or death. *(Cotran et al., pp. 109, 110)*

294. **(A)** Fractures of the major long bones or pelvis may produce fat embolization. Fatal fat embolism is rare, however, and is seen in only a small percentage of trauma cases. In fatal cases, microscopic fat and bone marrow globules are found in the small vessels of the brain, kidney, and lung. Brain microinfarcts and ischemia may result in confusion, decreased mental acuity, coma, or death. The lung emboli can produce adult respiratory distress syndrome and hypoxia. Kidney involvement may be documented by the premortem demonstration of fat globules in the urine. *(Cotran et al., p. 130)*

295. **(B)** Most pulmonary emboli arise from the large veins of the lower legs. Obesity, immobilization, estrogen usage, varicosities, and hypercoagulable states all predispose to venous thromboembolism. Most pulmonary emboli are too small to obstruct the main pulmonary artery and lodge further down the pulmonary arterial tree. Pulmonary infarction may complicate these smaller impacted emboli. The autopsy findings in this case revealed an obstructing saddle-type embolus in the main pulmonary artery. *(Cotran et al., p. 130)*

296. **(H)** The pleural effusion is a transudate. Transudates are typified as protein-poor collections of fluid devoid of inflammatory cells such as macrophages or neutrophils. The albumin levels are usually below 1 g/dL and the specific gravity is usually less than 1.010. Transudates are seen in states of increased hydrostatic pressure or decreased plasma oncotic pressure. Congestive heart failure commonly produces pleural effusions that are transudative in nature. *(Cotran et al., pp. 52–53)*

297. **(G)** The pleural effusion is an exudate. Exudates occur in inflammatory states. There is leakage of protein-rich fluid into body spaces with accompanying cellular elements. Usually the exudate has an albumin level greater than 2 g/dL and a specific gravity of more than 1.010. Neutrophils, red blood cells, macrophages, tumor cells, mast cells, and eosinophils may populate the exudate. Cellular disruption may produce elevations in clinically significant enzymes such as lactate dehydrogenase. Malignant tumors metastatic to the pleural cavity characteristically produce exudative effusions. *(Cotran et al., p. 53)*

REFERENCES

Chandrasoma P, Taylor CR. *Concise Pathology,* 3rd ed. Norwalk, CT: Appleton & Lange, 1998.

Cotran RS, Kumar V, Robbins SL. *Robbins Pathologic Basis of Disease,* 6th ed. Philadelphia: Saunders, 1999.

Guyton AC. *Textbook of Medical Physiology,* 8th ed. Philadelphia: Saunders, 1991.

Henry JB (ed). *Clinical Diagnosis and Management by Laboratory Methods,* 20th ed. Philadelphia: Saunders, 2001.

Rubin E, Farber JL. *Pathology.* Philadelphia: Lippincott, 1999.

CHAPTER 4

Immunopathology

Recent advances in the field of immunology have produced an explosion of knowledge about the immune system. This chapter deals with the basic concepts of immunology and the immunologic mechanisms involved in disease states of excess or deficient immunity.

BASIC FACTS AND CONCEPTS

The immune system is designed to produce humoral or cellular immunity. The salient features of both are shown in Table 4–1. The immunoglobulins (Ig) produced by plasma cells share a common double heavy-double light chain disulfide bonded structure with a Fab antibody end and an opposite Fc cell-binding end. The type of heavy chain involved defines the Ig into one of five major classes: IgG, IgM, IgA, IgE, or IgD. Each class has peculiarities (Table 4–2).

The hypersensitivity reactions are ordinary cellular or humoral immunity to foreign antigens carried to the point of damage to the person. The cogent features are listed in Table 4–3. Other instances of hyperimmunity are demonstrated by the autoimmune disorders (Table 4–4). In these diseases, the inciting antigen is a natural bodily substance, not an outside (nonself) antigen, as was the case in the hypersensitivity reactions. Some people suffer from deficient immune systems, either congenital or acquired. The major hereditary immunodeficiency states are shown in Table 4–5. Common acquired immunodeficiency states include acquired immunodeficiency syndrome (AIDS) and those resulting from immunosuppressive therapy for transplantation or neoplasia.

Table 4–1. FEATURES OF HUMORAL AND CELLULAR IMMUNITY

	Humoral Immunity	Cellular Immunity
Principal cell	B cell lymphocyte	T cell lymphocyte
Assisting cells	Macrophages	
	T helper cells	? Macrophages
End result	Immunoglobulin	Lymphokines
		Cytotoxic T cells
Effective against	Bacteria toxins	Viruses, fungi, transplants, tumor cells

Table 4–2. CHARACTERISTICS OF IMMUNOGLOBULINS

Class	Heavy Chain	Principal Location	Construction	Peculiar Function
gG	Gamma	Serum	Monomer	Secondary (anamnestic) immune response
gM	Mu	Serum	Pentamer	Primary immune response
gA	Alpha	Secretions	Dimer	Immunity against luminal antigens (?)
gE	Epsilon	Mast cells	Monomer	Type I hypersensitivity anaphylaxis
gD	Delta	B lymphocytes	Monomer	Immune modulation

Table 4–3. HYPERSENSITIVITY REACTIONS

Type of Reaction		Humoral or Cellular Immunity	Function
Type I	Anaphylactic	Humoral IgE	Antigen causes mast cell degranulation with resultant local or systemic anaphylaxis
Type II	Cytolytic (erythroblastosis)	Humoral IgG IgM complement	Antigen causes Ig and complement binding with cell lysis
Type III	Immune complex (systemic: serum sickness; localized: Arthus reaction)	Humoral IgG IgM + complement	Antigen–antibody complexes deposited at sites and via active intermediates produce tissue injury
Type IV	Cell-mediated (tuberculin reaction)	Cellular	Cell-mediated immunity produces lymphokines and cell-mediated cytotoxicity

Table 4–4. MAJOR AUTOIMMUNE DISEASES AND PRINCIPAL FEATURES

Disease	Probable Antigen	Symptoms
Systemic lupus erythematosus	Nuclear components	Facial rash, renal failure, serositis, arthritis
Rheumatoid arthritis	IgG	Arthritis
Scleroderma	Nuclear components	Cutaneous atrophy, dysphagia
Sjögren's syndrome	Salivary gland	Dry eyes, dry mouth, salivary destruction
Hashimoto's thyroiditis	Microsomes, thyroglobulin	Hypothyroidism
Myasthenia gravis	Acetylcholine receptors	Muscular weakness
Pemphigus vulgaris	Keratinocytes	Cutaneous bullae
Primary biliary cirrhosis	Mitochondria	Jaundice, cirrhosis

Table 4–5. MAJOR HEREDITARY IMMUNODEFICIENCY STATES

Type	Deficit	Characteristics
DiGeorge's immunodeficiency	Cellular	Thymic hypoplasia, tetany (parathyroid hypoplasia)
Bruton's immunodeficiency	Humoral	X-linked inheritance, agammaglobulinemia
Severe combined immunodeficiency	Cellular and humoral	Stem cell absence
Isolated IgA deficiency	IgA protein	Sinopulmonary infections
Wiskott–Aldrich syndrome	Cellular and humoral	X-linked inheritance, thrombocytopenia, eczema

Questions

DIRECTIONS (Questions 298 through 344): Each of the numbered items or incomplete statements in this section is followed by answers or by completions of the statement. Select the ONE lettered answer or completion that is BEST in each case.

298. The principal cell involved in immunity is

   (A) red blood cell
   (B) lymphocyte
   (C) endothelial cell
   (D) pancreatic acinar cell
   (E) adipose cell

299. B cell lymphocytes

   (A) are found in white pulp of spleen
   (B) are found in germinal follicles in lymph nodes
   (C) express surface immunoglobulin
   (D) express a receptor for complement 3b (C3b)
   (E) all of the above

300. T cell lymphocytes are

   (A) not found in the peripheral circulation
   (B) unable to bind to sheep erythrocytes
   (C) play a key role in cellular immunity
   (D) mature into plasma cells
   (E) have a receptor for Fc

301. Thymosin is

   (A) a pituitary hormone that regulates thymic development
   (B) a glycoprotein that confers passive immunity to nonsensitized hosts
   (C) an antiserum against thymocytes
   (D) a thymic hormone that induces maturation of pre-T cells
   (E) a lymphokine elaborated by activated thymocytes

302. Macrophages

   (A) help process and present antigen to immunocompetent cells
   (B) act as mediators in certain cell-mediated immune reactions
   (C) can have Fc receptors
   (D) can have complement 3 (C3) receptors
   (E) all of the above

303. Cell-mediated immunity is an important host defense mechanism against

   (A) deep-seated mycotic infections
   (B) measles
   (C) *Mycobacterium tuberculosis*
   (D) schistosomiasis
   (E) all of the above

304. The fusion of a myeloma cell with an antigensensitized B cell lymphocyte is termed

   (A) dendritic cell
   (B) opsonization
   (C) natural killer cell
   (D) null cell
   (E) hybridoma

305. Human leukocyte antigens are present in the cell membranes of

    (A) T lymphocytes
    (B) macrophages
    (C) B lymphocytes
    (D) endothelial cells
    (E) all of the above

306. Which human chromosome contains the human leukocyte antigen (HLA) complex?

    (A) chromosome 11
    (B) chromosome 23
    (C) chromosome 48
    (D) chromosome 6
    (E) sex chromosome

307. The chance that any two siblings will inherit an identical set of HLAs is

    (A) 100%
    (B) 25%
    (C) 50%
    (D) less than 1%
    (E) 33%

308. Mixed lymphocyte culture is useful in testing for

    (A) HLA-A
    (B) HLA-B
    (C) HLA-C
    (D) HLA-D
    (E) HLA-E

309. Specific HLAs have been associated with which disease?

    (A) Reiter's disease
    (B) ankylosing spondylitis
    (C) Addison's disease
    (D) acute anterior uveitis
    (E) all of the above

310. The immunoglobulin most likely to be found in secretions is

    (A) IgA
    (B) IgD
    (C) IgE
    (D) IgG
    (E) IgM

311. Immunoglobulins

    (A) are produced by plasma cells
    (B) can exist as monomers, dimers, and pentamers
    (C) have heavy and light chains
    (D) are antibodies with specific reactivity
    (E) all of the above

312. A delta heavy chain would be expected in

    (A) IgA
    (B) IgD
    (C) IgE
    (D) IgG
    (E) IgM

313. The major immunoglobulin produced in a primary immune response is

    (A) IgG
    (B) IgM
    (C) IgE
    (D) IgD
    (E) IgA

314. When pepsin acts on an immunoglobulin, the result is

    (A) Fc and heavy chains
    (B) heavy chains and light chains
    (C) Fc and Fab
    (D) Fab and light chains
    (E) Fc and light chains

315. An anamnestic immunologic response would be expected to occur with

    (A) immunodeficient populations
    (B) Bruton's hypogammaglobulinemia
    (C) rechallenge of a sensitized host with the sensitizing antigen
    (D) neurologically damaged patients with immune defects
    (E) common variable immunodeficiency

316. Anaphylactic reaction involve the following:

(A) IgE

(B) mast cells

(C) histamine release

(D) basophils

(E) all of the above

317. The complement (C) system

(A) may result in cell lysis

(B) is a classic pathway that starts at sites of immunoglobulin attachment

(C) has components that are mostly glycoproteins

(D) has a C3b fragment that is active in opsonization

(E) all of the above

318. Which cation is important to the function of complement 3 (C3) convertase?

(A) sodium

(B) chloride

(C) bicarbonate

(D) calcium

(E) magnesium

319. Identify the complement (C) factor with chemotactic activity.

(A) C5b67

(B) C9

(C) C8

(D) C3a

(E) C1

320. The ultimate function of the completed complement pathway onto a cell is to promote

(A) mitosis

(B) immunocompetency

(C) lysis

(D) immunoglobulin synthesis

(E) immune tolerance

321. Eight to 12 days after injection of a foreign antigen, an individual experiences fever, lymphadenopathy, glomerulonephritis, arthri-tis, and malaise. The most likely diagnosis would be

(A) type I hypersensitivity reaction

(B) type II hypersensitivity reaction

(C) type III localized hypersensitivity reaction

(D) type III generalized hypersensitivity reaction

(E) type IV hypersensitivity reaction

322. An example of type IV hypersensitivity is

(A) tuberculin reaction

(B) Arthus reaction

(C) serum sickness

(D) immune agranulocytosis

(E) hemolytic transfusion reaction

323. Which substance is not a lymphokine?

(A) macrophage migration-inhibiting factor (MMIF)

(B) interferon

(C) transfer factor

(D) interleukin II

(E) histamine

324. IgG is composed of

(A) kappa light chain

(B) Fc region

(C) variable region

(D) Fab region

(E) all of the above

325. Immune surveillance as a mechanism of host protection against tumorigenesis is best supported by

(A) increased levels of cancer in immuno-deficient populations

(B) low levels of immune complexes

(C) increased levels of antibody

(D) abnormal lymphocytes

(E) decreased levels of cancer in transplantation populations

326. An enlarged spleen is found to contain abundant acellular eosinophilic hyaline material by light microscopy. A Congo red stain demonstrates green birefringence. The most likely identity is

(A) amyloid
(B) edema fluid
(C) bacteria
(D) talc
(E) none of the above

327. On Southern blot examination the DNA of a malignant tumor is found to have a clonal immunoglobulin gene rearrangement. From what type of cell is the tumor derived?

(A) fibroblast
(B) T lymphocyte
(C) squamous epithelium cell
(D) cuboidal epithelium cell
(E) B lymphocyte

328. Goodpasture's syndrome is characterized by autoantibodies to

(A) basement membrane
(B) platelet surface antigens
(C) parietal cell antigens
(D) acetylcholine receptors
(E) colonic mucosal cells

329. Antimicrosomal antibodies are commonly seen in

(A) rheumatoid arthritis
(B) systemic lupus erythematosus (SLE)
(C) Hashimoto's thyroiditis
(D) scleroderma
(E) mixed connective tissue disease

330. Autoantibodies against acetylcholine receptors characterize

(A) pernicious anemia
(B) myasthenia gravis
(C) dermatomyositis
(D) rheumatoid arthritis
(E) scleroderma

331. A fluorescent antinuclear antibody (FANA) test may be helpful in diagnosing

(A) Hashimoto's thyroiditis
(B) primary biliary cirrhosis
(C) isolated IgA deficiency
(D) Wiskott–Aldrich syndrome
(E) systemic lupus erythematosus (SLE)

332. Nonbacterial verrucous endocarditis most commonly is associated with

(A) systemic lupus erythematosus (SLE)
(B) pneumocystis pneumonia
(C) complement 1 (C1) inhibitor deficiency
(D) Epstein–Barr virus (EBV) infection
(E) cytomegalovirus (CMV) infection

333. Identify the correct statement concerning Sjögren's syndrome.

(A) It may have keratoconjunctivitis sicca.
(B) It may have xerostomia.
(C) It has lymphocytic infiltration of salivary glands.
(D) It has an increased risk for malignant lymphoma.
(E) All of the above statements are correct.

334. A 35-year-old woman complains of dysphagia, symmetrical edema and thickening of the fingers, and Raynaud's phenomenon. Which immunologic disease is most likely?

(A) *Vibrio cholera* infection
(B) shigellosis
(C) polyarteritis nodosa
(D) scleroderma
(E) Hashimoto's thyroiditis

335. Severe combined immunodeficiency (SCID) can include all of the following EXCEPT

(A) poor cell-mediated immunity
(B) autosomal or sex-linked inheritance
(C) 80% 10-year survival
(D) low levels of adenosine deaminase
(E) poor humoral immunity

336. Chronic granulomatous disease includes

(A) poor bacterial killing by neutrophils
(B) usually afflicts males
(C) symptoms of pneumonia, lymphadenitis, or splenomegaly
(D) usually manifests in the first 2 years of life
(E) all of the above

337. Hereditary deficiency of complement 1 (C1) inhibitor is characterized by

(A) recurrent angioedema
(B) mild adolescent disease, crippling adult disease
(C) high levels of C1 inhibitor
(D) SLE
(E) sex-linked inheritance

338. A 6-year-old boy with a history of recurrent bacterial infections, partial albinism, and central nervous system disorders is found to have an unusual peripheral blood smear characterized by giant cytoplasmic granular inclusions in white cells and platelets. The most likely diagnosis is

(A) selective IgM deficiency
(B) selective IgA deficiency
(C) Wiskott–Aldrich syndrome
(D) Chediak–Higashi syndrome
(E) selective deficiency of IgG subclass

339. A marked decrease in T helper cells is a characteristic feature of

(A) SLE
(B) AIDS
(C) erythroblastosis fetalis
(D) autoimmune hemolytic anemia
(E) pernicious anemia

340. The causative agent of AIDS is

(A) a virus
(B) *Pneumocystis carinii*
(C) a protozoan parasite
(D) Kaposi's sarcoma
(E) lymphadenopathy

341. Usual findings in AIDS may include

(A) fever, weight loss, and lymphadenopathy
(B) *Pneumocystis carinii* infections
(C) Kaposi's sarcoma
(D) CMV infection
(E) all of the above

342. A transfer of immunocompetent cells into an antigenically different recipient who is immunocompromised is likely to produce

(A) Bruton's agammaglobulinemia
(B) graft-vs.-host disease
(C) type I hypersensitivity reactions
(D) clonal deletion
(E) DiGeorge's syndrome

343. Identify the statement that applies to hyperacute renal transplantation rejection.

(A) grossly appears as a flaccid, mottled, cyanotic kidney.
(B) usually occurs within minutes after transplantation.
(C) involves recipient's preformed circulating antibodies.
(D) early lesion are at vascular endothelium.
(E) all of the above are correct.

344. Joint pains, albuminuria and fever 10 days after an injection of horse serum occur because of

(A) histamine release
(B) circulating immune complexes
(C) cytokines produced by T-lymphocytes
(D) intravascular hemolysis
(E) cytotoxic horse antibodies

DIRECTIONS (Questions 345 through 396): Each group of items in this section consists of a list of lettered options followed by a set of numbered words or phrases. For each numbered word or phrase, select the ONE lettered option that is most closely associated with it. Each lettered option may be selected once, more than once, or not at all.

Questions 345 through 348

(A) HLA-B8
(B) HLA-Bw47
(C) HLA-B27
(D) HLA-C4
(E) HLA-C6

345. Ankylosing spondylitis

346. Celiac disease

347. Acute anterior uveitis

348. Reiter's disease

Questions 349 through 352

(A) type I hypersensitivity
(B) type II hypersensitivity
(C) type III hypersensitivity
(D) type IV hypersensitivity
(E) type V hypersensitivity

349. Cell-mediated type

350. Immune complex disease

351. Anaphylactic type

352. Cytotoxic type

Questions 353 through 356

(A) Hashimoto's thyroiditis
(B) autoimmune hemolytic anemia
(C) Goodpasture's syndrome
(D) SLE
(E) pemphigus vulgaris

353. Antibodies against red blood cells

354. Antibodies against microsomal components

355. Antibodies against basement membranes

356. Antibodies against nuclear antigens

Questions 357 through 360

(A) xenograft
(B) isograft
(C) autograft
(D) allograft
(E) avascular graft

357. Retransplantation of a host's own tissue

358. Transplantation from a genetically identical twin

359. Transplantation from a genetically dissimilar member of the same species

360. Transplantation from a different species

Questions 361 through 364

(A) platelets
(B) Langerhans' cells
(C) T cell lymphocytes
(D) B cell lymphocytes
(E) NK cells

361. Progenitor of plasma cells

362. Have helper (CD4) and suppressor (CD8) subsets

363. Antigen-processing cells usually found in skin

364. Cytotoxic cells lacking well-defined T or B cell markers

Questions 365 through 368

(A) IgM
(B) IgA
(C) IgG
(D) IgE
(E) IgD

365. Fc portion can bind to mast cells

366. Usually a dimer found in secretions

367. Gamma heavy chain

368. Usually found as pentamers

Questions 369 through 372

(A) DiGeorge's syndrome

(B) Bruton's agammaglobulinemia

(C) Wiskott–Aldrich syndrome

(D) myasthenia gravis

(E) isolated IgA deficiency

369. Thymic hypoplasia, tetany, and deficient cellular immunity

370. X-linked hereditary disorder of humoral and cellular immunity with thrombocytopenia and eczema

371. X-linked hereditary disorder of humoral immunity with absent gamma globulin

372. Reduced IgA levels with recurrent sinopulmonary infections

Questions 373 through 376

(A) class I major histocompatibility complex

(B) class II major histocompatibility complex

(C) class III major histocompatibility complex

(D) class IV major histocompatibility complex

(E) class V major histocompatibility complex

373. HLA-DR

374. HLA-A

375. Complement proteins

376. HLA-B

Questions 377 through 380

(A) type I hypersensitivity reaction

(B) type II hypersensitivity reaction

(C) type III hypersensitivity reaction

(D) type IV hypersensitivity reaction

377. Erythroblastosis fetalis

378. Tuberculin skin test

379. Anaphylaxis following an insect sting

380. Serum sickness

Questions 381 through 384

(A) SLE

(B) primary biliary cirrhosis

(C) pemphigus vulgaris

(D) myasthenia gravis

(E) Hashimoto's thyroiditis

381. Autoantibodies to thyroglobulin

382. Autoantibodies to mitochondria

383. Autoantibodies to keratinocytes

384. Autoantibodies to acetylcholine receptors

Questions 385 through 388

(A) properdin

(B) C3a

(C) C6

(D) C5b6789 complex

(E) C1

385. Causes focal cell membrane lysis

386. Binds to Fc initiating the classic pathway

387. Initiator of the alternative pathway

388. Anaphylatoxic

Questions 389 through 392

(A) SLE

(B) scleroderma

(C) Sezary's syndrome

(D) DiGeorge's syndrome

(E) rheumatoid arthritis

(F) myasthenia gravis

(G) secondary amyloidosis

(H) Hashimoto's thyroiditis

389. A 47-year-old female has noticed that in the mornings the small joints of her hands are swollen, painful, and stiff. Her rheumatoid factor is reported as strongly positive. What disease is she most likely to have?

390. A 51-year-old man has had a generalized erythroderma with intense itching for about 2 months. Numerous atypical lymphoid cells with cerebriform convoluted nuclei are evident in his peripheral blood. These atypical cells have T cell markers. What disease is he most likely to have?

391. A 76-year-old male with a long history of chronic osteomyelitis gradually develops cardiac arrhythmias and splenomegaly. A rectal biopsy shows abundant eosinophilic acellular material, which by polarized light examination, displays apple green birefringence after staining with Congo red. What disorder is he most likely to have?

392. A 32-year-old woman complains of diplopia and drooping eyelids. A trial dose of edrophonium produces an immediate transient improvement of her ocular muscle weakness. A serum assay for acetylcholine receptor antibodies is reported as positive. What disease is she most likely to have?

Questions 393 through 396

(A) neoplasm of B lymphocytes
(B) neoplasm of T lymphocytes
(C) tumor of Langerhans' cells
(D) neoplasm of myeloid cells
(E) neoplasm of erythroid cells
(F) neoplasm of thrombocytes
(G) neoplasm of epithelial cells
(H) neoplasm of muscle cells

393. A 77-year-old female is noted to be anemic. Her serum protein electrophoresis demonstrates a large monoclonal IgG kappa protein. In her bone marrow, are increased numbers of atypical plasma cells. Her skull x-rays show multiple lytic areas.

394. A 12-year-old African boy develops a large disfiguring tumor of the jaw. Histologically, the tumor is composed of small actively mitotic undifferentiated cells in a "starry sky" background. The scant cytoplasm of the cells is positive for Oil red O vacuoles. The majority of the cells have surface immunoglobulin.

395. A 45-year-old male has noticed an erythematous skin rash for about 2 months. On biopsy, the skin demonstrates Pautrier's microabscesses and tumor cells. The tumor cells are positive for CD4 and CD3. No surface immunoglobin is present on the tumor cells.

396. A 15-year-old female complains of rib pain. An x-ray demonstrates a solitary lytic rib lesion. The biopsy contains eosinophils and tumor cells. The tumor cells are large, have nuclear groves, contain S100 antigen, and on electron microscopy are shown to possess Birbeck bodies.

DIRECTIONS (Questions 397 through 399): Each of the numbered items or incomplete statements in this section is followed by answers or by completions of the statement. Select the ONE lettered answer or completion that is BEST in each case.

397. What is required for a killer cell to lyse another cell?

(A) It must be coated with IgE.
(B) It must be coated with IgG.
(C) It must be coated with IgM.
(D) It has bound histamine.
(E) It expresses CD3.

398. What action is more pertinent of Interleukin-2?

(A) It induces T cell proliferation.
(B) It activates macrophages.
(C) It increases immunoglobulin secretion.
(D) It promotes B cell differentiation.
(E) It increases chemotaxis of eosinophils.

399. An increase of interferon gamma in delayed hypersensitivity will promote

(A) killing of microorganism and neoplastic cells by macrophages
(B) expression of α_2 macroglobulin on all cells
(C) chemotaxis and phagocytosis by neutrophils
(D) activation of the alternate complement pathway
(E) prostacyclin secretion by endothelial cells

DIRECTIONS (Questions 400 through 402): For each numbered word or phrase, select the ONE lettered option that is most closely associated with it. Each lettered option may be selected once, more than once, or not at all.

(A) activated macrophage

(B) T$_4$ lymphocyte

(C) neutrophil

(D) cytotoxic T cell

(E) B lymphocyte

400. Mediator of injury in serum sickness

401. Characteristic cell of delayed type hypersensitivity to persistent antigens

402. Recognize viral antigens presented with class I major histocompatibility molecules

DIRECTIONS (Questions 403 through 410): Each of the numbered items or incomplete statements in this section is followed by answers or by completions of the statement. Select the ONE lettered answer or completion that is BEST in each case.

403. Select the most important function of the dendritic and Langerhans' cells.

(A) processing and presentation of antigen to immunocompetent T lymphocytes

(B) phagocytosis of bacteria and necrotic debris

(C) secretion of interleukin-2

(D) secretion of immunoglobulins

(E) killing of virally infected cells

404. Allergic reactions on tissue sections may show

(A) giant cells

(B) neutrophils

(C) eosinophils

(D) monocytes

(E) epithelioid cells

405. How would you describe Arthus reaction?

(A) phagocytosis of antigen by neutrophils

(B) antigen–antibody complexes activate complement with the release of chemotactic factors for neutrophils

(C) antigen couple with complement to cause the release of prostaglandins

(D) activation of sensitized lymphocytes which lead to production of chemotactic factors

(E) antigen–antibody complexes activate complement

406. In SLE, which is the most common antigen?

(A) histone

(B) DNA ribonucleoprotein

(C) RNA

(D) rheumatoid factor

407. The histological change seen in a hypersensitivity reaction involves

(A) deposits of immunoglobulin and complement in the arterial wall

(B) neutrophilic infiltrates around arterioles

(C) vascular stasis and pavementing of neutrophils

(D) mononuclear cell infiltrates surrounding small vessels

(E) necrosis of the epidermis

408. Cell-mediated type of hypersensitivity is initiated by

(A) B lymphocytes

(B) T lymphocytes

(C) macrophages

(D) polymorphonuclear cells

(E) eosinophils

409. Approximately 20% of all peripheral lymphocytes are composed of natural killer (NK) cells. The function of these cells is

(A) to secrete immunoglobulins

(B) to require prior sensitization to cellular antigens

(C) to lyse transplanted cells only

(D) to lyse neoplastic or virus-infected cells

(E) important in type III hypersensitivity

410. Hyperacute graft rejection occurs

(A) during the graft versus host reaction

(B) when cytotoxic lymphocytes react with donor cells

(C) where there is HLA compatibility

(D) if the recipient has preformed antibodies to donor cellular antigens

(E) if the recipient is not properly immunosuppressed

Answers and Explanations

298. **(B)** Lymphocytes (both T and B cell types) are the principal cells involved in immunity. Macrophages and neutrophils also are helpful in modulating the immune response. Red cells, endothelial cells, pancreatic acinar cells, and adipose cells are not significantly involved in immunity. *(Cotran et al., pp. 189–190)*

299. **(E)** B lymphocytes make up only about 10–20% of lymphocytes in the peripheral blood. T lymphocytes are the subset that constitute 79–80% of circulating lymphocytes. *(Cotran et al., pp. 189–191)*

300. **(C)** T cells play a pivotal role in cellular immunity. They are present in the peripheral blood and readily bind sheep erythrocytes (rosetting). B cells, not T cells, have Fc receptors and mature into plasma cells. *(Cotran et al., pp. 189–191)*

301. **(D)** Thymosin is a thymic hormone that regulates pre-T cell development. It is not released from the pituitary. Antithymocyte antibodies are not thymosin but are useful in transplantation rejection therapy. Lymphokines are released from T cells, but thymosin is a thymic hormone, not a lymphokine. *(Cotran et al., p. 305)*

302. **(E)** Macrophages are crucial effectors and affectors of immunity. They can produce soluble factors to influence the growth and function of lymphoid and nonlymphoid tissue, as well as responding to certain lymphokines. *(Cotran et al., pp. 190, 191)*

303. **(E)** Cell-mediated immunity is an important host mechanism against infection by obliga-tory intracellular pathogens, fungi, and parasites. *(Cotran et al., pp. 207–211)*

304. **(E)** The usefulness of hybridomas arises from their ability to produce abundant monoclonal antibody to specific antigens. Natural killer and null cells are types of lymphoid cells. Dendritic cells may possess weak phagocytic activity and may be helpful in antigen presentation. Opsonization is the coating of antigens, usually bacterial, with complement fragments to enhance phagocytosis. *(Henry, p. 852)*

305. **(E)** The human leukocyte antigens (HLA) are glycoproteins present on the surface of virtually all nucleated cells. *(Henry, 999)*

306. **(D)** The HLA system is present on chromosome 6. Beta-hemoglobin production is present on chromosome 11, making it the site of thalassemias and beta-hemoglobinopathies. Chromosome 23 and the sex chromosome are identical. Because humans have only 23 chromosome pairs, there is no chromosome 48. *(Rubin and Farber, pp. 112, 113)*

307. **(B)** Half of each parental HLA genotype is transmitted to each offspring. Because each child possesses half of the mother's and half of the father's HLA antigens, the chance of any two siblings possessing the same HLA genotype (identical HLA antigens), is 0.5 × 0.5, or 25%. *(Rubin and Farber, pp. 112–114)*

308. **(D)** Mixed lymphocyte cultures demonstrate the approximately 12 subsets of HLA-D. Mixing non-D identical lymphocytes will result in a proliferation of the lymphocytes indicating nonidentity. HLA-A, HLA-B, and HLA-C usually are determined by serologic procedures. There is no HLA-E. *(Henry, p. 940)*

309. **(E)** Ankylosing spondylitis, Reiter's disease, and acute anterior uveitis are all associated with HLA-B27. Addison's disease is associated with HLA-B8. *(Cotran et al., pp. 195–206)*

310. **(A)** IgA has its major role in secretions. It is secreted as a dimer with some linking pieces and a secretory piece made by epithelial cells in the vicinity of the plasma cells in which IgA is made. IgM is predominantly intravascular. IgG is both intravascular and extravascular. IgE is bound to mast cells or basophils. IgD is present throughout the body in very scant quantity. *(Henry, pp. 883–886)*

311. **(E)** The Fc portion is the site of macrophage receptor binding. Immunoglobulins are Y-shaped and occur as monomers, dimers, and pentamers. They consist of both light and heavy chains. Reagin antibodies are another term for immunoglobulins of the IgE class. *(Henry, pp. 883–886)*

312. **(B)** The heavy chains are specific for each of the five major classes of immunoglobulins. The heavy chains are alpha, delta, epsilon, gamma, and mu for IgA, IgD, IgE, IgG, and IgM, respectively. *(Henry, pp. 883–886)*

313. **(B)** IgM is the effector of the primary immune response. The primary response follows the antigen encounter by 4–7 days and results in sensitization in the immunocompetent host. Rechallenge by the same antigen in a sensitized host will produce a secondary immune response with IgG. *(Henry, pp. 883–916)*

314. **(C)** An immunoglobulin is composed of four peptide chains linked by disulfide bonds. Pepsin splits the immunoglobulin into Fc (crystallizable) and Fab (antigen-binding) fragments. Free heavy or free light chains are not produced by pepsinolytic activity. *(Chandrasoma and Taylor, pp. 59–63)*

315. **(C)** An anamnestic immune response, also called the "secondary immune response," occurs in immunocompetent and sensitized individuals rechallenged by the sensitizing antigen. The word *anamnestic* has origin from the Greek, meaning to recall or recollect. The other four listed choices are states of immunodeficiency and would be unlikely to mount an anamnestic response. *(Chandrasoma and Taylor, pp. 63–65)*

316. **(E)** Anaphylactic (type I hypersensitivity) reactions involve formation of IgE cytotropic antigen binding to mast cells or basophils. Appropriate antigens react with the IgE antibodies to cause cell degranulation, histamine release, and anaphylaxis. *(Cotran et al., pp. 196–201)*

317. **(E)** The complement system is composed predominantly of glycoproteins. It can be activated by either antigen–antibody reactions (classic pathway) or by properdin stabilization (alternate pathway). Fragments generated in the pathway may become chemical mediators, such as C3b for opsonization. The ultimate goal of the complement system, when fully activated, is to produce cellular lysis. *(Cotran et al., pp. 67–69)*

318. **(E)** Magnesium is a cofactor in C3 convertase, allowing cleavage of C3 and yielding C3a and C3b fragments. Cations must have positive electrical charges. HCO_3 and chloride are anions. *(Cotran et al., pp. 67–69)*

319. **(A)** The complement factor C5b67 is chemotactic and induces migration of neutrophils and monocytes. The C3a and C5a factors are anaphylatoxins, increasing vascular permeability and causing smooth muscle contraction. C9 and C8 are final proteins in the complement pathway and are needed for complement-mediated cell lysis. *(Cotran et al., pp. 67–69)*

320. **(C)** The complement pathway has cell lysis as its ultimate goal. In the process, numerous chemotactic, opsonin, and spasmogenic products are produced. *(Cotran et al., pp. 67–69)*

321. **(D)** The clinical history is a classic description of one-shot serum sickness, a generalized type III hypersensitivity reaction. The localized type III hypersensitivity reaction is the

Arthus complex and usually is characterized by swelling and fibrinoid vasculitis at a subcutaneal injection site. *(Cotran et al., pp. 201–204)*

322. **(A)** Type IV hypersensitivity reactions involve cellmediated immunity, with the tuberculin reaction being the classic example. Serum sickness and the Arthus reaction are examples of generalized and localized type III hypersensitivity, respectively. Immune agranulocytosis and hemolytic transfusion reactions are examples of type II hypersensitivity. *(Cotran et al., pp. 204–207)*

323. **(E)** Lymphokines are substances produced by lymphocytes to assist in cell-mediated immunity and type IV hypersensitivity reactions. They include MMIF, interferon, chemotactic factors, interleukin II, and transfer factor. Histamine is not a lymphokine. It is present in basophils and mast cells and plays a major role in anaphylaxis (type I hypersensitivity). *(Cotran et al., p. 82)*

324. **(E)** The IgG molecule is composed of either two gamma heavy chains and two kappa light chains, or two gamma heavy chains and two lambda light chains. The heavy chains are located centrally within the molecule and bound together by disulfide linkages. The two identical light chains are located peripherally and opposite each other: one bound to each heavy chain by disulfide linkages. Conceptually, the immunoglobulin molecule can be viewed as a "Y." The open branched end contains variable regions of the heavy and light chains that are termed "Fab." The Fab portion of the molecule is the site of antigen recognition and antibody–antigen binding. The other end of the immunoglobulin molecule contains the Fc region, constructed only by the two heavy chains. The Fc component can fix complement and has chemotactic properties. The intact whole immunoglobulin molecule can be split into Fab (fragment antibody) and Fc (fragment complement) by enzymatic digestion. *(Henry, pp. 878, 879)*

325. **(A)** Immune surveillance is the mechanism whereby a host mounts an immune response against antigens expressed by the tumor. The increased level of tumorigenesis seen in immunodeficient populations supports the concept of immune surveillance. Low levels of immune complexes, increased levels of antibody, and abnormal lymphocytes are not central concepts to immune surveillance. There are increased, not decreased, levels of tumorigenesis in transplant populations. *(Cotran et al., pp. 231–236)*

326. **(A)** Amyloid is acellular material that by routine light microscopy appears eosinophilic and hyaline. Special stains, such as Congo red, produce a diagnostic green birefringence. An additional aid is that the spleen is a likely systemic site for amyloid deposition. *(Cotran et al., p. 252)*

327. **(E)** The Southern blot technique is a very potent laboratory test for identifying the lineage of lymphomatous tumor cells. Very early in their ancestry B lymphocytes and T lymphocytes undergo physical rearrangement of their immunoglobulin genes and T cell receptor genes, respectively. Identification of rearranged monoclonal immunoglobulin genes in a tumor points to a B cell lineage. Likewise, tumors that demonstrate monoclonal T cell receptor genes are T lymphocyte derived. The Southern blot technique involves the initial fragmentation of tumor DNA by endonucleases. The fragmented DNA is then sorted by size through electrophoresis. Labeled complementary DNA probes to immunoglobulin genes or T cell receptor genes are then hybridized with the tumor sample. Monoclonal binding indicates the appropriate lineage. If there is binding only to the germline (nonrearranged) DNA component, then the tumor cells are of nonlymphoid origin, such as fibroblasts or epithelial cells, or the tumor is not a clonal proliferation (benign). *(Henry, pp. 1349–1350)*

328. **(A)** Goodpasture's disease is characterized by antibasement antibodies, with the lung and kidneys bearing the brunt of the damage. Antibodies against platelet surface antigens, parietal cells, acetylcholine receptors, and colonic mucosal cells are seen in autoimmune thrombocytopenia, pernicious anemia, myasthenia gravis, and ulcerative colitis, respectively. *(Chandrasoma and Taylor, pp. 538, 539)*

329. (C) Antimicrosomal antibodies are commonly seen in Hashimoto's thyroiditis. Parenchymal immune destruction of the thyroid gland can produce clinical hypothyroidism. Antinuclear antibodies are associated with SLE, scleroderma, and Sjögren's syndrome. Mixed connective tissue disease is characterized by antiribonuclear protein antibodies. *(Cotran et al., pp. 1134–1136)*

330. (B) Autoantibodies against acetylcholine receptors characterize myasthenia gravis. Antinuclear antibodies are found in scleroderma and dermatomyositis. Pernicious anemia is the result of antiparietal and anti-intrinsic factor antibodies. Rheumatoid arthritis is characterized by anti-Ig antibodies, usually of the IgM type. *(Chandrasoma and Taylor, pp. 956–958)*

331. (E) A FANA test is used to detect antibodies against nuclear cellular components. Only SLE of the choices listed characteristically has a positive FANA. Antibodies against thyroglobulin and microsomal antigens characterize Hashimoto's thyroiditis. Antibodies against mitochondria are seen in primary biliary cirrhosis. Wiscott–Aldrich syndrome and isolated IgA deficiency are immunodeficiency states. *(Cotran et al., pp. 216–224)*

332. (A) Nonbacterial verrucous endocarditis, also called Libman–Sacks endocarditis, is associated with SLE and is characterized by sterile excrescences on the mitral and tricuspid valves with fibrinoid necrosis. C1 inhibitor deficiency is characterized by bouts of episodic angioedema. Pneumocystis, EBV, and CMV infections are features of acquired immunodeficiency syndrome (AIDS). Neither AIDS nor C1 inhibitor deficiency has a strong association with nonbacterial verrucous endocarditis. *(Cotran et al., pp. 216–224)*

333. (E) Sjögren's syndrome is characterized by lymphocytic infiltration and fibrosis of lacrimal and salivary gland tissue, producing a clinical picture of dry eyes (keratoconjunctivitis) and dry mouth (xerostomia). Other autoimmune diseases, such as rheumatoid arthritis, systemic lupus erythematosus, polymyositis, scleroderma, vasculitis, and thyroiditis, are seen in a fair number of Sjögren's patients. Because of this, many patients have positive rheumatoid factor, ANA, and LE cell preparations. The risk factor for subsequent lymphoma is estimated as 40 times higher in Sjögren's patients. *(Cotran et al., pp. 225–226)*

334. (D) The clinical history provides the classic presentation of scleroderma, also called progressive systemic sclerosis. Hashimoto's thyroiditis, an autoimmune disorder, usually occurs with hypothyroidism and goiter. Cholera and shigellosis are bacterial infections with severe diarrhea. Polyarteritis nodosa is a noninfectious necrotizing vasculitis of possible autoimmune origin, with a protean clinical appearance. *(Cotran et al., pp. 226–229)*

335. (C) Most children with SCID die in the first 2 years of life; long-term survival is exceptional. SCID results in impaired cellular and humoral immunity. Autosomal recessive and sex-linked inheritance have been described. In the autosomal recessive form, adenosine deaminase levels are markedly reduced in some patients. *(Rubin and Farber, pp. 123–124)*

336. (E) Chronic granulomatous disease is most often X-linked and associated with a decreased ability of neutrophils and other phagocytic cells to kill bacteria. As a result, by 2 years of age, signs of chronic low-grade infections appear, such as lymphadenopathy, splenomegaly, pneumonia, and sinusitis. The NBT test shows markedly decreased, chemical reduction and helps confirm the diagnosis, because lack of NBT reductive capacity correlates with poor bactericidal activity. *(Cotran et al., pp. 235–236)*

337. (A) Hereditary deficiency of C1 inhibitor is characterized by angioedema. The mode of inheritance is autosomal dominant, not sex-linked. There is a marked decrease in the levels of C1 inhibitor, which is worse in adolescents and gradually subsides in about the fifth decade. SLE is associated with genetic deficiency of C2 inhibitor. *(Cotran et al., p. 236)*

338. (D) The clinical description as well as the peripheral blood findings are classic for

Chediak–Higashi syndrome. Selective immunoglobulin deficiencies are not associated with albinism, and the leukocytes and platelets both are morphologically normal. Wiskott–Aldrich syndrome is immunodeficiency with eczema and thrombocytopenia. *(Cotran et al., pp. 64, 65)*

339. **(B)** AIDS is characterized by a relative decrease in T helper cells. The usual ratio of helper/suppressor cells is about 2. In AIDS patients, ratios of 0.7–0.4 are not uncommon. *(Rubin and Farber, pp. 133–140)*

340. **(A)** AIDS is caused by the human immunodeficiency virus (HIV, formerly called HTLV III). The other listed choices are opportunistic infections, neoplasms, or symptoms associated with AIDS. *(Rubin and Farber, pp. 133–140)*

341. **(E)** The basic problem in AIDS is decreased cellular immunity, due in part to destruction of T helper (T4) cells. As a result of poor cellular immunity, opportunistic infections and exotic tumors, such as *Pneumocystis carinii*, CMV, and Kaposi's sarcoma are common. Usual findings in the AIDS patient include weight loss, fever, diarrhea, and generalized lymphadenopathy. *(Rubin and Farber, pp. 133–140)*

342. **(B)** A transfer of immunocompetent cells into an antigenically different immunodeficient host is likely to produce graft-vs.-host disease. The term "clonal deletion" refers to Burnet's theory of how self-antigens are eliminated from the lymphoid system during development. Bruton's agammaglobulinemia and DiGeorge's syndrome are genetic immunodeficiency states. *(Cotran et al., pp. 234–236)*

343. **(E)** Hyperacute renal transplantation rejection usually occurs minutes after reestablishing blood flow to the organ. Preformed circulating antibodies attach to sites, causing vascular injury. This is reflected grossly by cyanotic, mottled, flaccid kidney. There is no involvement of mediated immunity, as in type IV hypersensitivity reactions, hyperacute rejection. *(Rubin, pp. 910–912)*

344. **(B)** Type III hypersensitivity reaction is induced by antigen–antibody complexes that produce tissue damage as a of their capacity to activate the complement system. The is initiated when the antigen combines with the antibody within the circulation or in extravascular sites. The formed in the circulation produce damage, particularly as localize within blood vessel walls. The antigen may be or endogenous. In this type of reaction the mediated disease be generalized affecting many organs, or localized to some such as kidney. The other options sited on this question are Type III hypersensitivity reaction. *(Cotran et al., p. 201)*

345–348. **(345-C, 346-A, 347-C, 348-C)** Some autoimmune and immunologic disorders have been associated with certain HLA types. The close spatial relationship of the Ir genes and the HLA locus may be the operative factor. HLA-B27 is strongly associated with ankylosing spondylitis, Reiter's disease, and acute anterior uveitis. HLA-B8 and HLA-DR3 are associated with celiac disease (gluten-induced enteropathy). The HLA-DR3 locus is also linked to myasthenia gravis, systemic lupus erythematosus, and insulin-dependent diabetes mellitus. HLA-DR2 is associated with multiple sclerosis and Goodpasture's syndrome. HLA-DR4 is seen with rheumatoid arthritis and pemphigus vulgaris. HLA-DR5 occurs in many individuals with Hashimoto's thyroiditis, pernicious anemia, and juvenile rheumatoid arthritis. *(Chandrasoma and Taylor, pp. 498, 976, 590, 591)*

349–352. **(349-D, 350-C, 351-A, 352-B)** Type I, or anaphylactic, hypersensitivity involves a rapid release of vasoactive amines from cytotropic mast cells and basophils. Type II, or cytotoxic, hypersensitivity involves immune-facilitated phagocytosis or cell lysis. Type III, or immune complex, hypersensitivity involves the activation of neutrophils through antigen–antibody complexes and complement. Type IV, or cell-mediated, hypersensitivity involves sensitized T lymphocytes. *(Cotran et al., pp. 196–207)*

353–356. **(353-B, 354-A, 355-C, 356-D)** A number of disease states are characterized by autoantibodies against specific cellular components. Antibodies against red blood cells are the characteristic alteration in autoimmune hemolytic anemia. Hashimoto's thyroiditis has autoantibodies against thyroglobulin and microsomal antigens. Autoantibodies against lung and kidney basement membranes are features of Goodpasture's syndrome. SLE produces antibodies against numerous nuclear components. *(Chandrasoma and Taylor, pp. 107–115)*

357–360. (357-C, 358-B, 359-D, 360-A) The body's acceptance or rejection of transplanted tissue is determined by the antigenic similarity of the transplanted tissue to the host's native tissue as well as the host's immune competency. Autotransplantation involves retransplantation of a host's own tissue, such as using an individual's own saphenous leg vein in a coronary bypass operation. Isografts are transplants between genetically identical twins. Autografts and isografts do not evoke an immune rejection response. Allografts are transplants derived from genetically dissimilar individuals of the same species, such as a human cadaveric kidney transplantation. The degree of rejection is dependent on the antigenic dissimilarity between donor and host, and the immune status of the host. Xenografts are transplants between species. They evoke a strong immune rejection response. Avascular grafts refer to sites, such as the cornea, that are unable to mount an immune rejection response to antigenically foreign material because immunocompetent cells have no vascular access to the site. *(Chandrasoma and Taylor, pp. 116–117)*

361–364. (361-D, 362-C, 363-B, 364-E) A wide variety of cells are involved in the immune system. T cell lymphocytes constitute about 75% of the circulating peripheral blood lymphocytes. T cells are a critical element in cellular immunity. Furthermore, the helper and suppressor subsets of T lymphocytes help to modulate varied immune processes. B cell lymphocytes are the progenitors of plasma cells. Plasma cells secrete immunoglobulin, the effector protein of humoral immunity. The Langerhans' cells are usually found scattered in the middle strata of the epidermis. These bone marrow derived dendritic cells have

monocytic–macrophagic properties, are S100 antigen positive, and by electron microscopy possess a unique racquet-shaped pentalaminar Birbeck body. The Langerhans' cells are believed to play a role in antigen processing. The NK cells are large granular lymphocytes which lack well-defined mature T cell or B cell markers. Many NK (natural killer) cells have cytotoxic ability. Platelets are bone marrow derived elements and are a vital component of blood clotting. They are not believed to have any immune function. *(Cotran et al., pp. 189–192)*

365–368. (365-D, 366-B, 367-C, 368-A) There are five major classes of immunoglobulins synthesized by plasma cells. Their characteristics are outlined in Table 4–2 at the beginning of this chapter. The IgA molecule is unusual in that it is first synthesized as a monomer by plasma cells located in luminal mucosa and submucosa. As the monomer travels through the surface epithelium, a dimer is formed by joining two IgA molecules with an epithelial synthesized J (joining) protein. The dimer is then bound additionally to a secretory component, also produced by epithelial cells, to facilitate passage of the dimer complex out into the lumen. The IgE class of immunoglobulins is avidly bound to mast cells and basophils so that the free (nonbound) serum IgE concentration is usually very low. In states of prolonged allergenic challenge, such as asthma, free serum IgE levels may be markedly elevated. In these cases, the specific offending allergen may be identified by radioallergosorbent testing (RAST). *(Chandrasoma and Taylor, pp. 59–61)*

369–372. (369-A, 370-C, 371-B, 372-E) DiGeorge's syndrome is characterized by disembryogenesis of the third and fourth brachial pouch. This developmental failure usually results in an absence of the parathyroids and thymus gland. Hypocalcemic tetany can result from hypoparathyroidism. There is deficient T cell immune function because of thymic aplasia. The mode of inheritance is autosomal recessive. Bruton's agammaglobulinemia is an x-linked hereditary disorder in which there are no B cells or their B cell precursors. Repeated bacterial infections develop due to the lack of immunoglobulin production. Most of the offending bacterial organisms are pyogenic (streptococci, staphylococci) and the common sites of infection include pharynx, conjuctiva, inner ear, lung, and skin. Wiskott–Aldrich syndrome is an x-linked recessive hereditary disorder characterized by decreased platelet aggregation, thrombocytopenia, eczema, and a combined deficiency of antibody production and cellular immunity. Clinically, there are repeated infections with bacterial and viral organisms. Most Wiskott–Aldrich individuals die before age 5. Selective IgA deficiency is the most common of the isolated immunoglobulin deficiencies. Patients lacking IgA suffer from recurrent sinopulmonary bacterial infections. Isolated IgA deficiency is also associated with glutensensitive enteropathy, allergies, and arthritis. *(Cotran et al., pp. 231–236)*

373–376. (373-B, 374-A, 375-C, 376-A) The major histocompatibility complex (MHC) in humans is located on the short arm of chromosome 6. The MHC is presently divided into three classes. Class I antigens include HLA-A, HLA-B, and HLA-C. These genes code for transmembrane glycoproteins that are noncovalently linked to beta$_2$-microglobulin. These class I antigens are present on almost all nucleated cells in the body. Because of their highly polymorphic nature, they provide a unique immunologic marker for "selfness." The class II MHC genes code for HLA-DR, HLA-DQ, and HLA-DP molecules. These molecules are found mainly on macrophages and B cell lymphocytes. Class II antigens consist of two noncovalently linked transmembrane glycoprotein chains. The larger is termed "alpha" and is about 34,000 daltons. The smaller is termed "beta" and is about 29,000 daltons. Class II molecules help with antigen presentation to the T cells. The class III MHC region codes for complement proteins C2, factor B, and C4. At present, there are no class IV or class V MHC antigens. *(Henry, pp. 959–973)*

377–380. (377-B, 378-D, 379-A, 380-C) Erythroblastosis fetalis (hemolytic disease of the newborn) is a type II hypersensitivity reaction in which maternal IgG antibodies cross the placenta to lyse fetal erythrocytes. The provoking fetal antigen is usually Rh D (Rh positive) reoccurring in a previously sensitized mother. In the most severe instances, there is fetal hydrops with intrauterine demise, anasarca, and maceration. The tuberculin skin test is an example of a type IV hypersensitivity reaction. Immunologically competent and sensitized lymphocytes produce a granulomatous response to the tuberculin antigen. Anaphylaxis following an insect bite is an example of a type I hypersensitivity reaction. The insect venom antigens reacting with IgE antibodies bound to basophils and mast cells stimulate these cells to release vasoactive amines into the peripheral circulation. These vasoactive amines can bring about circulatory collapse and anaphylactic shock through generalized vasodilation, increased vascular permeability, and reduced intravascular volume. Serum sickness is an example of an immune complex injury. Following exposure to a large dose of foreign antigen circulating immune complexes form in the blood. These immune complexes may be trapped in the endothelial pores in blood vessels causing vasculitis, or in the kidney causing glomerulonephritis. Complement may exacerbate the tissue damage by recruiting inflammatory cells. Serum sickness is a Type II hypersensitivity reaction. *(Cotran et al., pp. 196–206)*

381–384. (381-E, 382-B, 383-C, 384-D) Autoantibodies directed against native components of the body can produce a wide range of clinical disease states. Hashimoto's thyroiditis is an autoimmune disorder in which there is immunologic destruction of the thyroid gland with resultant hypothyroidism. The antibodies produced act against thyroglobulin and microsomal follicular cell fractions. Histologically, the thyroid gland demonstrates a mixed lymphocytic and plasmacytic inflammatory infiltrate, germinal follicle formation, and reactive epithelial changes. Another autoimmune disorder, primary biliary cirrhosis, typically has high titers of antibodies that react with mitochondria. In this disorder, there is immune-mediated destruction of hepatic bile ductules, with subsequent cirrhosis. Pemphigus vulgaris is a disease of autoimmunity in which there are antibodies produced against keratinocytes and their desmosomal attachment sites. Clinically, skin bullae occur because of autoimmune-mediated disattachment of affected keratinocytes. Myasthenia gravis is an autoimmune disorder in which acetylcholine receptor autoantibodies are produced. The immunologic impairment of the acetylcholine receptors is observed clinically as diminished muscular endurance, particularly noticeable in the periorbital and eyelid muscles. *(Cotran et al., pp. 216–235, 877, 1135, 1289)*

385–388. (385-D, 386-E, 387-A, 388-B) Complement may be activated either through the classical pathway or through the properdin alternative pathway. In the classic pathway IgG or IgM first binds to an antigen. The C1 fraction of complement then attaches to the Fc portion of the immunoglobulin molecule. Cleavage of bound C1 initiates the complement cascade. In the alternative pathway properdin and other cofactors (D, B, and magnesium) can cleave C3 independent of antibody binding and independent of the early classic pathway complement proteins (C1, C2, and C4). As the complement cascade builds, a number of biologically active fractions are released. For example, the C3a and C5a fragments are anaphylatoxins. C3b encourages immune phagocytosis by macrophages and neutrophils because of its opsonic properties. C5b67 is chemotactic. The final product of the complement cascade is a C5b6789 complex capable of inducing focal cell membrane lysis. *(Chandrasoma and Taylor, pp. 67–69)*

389. **(E)** In this scenario, the patient most likely has rheumatoid arthritis, an immunologic disorder of the joints. The disease is usually seen in Western European and North American white females between the ages of 30 and 50 years old. The clinical hallmark of the disease is symmetric swelling of the small joints of the hands and feet, particularly at the proximal interphalangeal joint. Swelling, pain, and stiffness is most severe in the morning. Pathologically, a pannus of hypertrophic inflamed synovium is produced that may eventually erode the articular cartilage with subsequent fibrosis, restriction of movement, and deformity. Most individuals with rheumatoid arthritis demonstrate a serum rheumatoid factor, an IgM molecule with anti-IgG specificity. *(Rubin and Farber, pp. 141, 142)*

390. **(C)** Sezary's syndrome is a lymphoproliferative disorder of T cell lymphocytes. Sezary cells are found circulating in the peripheral blood and are characterized as convoluted lymphocytic cells with cerebriform nuclei. T cell markers are invariable present on these cells, usually of the helper (T4, CD4) subset. Most individuals have erythroderma or eczema concomitant with the circulating cerebriform lymphocytes. The median survival rate is about 9 years. In the late stages of the disorder, there is extensive involvement of the visceral organs and lymph nodes by lymphomatous cells. *(Rubin and Farber, pp. 1139–1296)*

391. **(G)** The elderly gentleman in this scenario is most likely to have secondary amyloidosis. Amyloid is a pathologic proteinaceous material deposited in the interstitial spaces. It is an acellular eosinophilic material with the biochemical ability to produce apple green birefringence when examined under polarized light in Congo red stained histologic material. This peculiar optical feature is due to the beta-pleated sheet arrangement of the amyloid molecules. Clinically, amyloidosis occurs in both localized and systemic forms. It is not uncommon to see amyloidosis follow longstanding inflammatory or infectious disorders, such as chronic osteomyelitis or tuberculosis. In these cases, the amyloidosis is almost always systemic in nature and deposited throughout the body. The heart interstitium, spleen interstitium, and perirectal blood vessels are preferential sites of systemic amyloid deposition. *(Rubin and Farber, pp. 1232–1233)*

392. **(F)** The woman most likely has myasthenia gravis. This is an immunologic disorder most commonly occurring in women between the ages of 20 and 40 years old. Individuals with myasthenia gravis have muscle weakness that worsens as the muscle is exercised. The periorbital and lid muscles are likely to be involved, with affected individuals complaining of drooping eyelids and double vision (diplopia). Antibodies to acetylcholine receptors are present in myasthenia gravis and thought to be the most sensitive and specific method of diagnosing the disorder in patients with the appropriate clinical symptoms. Another diagnostic technique is to administer edrophonium, a short-acting anticholinesterase drug, to suspected myasthenic individuals. Those with myasthenia gravis will demonstrate a transient immediate improvement of muscular endurance and strength. Untreated, about 40% of myasthenic patients will die of their disease within 10 years, usually due to respiratory complications. Thymic abnormalities (hyperplasia and thymomas) may be seen in association with myasthenia gravis. *(Rubin and Farber, pp. 118–119)*

393. **(A)** The elderly woman has multiple myeloma, a malignant tumor of plasma cells. Plasma cells are derived from B cell lymphocytes. Multiple myeloma is a disease rarely seen before age 50. The clinical features include anemia, bone pain, renal disease, hypercalcemia, infections, bleeding diatheses, and neuropathy. The bones may demonstrate multiple lytic defects when examined radiographically. The bone marrow contains increased numbers of atypical plasma cells. A monoclonal intact immunoglobulin, heavy chain, or light chain can be found in serum, urine, or both serum and urine. The mean survival is about 3 years. Death is usually due to hemorrhagic or infectious complications. *(Rubin and Farber, pp. 1222–1224)*

394. **(A)** The child has Burkitt's lymphoma (small noncleaved cell lymphoma), a malignancy of B cell lymphocytes. Burkitt's lymphoma is a common tumor of African children. It usually occurs as a large disfiguring mass of the jaw. In North America, the disease is infrequent. The North American variety is characterized by abdominal masses in childhood. Both the tropical and temperature varieties share similar histology: sheets of small undifferentiated cells with an elevated mitotic rate and

a "starry sky" background of phagocytic macrophages filled with debris. Histochemically, the cytoplasm of the tumor cells contains Oil red O vacuoles. There is surface immunoglobulin on the Burkitt's cells confirming their B cell lineage. Burkitt's lymphoma is an aggressive high grade lymphoma. *(Rubin and Farber, pp. 1131–1134)*

395. **(B)** The man has mycosis fungoides (cutaneous T cell lymphoma), a malignancy of T cell lymphocytes. This neoplasm is a primary lymphoreticular malignancy that originates in the skin. The early stages of the disease may have only nonspecific erythroderma. Later stages of the disorder are plaque-like and demonstrate the diagnostic histology of Pautrier's microabscesses and Sezary–Lutzner tumor cells. The tumor cells are CD4 positive (T-helper subset) and have a folded cerebriform nucleus. A leukemic variety of this disorder is termed "Sezary's syndrome." Most individuals with mycosis fungoides eventually die from widespread visceral lymphoma, hemorrhagic complications, or infections. *(Rubin and Farber, pp. 1134–1139)*

396. **(C)** The adolescent has an eosinophic granuloma, a tumor of Langerhans' cells. The disorder usually occurs in individuals under the age of 20. There is bone pain with one or two lytic areas noted radiographically. The ribs and vertebral bones are most commonly affected. If these lytic areas are biopsied, they are found to contain a polymorphous mixture of inflammatory cells, eosinophils, fibrous tissue, and Langerhans' cells. The Langerhans' cells can be identified with certainty by demonstrating their S100 protein positivity and the presence of pentalaminar Birbeck bodies. Eosinophilic granuloma is a benign self-limited disorder in the bones. Biopsy or curretage is usually curative. More aggressive diseases of Langerhans' cells include Hand–Schuller–Christian disease and Letterer–Siwe disease. *(Cotran et al., pp. 685, 686)*

397. **(B)** Natural killer cells are a subset of T cells that can kill another cell whether neoplastic, transplanted tissue, or virus-infected cell. The

lysis of cells (cytolytic action) is produced by producing holes in the surface membrane of an antigen-positive cells, particularly if it is coated with IgG. *(Chandrasoma and Taylor, p. 55)*

398. **(A)** Interleukin-2 causes autocrine and paracrine proliferation of T cells. The activated T cells by interleukin-2 tend to accumulate on the sites of delayed hypersensitivity. *(Cotran et al., p. 206)*

399. **(A)** A macrophage activation is obtained by secretion of cytokines (lymphokines) secreted by T cells, fibroblasts, and macrophages. The activation of the macrophages stimulates lysis of either microorganisms or neoplastic cells. Gamma interferon does not produce any activity. *(Cotran et al., pp. 80, 81)*

400–402. **(400-C, 401-A, 402-D)** Acute serum sickness is a prototype of a systemic immune complex disease. It was seen in the past when the horse antitetanus serum was used for passive immunization. At the present time, it may occur after administration of horse antithymocytic globulin for treatment of aplastic anemia or antibiotic therapy for microbial diseases. The delayed-type of hypersensitivity the classic example is the tuberculin reaction that is produced by the intracutaneous injection of tuberculin. In a previously sensitized individual, reddening and induration of the site appears in 8–12 hours. The cytotoxic T cell recognize antigens present with the class I major histocompatibility molecules. This action facilitates their cytotoxic effect. *(Cotran et al., pp. 202–206)*

403. **(A)** Dendritic cells are one of the most important functions is to process and present the antigen to immunocompetent T cells. Because the T cells cannot be activated by soluble antigens, the presentation of processed antigens is mandatory for the induction of the cell-mediated immunity. *(Cotran et al., pp. 190, 191)*

404. **(C)** Eosinophils are particularly important in a late-phase reaction, and they are recruited by cytokines and chemokines released from activated epithelial cells under the influence of mediators such as TNF-α. The activated eosinophils and other leukocytes can produce leukotriene, and the recruited cells amplified and sustain the inflammatory response without additional exposure to the triggering antigen. *(Cotran et al., pp. 198, 199)*

405. **(B)** Arthus reaction is defined as a localized tissue necrosis resulting from acute immune complex vasculitis. The reaction can be produce experimentally by intracutaneous injection of antigen in an immune animal having circulating antibodies against the antigen. These antigen–antibody complexes will eventually activate the complement system, and the release of chemotactic factors will attract the polymorphonuclear cells. Moreover, also at the area of injection, there will be a central area of fibrinoid necrosis, with rupture of vessels, with secondary hemorrhage, and more often the vascular lumens undergo thrombosis. *(Cotran et al., p. 204)*

406. **(B)** The pathogenesis of systemic lupus erythematosus remains unknown, however, a number of antibodies against self-constituents indicates the failure of a regulatory mechanism to sustain self-tolerance. The most common antibodies are identified against the nuclear component, as well as the cytoplasmic components. The antibodies to DNA are the most commonly found in lupus erythematosus. However, antibodies to double-stranded DNA and the so-called Smith (Sm antigen) are virtually diagnostic of systemic lupus erythematosus. *(Cotran et al., pp. 216–225)*

407. **(D)** Morphologically delayed-type sensitivity is characterized by the accumulation of mononuclear cells around the small veins and venules producing a perivascular "cuffing." Moreover, an associated increase in microvascular permeability causing edema of the soft tissues is present. *(Cotran et al., p. 204)*

408. **(B)** The cell mediator of hypersensitivity is initiated specifically by sensitized T lymphocytes. The classic example of delayed hypersensitivity is tuberculin reaction. Histologically, the small veins show a perivascular cuffing with an increase in permeability that causes edema and inflammation of the surrounding tissues. After some time, these perivascular lymphocytic infiltrates is replaced by macrophages, which accumulate and transform into epithelial-like cells referred as epithelioid cells. Some of these cell share the same cytoplasm, and form multinucleated giant cells, and these structures surrounded by lymphocytes is known as a granulomatous reaction. *(Cotran et al., p. 204)*

409. **(D)** Natural killer cells make up approximately 10–15% of the peripheral lymphocytes. They are somehow larger than the common lymphocytes and contain abundant azurophilic granules. Natural killer cells have the function and ability to lyse a variety of tumor cells and viral-infected cells. Another name for these cells is large granular lymphocytes. *(Cotran et al., p. 191)*

410. **(D)** This type of graft rejection occurs only minutes or hours after transplantation and can happen only if the recipient has circulating antibodies to donor cellular antigens. The histological lesions are characterized by a classic Arthus reaction. There is a rapid accumulation of neutrophils and immunoglobulins and complement deposit in the vessel wall. The earliest lesion point out to an antigen–antibody reaction at the level of vascular endothelium. *(Cotran et al., pp. 207, 208)*

REFERENCES

Chandrasoma P, Taylor CR. *Concise Pathology,* 3rd ed. Norwalk, CT: Appleton & Lange, 1998.

Cotran RS, Kumar V, Robbins SL. *Robbins Pathologic Basis of Disease,* 6th ed. Philadelphia: Saunders, 1999.

Henry JB (ed.). *Clinical Diagnosis and Management by Laboratory Methods,* 20th ed. Philadelphia: Saunders, 2001.

Rubin E, Farber JL. *Pathology.* Philadelphia: Lippincott, 1999.

CHAPTER 5

Infectious Diseases

Although man can build a better mousetrap, nature always seems to build a better mouse.
—Alto E. Feller (1953)

BASIC FACTS AND DEFINITIONS

This chapter emphasizes the interactions and the host responses to invasion by microbiologic organisms. There are complicated interactions between host and parasite mediated through the immune system. There is an important distinction among symbiosis, commensalism, and parasitism.

The outcome and resultant disease processes that occur in response to invasion by pathogenic organisms depend on the balance between host factors and properties of the organism (Figure 5–1). Some examples of defense mechanisms and their failure to prevent microorganism-related diseases are seen in Table 5–1. Table 5–2 summarizes some of the more important characteristics of the various types of pathogenic organisms in human disease.

An important aspect of disease associated with protozoa and metazoa is the life cycle of the parasites. Examples are shown in Figure 5–2 and Table 5–3 to demonstrate how humans may occupy different positions in such life cycles.

Examples of bacteria that produce some of their effects through the production of toxins are shown in Table 5–4. Fungal or mycotic infections can produce superficial (most frequent) or deep and widespread lesions. Table 5–5 summarizes some of the more important causes of deep fungal infections for quick reference. There are many more fungal infections, with specialized geographic distribution.

Many and varied types of protozoa are pathogenic to humans. Table 5–6 summarizes some of these.

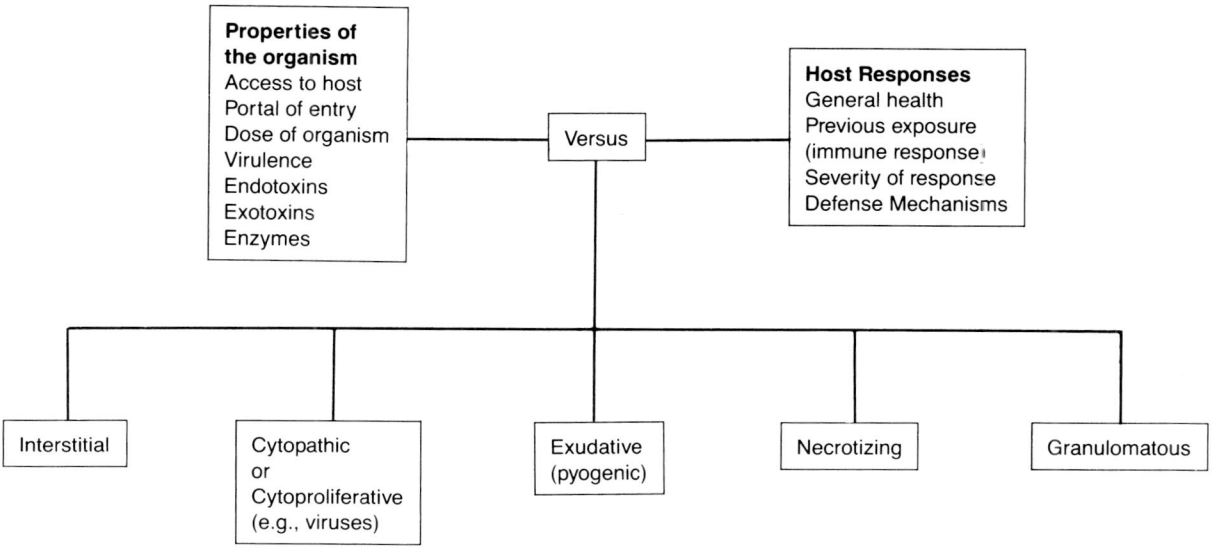

Figure 5–1. Pathogenesis of infectious diseases.

Table 5–1. SOME EXAMPLES OF DEFENSE MECHANISMS IN INFECTIOUS DISEASES

Portal of Entry	Defense Mechanisms	Examples of Failure or Breakdown of Defenses
Skin	Layers of stratified squamous epithelium Antimicrobial effects of secretions	Wounds, abrasions, burns, ulceration, pre-existing dermatoses
Respiratory tract	Nasal–oral secretions, pharyngeal lymphoid ring Mucociliary mechanism, cough reflex	Trauma, aspiration of material, obstruction, loss of cough reflex, failure of mucociliary action, low temperature, noxious gases, viral infection, destruction of epithelium
Gastrointestinal tract	Oral secretions, pharyngeal lymphoid ring, epithelium of esophagus and stomach acid, lymphoid tissue with secretion IgA of intestine, resident normal bacterial flora	Ingestion of infected material, food in nasopharynx or sputum, loss of gastric acid, ulceration of mucosa, obstruction, trauma, perforation, loss of flora due to stagnation or broad-spectrum antibiotics
Urinary tract	Flow of urine, pH of urine, transitional epithelium	Obstruction, stagnation of urine, stones, catheters, alteration of pH, penetrating injuries, ulceration
Female genital tract	Stratified squamous epithelium of vagina, acid and normal flora of vagina, mucous plugs of cervix	Hormonal loss with epithelial regressive changes, lowering of acidity and flora, trauma, parturition, foreign bodies (tampons), tumors, ulceration
Eyes (conjunctiva)	Secretions, tears, intact epithelium	Direct inoculation with infected material, lack of tears and secretions, trauma
Bloodstream and lymphatics	Usual inaccessibility and immune factors	Extension from any of the above mechanisms, direct inoculation—intravenous or intra-arterial fluids, failure of immune mechanism, loss of leukocytes of various types

Table 5–2. SUMMARY OF IMPORTANT CHARACTERISTICS OF SOME PATHOGENIC ORGANISMS

Bacteria (0.8–15 μm)	Viruses (20–30 nm)	Rickettsia (300–1,200 nm)	Mycoplasma (25–35 μm)	Fungi (2–200 μm)	Metazoa (including Protozoa (1–50 mm)	helminth) (3–10 mm)	Chlamydiae (20–1,000 nm)
Facultative, Intracellular, or extracellular	Mostly obligate Intracellular	Mostly obligate Intracellular	Extracellular	Facultative, Intracellular, or extracellular	Variable, Extracellular, or intracellular	Variable, intracellular, or extracellular	Mostly obligate Intracellular

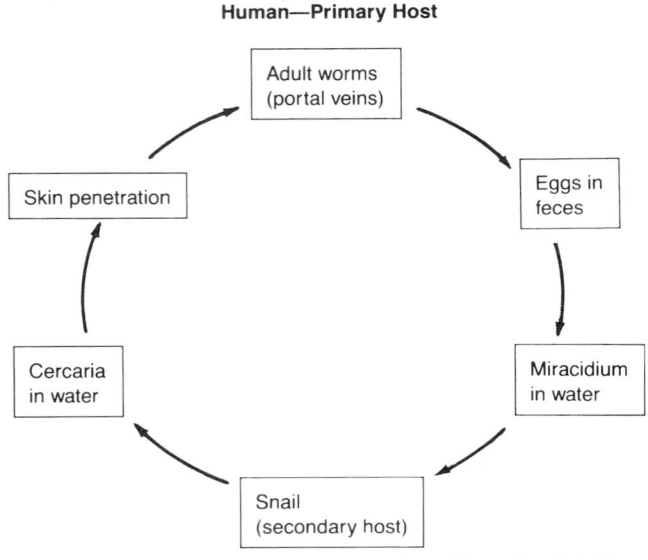

Human—Primary Host

Adult worms (portal veins)

Skin penetration

Eggs in feces

Cercaria in water

Miracidium in water

Snail (secondary host)

Figure 5–2. Schematic representation of the life cycle of *Schistosoma mansoni.*

Table 5–3. TYPES OF PARASITIC LIFE CYCLES

Parasite	Primary Host (Adult Form of Parasite)	Secondary Host	Intermediate Host (Often Accidental)
Schistosoma	Human	Snail	—
Plasmodium (malaria)	Mosquito	Human	—
Taenia solium (pig tapeworm)	Human	Pig	—
Echinococcus	Dog	Sheep	Human
Hookworm	Human	—	—

Table 5-4. EXAMPLES OF BACTERIAL TOXINS AND THEIR EFFECTS ON THE HOST

Type of Organism	Type of Toxin	Effect
Staphylococcus aureus	Enterotoxin	Gastrointestinal tract, food poisoning
	Alpha toxin	Necrosis of tissue, abscess formation
	Exfoliation	Exfoliation of skin
	Pyrogens	Fever
Streptococcus pyogenes	Streptolysins	Cellulitis
	Erythrogenic toxin	Vascular injuries, scarlet fever
Escherichia coli	Enterotoxin	Damage to intestinal epithelium, diarrhea, dehydration
Vibrio cholerae	Enterotoxin	Damage to intestinal epithelium, diarrhea, dehydration
Clostridium difficile	Enterotoxin	Epithelial damage: pseudomembranous colitis
Clostridium perfringens	Alpha toxin	Necrosis and hemolysis
Clostridium botulinum	Botulinus toxin	Neurotoxic, causes paralysis
Clostridium tetani	Tetanus toxin	Neurotoxic
Corynebacterium diphtheriae	Diphtheria toxin	Neurotoxic

Table 5-5. SUMMARY OF DEEP MYCOTIC INFECTIONS

Species of Fungus	Usual Port of Entry	Distribution of Lesions in Body
Sporothrix schenckii	Skin	Skin, occasionally lymph nodes
Torulopsis glabrata	Oral	Systemic
Candida subspecies	Skin, gastrointestinal tract, intravenous	Skin or mucus membranes, systemic: various organs
Cryptococcus neoformans	Respiratory tract	Lung, meninges, systemic
Aspergillus subspecies	Respiratory tract	Lung localized, lung diffuse, systemic
Mucor species	Respiratory tract	Upper respiratory, lung, systemic
Blastomyces dermatitidis	Respiratory tract	Lung, systemic with skin lesions
Coccidioides	Respiratory tract	Lung, systemic with meninges
Histoplasma capsulatum	Respiratory tract	Lung, systemic with widespread locations

Table 5-6. EXAMPLES OF PATHOGENIC PROTOZOA

Species	Usual Site of Disease	Usual Pathologic Disorder
Luminal		
Entamoeba histolytica	Colon	Amebic dysentery, liver or lung abscess
Balantidium coli	Colon	Dysentery
Giardia lamblia	Small intestine	Diarrhea with malabsorption
Cryptosporidium	Small and large intestine	Enterocolitis with malabsorption
Trichomonas vaginalis	Vagina and urethra	Vaginitis and urethritis
Pneumocystis carinii	Bronchial tree	Opportunistic lung infections
Bloodstream		
Plasmodium species	Red cells and blood stream, some in liver	Malaria
Trypanosoma species	Bloodstream	African sleeping sickness
Intracellular		
Trypanosoma cruzi	Various parenchymal cells, including myocardial cells	Chagas disease
Leishmania donovani	Macrophages	Kala-azar
Leishmania species	Macrophages	Cutaneous and mucocutaneous leishmaniasis
Toxoplasma gondii	Various parenchymal cells	Toxoplasmosis

Questions

DIRECTIONS (Questions 411 through 427): Each of the numbered items or incomplete statements in this section is followed by answers or by completions of the statement. Select the ONE lettered answer or completion that is BEST in each case.

411. The relationship between the human host organism and the normal bacterial flora (indigenous microbiota) is best called

 (A) saphrophytic
 (B) commensal
 (C) symbiotic
 (D) parasitic
 (E) facultative

412. Which organism produces chronic rhinitis?

 (A) rotavirus
 (B) enteropathogenic *Escherichia coli*
 (C) *Shigella dysenteriae*
 (D) *Vibrio cholerae*
 (E) *Klebsiella rhinoscleromatis*

413. Which organism is an obligate intracellular parasite?

 (A) *Mycobacterium tuberculosis*
 (B) *Mycobacterium kansasii*
 (C) *Mycobacterium leprae*
 (D) *Histoplasma capsulatum*
 (E) *Legionella pneumophila*

414. Which organism does not involve endothelial or mural vascular invasion?

 (A) rickettsiae
 (B) *Pseudomonas*
 (C) *Aspergillus*
 (D) *Treponema pallidum*
 (E) *Actinobacillus*

415. Which of the following ectoparasites has no intermediate host?

 (A) *Loa loa*
 (B) *Trichuris trichiura*
 (C) *Paragonimus westermani*
 (D) *Dracunculus medinensis*
 (E) *Clonorchis sinensis*

416. Stellate microabscesses with a granulomatous rim of epithelioid histiocytes may be seen in biopsies of lymphoid tissue from patients with

 (A) *Yersinia enterocolitica* infection
 (B) lymphogranuloma venereum (LGV)
 (C) *Brucella suis* infection
 (D) cat-scratch disease
 (E) all of the above

417. Genital skin ulcers are common in the acute presentation of which of the following venereal diseases

 (A) syphilis
 (B) granuloma inguinale
 (C) herpes simplex virus type 2 infection
 (D) chancroid
 (E) all of the above

418. Acute inflammation, suppuration, and abscess formation are common features of infections caused by which organism?

(A) *Staphylococcus aureus*
(B) *Sporothrix schenckii*
(C) *Blastomyces dermatiditis*
(D) *Coccidiodes immitis*
(E) *Cryptococcus neoformans*

419. The prognosis is best in rapidly progressive (crescentic) glomerulonephritis associated with

(A) poststreptococcal glomerulonephritis
(B) systemic lupus erythematosus (SLE)
(C) Henoch–Schoenlein purpura
(D) polyarteritis nodosa
(E) Goodpasture's syndrome

420. The most common cause of parasitic endophthalmitis is

(A) *Cysticercus cellulosae*
(B) *Toxacara* species
(C) *Toxoplasma gondii*
(D) *Oncocerca volvulus*
(E) *Loa loa*

421. The only ciliated pathogen of humans is

(A) *Giardia lamblia*
(B) *Trichomonas vaginalis*
(C) *Chilomastix mesnili*
(D) *Balantidium coli*
(E) *Acanthamoeba culbertsoni*

422. Which of the following diseases is transmitted by *Culex* mosquitoes?

(A) filariasis caused by *Onchocerca volvulus*
(B) filariasis caused by *Wuchereria bancrofti*
(C) leishmaniasis
(D) malaria
(E) all of the above

423. Which of the following is true of mumps?

(A) humans are the only natural host
(B) commonly occurs in infants

(C) commonly causes orchitis and consequent sterility
(D) produces intracellular inclusions in vivo in infected parotid acinar cells
(E) optimum prevention is by administration of killed mumps virus

424. The fungus most frequently isolated by the clinical laboratory from patient blood cultures is

(A) *Aspergillus* species
(B) *Actinomyces* species
(C) *Cryptococcus* species
(D) *Candidia* species
(E) *Mucor* species

425. Each of the following descriptions is true of *Plasmodium falciparum* is better described as

(A) the sporozoites form more merozoites than the sporozcites of other malarial plasmodia
(B) the merozoites parasitize both young and old red blood cells (RBC)
(C) parasitized erythrocytes have increased adherence to vascular endothelium
(D) infection is more frequently fatal than is infection with the other malarial plasmodia
(E) all of the above

426. The adult population groups that currently have a greatly increased risk of infection with human immunodeficiency virus (HIV) are homosexual or bisexual men, intravenous drug abusers, and their sexual contacts. What percentage of adult acquired immunodeficiency syndrome (AIDS) patients in the United States is classified as having none of these risk factors?

(A) 3%
(B) 10%
(C) 15%
(D) 20%
(E) 25%

427. Enzyme immunoassay (EIA) screening tests are the standard method used to detect the presence of serum antibody to human immunodeficiency virus (anti-HIV). The sensitivity and specificity of EIA for anti-HIV are both

(A) 1%
(B) 10%
(C) 50%
(D) 90%
(E) 99%

DIRECTIONS (Questions 428 through 486): Each group of items in this section consists of a list of lettered options followed by a set of numbered words or phrases. For each numbered word or phrase, select the ONE lettered option that is most closely associated with it. Each lettered option may be selected once, more than once, or not at all.

Questions 428 through 432

(A) pathogenicity does not involve mucosal invasion but is caused by an enterotoxin
(B) an enteroinvasive, flagellated gram-negative bacillus
(C) recovery from stool culture enhanced by cold enrichment
(D) pulmonary and cutaneous transmission by spores
(E) pathogenicity involves attachment of surface pili to host mucosal cell surface

428. *Neisseria gonorrhoeae*

429. *Vibrio cholerae*

430. *Campylobacter jejuni*

431. *Yersinia enterocolitica*

432. *Bacillus anthracis*

Questions 433 through 435

(A) the mature egg is an infective agent
(B) infective larvae are injected into humans by infected black fly or buffalo gnat
(C) larvae reaching soil via human feces may develop into a parasitic infective phase or a nonparasitic free-living phase

(D) the only tapeworm with humans as both intermediate and definitive hosts
(E) larvae become encysted in muscles of pigs or carnivores

433. *Onchocerca volvulus*

434. *Hymenolepis nana*

435. *Ascaris lumbricoides*

Questions 436 through 439

(A) entry into host cell involves fusion of viral coat with cell membrane
(B) entry into host cell involves release of nucleocapsid from endosome into cytosol
(C) entry into host cell involves release of nucleocaspid from endosome into cell nucleus
(D) entry into cell host involves fusion with T4 receptor on host cell surface
(E) an enveloped double-stranded DNA virus that replicates in the host cell cytoplasm

436. Influenza A virus

437. Polyoma virus

438. Human immunodeficiency virus (HIV)

439. *Paramyxovirus*

Questions 440 through 445

These questions refer to the microscopic examination of a stained smear of stool or diarrhea contents from a patient to ascertain the presence and type of inflammatory cells as a diagnostic test for pathogenesis of enteritis.

(A) many basophils
(B) many mononuclear leukocytes
(C) no (or rare) leukocytes
(D) many polymorphonuclear leukocytes
(E) many multinucleated giant cells

440. Typhoid fever

441. Shigellosis

442. Cholera

443. Enterotoxigenic *Escherichia coli*

444. Salmonellosis

445. Ulcerative colitis

Questions 446 through 449

Studies have shown that most patients in the United States with acquired immunodeficiency syndrome (AIDS) fall into four common categories. What is the approximate percentage of AIDS patients in each numbered category?

- (A) 17%
- (B) 1%
- (C) 4%
- (D) 73%
- (E) 100%

446. Homosexual or bisexual men

447. Hemophiliacs

448. Intravenous drug abusers

449. Haitians living in the United States

Questions 450 through 454

- (A) *Streptococcus pyogenes*
- (B) *Clostridium perfringens*
- (C) *Clostridium botulinum*
- (D) *Clostridium tetani*
- (E) *Clostridium difficile*

450. Tetanus

451. Scarlet fever

452. Pseudomembranous enterocolitis

453. Gas gangrene

454. Botulism

Questions 455 through 459

- (A) *Coxiella burnetti*
- (B) *Rickettsia rickettsii*
- (C) *Chlamydia psittaci*
- (D) *Chlamydia trachomatis*
- (E) *Rickettsia prowazekii*

455. Epidemic typhus

456. Rocky Mountain spotted fever

457. Blindness

458. Q fever

459. Ornithosis

Questions 460 through 464

- (A) *Trypanosoma cruzi*
- (B) *Entamoeba histolytica*
- (C) *Borrelia burgdoferi*
- (D) *Leishmania donovani*
- (E) *Plasmodium* species

460. Chagas' disease

461. Malaria

462. Lyme disease

463. Amebiasis

464. Kala-azar

Questions 465 through 469

- (A) *Wuchereria bancrofti*
- (B) *Enterobius vermicularis*
- (C) *Taenia solium*
- (D) *Necator americanus*
- (E) *Toxocara canis*

465. Filariasis

466. Visceral larva migrans

467. Hookworm

468. Pork tapeworm

469. Pinworm

Questions 470 through 474

- (A) Epstein–Barr virus
- (B) human papillomavirus
- (C) rubella virus
- (D) coxsackievirus type A
- (E) rhinovirus

470. Common cold

471. Infectious mononucleosis

472. Herpangina

473. Infection in the female genital tract may be associated with cervical dysplasia.

474. German measles

Questions 475 through 479

  (A) Anopheles mosquitoes
  (B) fleas
  (C) ixodid ticks
  (D) tsetse flies
  (E) no insect vector known

475. Vector of sleeping sickness

476. Vector of Lyme disease

477. Vector of plague

478. Vector of smallpox

479. Vector of malaria

Questions 480 through 482

  (A) aerobic bacteria
  (B) anaerobic bacteria
  (C) toxigenic bacteria
  (D) fungal organism
  (E) obligate intracellular virus
  (F) obligate extracellular virus
  (G) protozoan organism
  (H) blastogenic infection

480. A 45-year-old insulin-dependent diabetic male develops a sore throat. On examination the pharynx is coated by a superficial white, curdy membrane that can be readily scraped off to reveal an underlying reddened and swollen oropharyngeal mucosa. The physician's diagnosis is thrush, confirmed 2 days later by the laboratory's report of a pure culture of *C. albicans*. What kind of organism causes thrush?

481. A 2-month-old infant dies, and an autopsy is requested. Premortem history included seizures since birth, hydrocephalus, myocarditis, endocarditis, and jaundice. The most striking autopsy finding is the presence of multiple cysts of *Toxoplasma gondii* throughout the body. What kind of organism caused this infant's death?

482. A 32-year-old sexually active, healthy male donates blood at a local blood drive. Several weeks later he is asked to return to the blood bank and is informed that he has antibodies to HIV. A confirmatory Western blot is positive. What kind of organism has the man developed antibodies against?

Questions 483 through 486

  (A) bunyavirus
  (B) *Wuchereria bancrofti*
  (C) herpes simplex virus
  (D) *Onchocerca volvulus*
  (E) *Treponema pallidum*
  (F) *Mycobacterium leprae*
  (G) *Aspergillus fumigatus*
  (H) *Plasmodium vivax*

483. A 54-year-old sexually active male notices a painless, shallow ulceration on his penis. A darkfield examination reveals numerous corkscrew-shaped spirochetes. Which organism is most likely to have caused this ulcer?

484. A 43-year-old Malaysian woman has several hypopigmented nodules on her face that have been slowly enlarging. These nodules have no sensation to touch (hypoesthetic). A biopsy of one of these nodules is remarkable for the presence of numerous acid-fast bacilli. What organism is most likely to have caused these nodules?

485. A 21-year-old sexually active female suddenly develops numerous painful vesicles on her perineum, introitus, and labia. A smear of fluid and cells taken from the base of a vesicle is examined microscopically and is found to contain several multinucleate giant cells with prominent macronucleoli. What organism is most likely to have caused these vesicles?

486. A 56-year-old East Indian develops massive scrotal swelling over a period of several years. A biopsy of the scrotum demonstrates numerous microfilaria in the lymphatics and abundant reactive lymphatic fibrosis. What organism is most likely to have caused this lymphatic obstruction?

DIRECTIONS (Questions 487 through 496): Each of the numbered items or incomplete statements in this section is followed by answers or by completions of the statement. Select the ONE lettered answer or completion that is BEST in each case.

487. What are the cells that are markedly depleted in HIV?

(A) cells of the monocyte/macrophage lineage
(B) cytotoxic/suppressor T lymphocytes
(C) helper/inducer T lymphocytes
(D) mature plasma cells
(E) pre-B lymphocytes

488. What is the cell that harbors the immunodeficiency virus as a reservoir?

(A) epithelial cell
(B) B lymphocyte
(C) fibroblast
(D) monocyte
(E) T lymphocyte

489. Select the cell that has a high-affinity receptor for human immunodeficiency virus (a surface glycoprotein).

(A) gp120
(B) gp62
(C) OK-T8
(D) gp41
(E) CD4

490. Name the mechanism for which lymphoid hyperplasia occurs in patients with HIV.

(A) direct activation of B lymphocytes by HIV
(B) productive infection of T4 lymphocytes by HIV

(C) productive infection of T8 lymphocytes by HIV
(D) destruction of polymorphonuclear leukocytes
(E) productive infection of monocyte–macrophage by HIV

491. The central nervous system symptomatology, and the destruction of neurons and glial cells in patients with AIDS is most likely due to

(A) direct infection by HIV
(B) monokines and enzymes released by HIV-infected monocyte macrophages
(C) immune complex deposition
(D) cytotoxic effect of the T8 lymphocyte
(E) development of an astrocytoma

492. Common routes of transmission of HIV (Human immunodeficiency virus) include

(A) needle stick
(B) homosexual contact (male to male)
(C) heterosexual contact
(D) transplacental passage, from mother to fetus
(E) all of the above

493. In an HIV-infected individual, the monocytes/macrophages will

(A) serve as reservoirs and carriers
(B) form caseating granulomas
(C) be immediately killed by the HIV
(D) become a highly malignant neoplasm
(E) directly lyse T4 lymphocytes

494. The patients with AIDS commonly show respiratory symptoms which are secondary to

(A) pulmonary thromboembolism
(B) bronchogenic carcinoma
(C) metastatic carcinoma to the lung
(D) infection(s)
(E) rupture of the lung parenchyma into the pleural cavity

495. The drug 3′-azido-3-dioxythymidine (AZT) inhibits

(A) gp 120 protein expression
(B) viral reverse transcription
(C) viral envelope (ENV) gene expression
(D) CD4 receptor expression
(E) viral GAG core protein expression

496. Cells that are specifically infected by human immunodeficiency virus (type 1) are

(A) macrophages
(B) plasma cells
(C) CD8+ T lymphocytes
(D) polymorphonuclear leukocytes
(E) CD4+ T lymphocytes

Answers and Explanations

411. **(C)** The relationship of the human host and its normal flora is one of a vast number of examples of symbiosis in the animal and plant kingdoms. Symbiosis is the intimate living together of two dissimilar organisms in a mutually beneficial relationship. This evolutionarily conserved relationship is of immense importance, and its delicate balance may be easily disturbed by many factors, such as drug therapy, primary or secondary immunodeficiency, infection, and trauma, with harmful consequences for both symbionts. Commensalism is a relationship between organisms in which one obtains benefits (especially food intake) from the other without benefiting or harming it. A saprophyte lives on dead or decaying organic matter, such as human excreta. Facultative means optional, e.g., a facultative pathogen is an organism that is sometimes, but not invariably, pathogenic. A facultative intracellular parasite is one that can survive and reproduce either within or outside of cells. Parasites have a harmful effect on their hosts. Microorganisms of the normal flora (nonparasites) may become parasites in the compromised host and are then called opportunists. *(Chandrasoma and Taylor, pp. 189–195)*

412. **(E)** Gastrointestinal pathogens capable of producing diarrhea in infected human hosts are usually acquired through the ingestion of food or drink contaminated by the organisms. The defense mechanisms employed by gut to thwart these invaders include the physical barrier of the mucosa, the acidity of the stomach, the continuous flow of the lumenal contents, secreted mucus and IgA, and competition by commensal organisms. *Klebsiella rhinoscleromatis* infections produce chronic rhinitis, not diarrhea. *(Chandrasoma and Taylor, pp. 219, 435)*

413. **(C)** *Mycobacterium leprae,* an acid-fast bacillus, is an obligate intracellular parasite with a strong tropism for macrophages and Schwann cells. It is the cause of Hansen's disease (leprosy), a chronic, indolent infection primarily of skin, peripheral nerves, mucous membranes, and eyes. Leprosy usually begins as a hypopigmented macule (indeterminate leprosy) that gradually progresses to more macules and plaques, which contain granulomas (tuberculoid leprosy) in patients with a cell-mediated immune reaction against the organism. If cell-mediated immunity is lost or becomes weak, the infection becomes much more extensive, and there is less granulomatous reaction (lepromatous leprosy). There is a range of disease severity between the tuberculoid and lepromatous forms (borderline or dimorphous leprosy). The other organisms listed are facultative intracellular parasites. *(Cotran et al., pp. 385, 386)*

414. **(E)** The actinobacilli are fastidious gram-negative bacilli and coccobacilli that cause disease in humans and some herbivores. The only species usually associated with human infections is *Actinobacillus actinomycetemcomitans,* which may cause localized purulent granulomas and abscesses, septicemia, endocarditis, and meningitis. It probably is a factor in periodontosis (juvenile periodontitis). Rickettsiae are obligate intracellular parasites of humans and lower animals and are more closely related to bacteria than to viruses. They invade and multiply within endothelial cells, causing vasculitis. *Pseudomonas aeruginosa* can invade extensively both small and large blood vessels in patients with decreased resistance. Another opportunist, *Aspergillus,* also invades blood vessels. *T. pallidum* causes obliterative endarteritis by invading small blood vessels, e.g., in skin, liver, bones, central nervous system, and vasa vasorum of the aorta. Infections with organisms that invade blood vessels usually cause proliferative or thrombotic vascular obstruction with ischemic damage or hemorrhage (Table 5–2). *(Chandrasoma and Taylor, pp. 193–212)*

415. **(B)** *Trichuris* has no intermediate host. The eggs are hatched, and the larval forms enter the primary host again. *(Chandrasoma and Taylor, p. 609)*

416. **(E)** *Y. enterocolitica* causes enterocolitis and mesenteric lymphadenitis, which may range from mild to severe (pseudoappendicitis or pseudo-Crohn's disease). *Y. pseudotuberculosis* also causes acute mesenteric lymphadenitis but is less likely to cause enterocolitis. The I, II, and III serotypes of *Chlamydia trachomatis* cause LGV, a venereal disease characterized by the occurrence (in stages) of genital vesicles, ulcers, lymphadenopathy, and fibrous rectal stricture. *B. suis, B. abortus,* and *B. canis* may colonize the lymphoreticular system and cause an acute or chronic syndrome, with fever, pain, lassitude, lymphadenopathy, hepatosplenomegaly, infarcts, and (infrequently) pneumonia. Cat-scratch disease is an acute, self-limited disease characterized by mild fever and regional lymphadenopathy and probably is caused by an incompletely identified delicate pleomorphic gram-negative bacillus. All of these organisms may cause stellate microabscesses with a granulomatous rim. These may be seen also with some fungal infections and tularemia, but the granulomas in these diseases are more often tuberculoid. Brucellae may cause sarcoid-like granulomas. *(Cotran et al., pp. 83, 334, 361, 362, 376, 377)*

417. **(C)** The primary chancre is the earliest lesion of venereal syphilis and appears after a 2- to 3-week incubation period as a firm papule that superficially erodes to form an indurated, clean-based ulcer that heals spontaneously. It is characterized by obliterative endarteritis and marked plasma cell infiltration. Granuloma inguinale is caused by *Calymmatobacterium granulomatis (donovani),* a tiny, fastidious gram-negative bacillus that causes indolent, gradually progressive cutaneous and mucocutaneous ulcers of the external genitalia, inguinal region, anus, and perianal region. The ulcers are painless or mildly painful and are characterized by proliferation of chronically inflamed granulation tissue and squamous epithelium. *Haemophilus ducreyi* causes an acute venereal disease characterized by ulcers that are chancroid but differ from the primary ulcer of syphilis in that they are not indurated (soft chancre) and are covered by a superficial layer of acute inflammatory exudate. Genital infection with herpes simplex viruses, types 1 and 2, result in multiple, small, grouped vesicles that coalesce into ulcers, especially in moist areas. The virus replicates in the epithelium, causing ballooning degeneration with loss of intercellular bridges (acantholysis), edema, multinucleated cells, and viral inclusions. *(Rubin and Farber, pp. 408–413, 385, 386)*

418. **(A)** *Staphylococcus aureus* infections characteristically produce acute inflammatory infiltrates, suppuration, and abscess formation. Bacteria that evoke this suppurative pattern of host response possess an ability to resist immediate phagocytosis by neutrophils, monocytes, and macrophages. The initial failure to phagocytize the invading organisms leads to an overabundance of these cellular defenders, producing the associated suppurative pattern. The other listed choices are fungi that produce granulomatous inflammation in sensitized hosts with intact cellular immunity. *(Rubin and Farber, pp. 374–376)*

419. **(A)** Rapidly progressive glomerulonephritis may occur in association with the five diseases mentioned and also with periarteritis (polyarteritis) nodosa, Wegener's granulomatosis, and essential cryoglobulinemia. Some cases arise without a known antecedent disease (idiopathic). Although the prognosis is poor in all types of rapidly progressive glomerulonephritis, poststreptococcal disease has a better prognosis than the other types, and up to 50% of patients may recover sufficient renal function to avoid chronic dialysis or transplantation. (*Rubin and Farber, pp. 882–884*)

420. **(B)** The definitive host of the ascarid nematode *Toxocara canis* is the dog and its canine relatives. Many lactating bitches and more than 80% of puppies pass large numbers of infective fertilized eggs in feces for about 6 months after parturition. The fertilized eggs can remain infective for months to years in moist soil. *Toxocara* eggs have been found contaminating 10–30% of soil samples taken from public playgrounds and parks in the United States and 24% of soil samples from public places in Britain. A human who ingests infective *T. canis* eggs becomes an accidental host for the larvae. The larvae hatch in the proximal small bowel, penetrate the mucosa, and migrate through the portal circulation to the liver, where they cause granulomatous inflammation. Some migrate on through the systemic circulation to lungs, heart, kidney, central nervous system, and muscles. The larvae do not complete their life cycle. Most infections are mild, but clinically apparent infection generally occurs in one of two patterns, visceral or ocular. The visceral larva migrans syndrome (VLM) is most common in children 1–5 years old with geophagous pica and is characterized by fever, malaise, weight loss, marked eosinophilia, hepatomegaly, wheezing, abdominal pain, myalgia, and neurologic signs. The mean age of children with ocular larva migrans (OLM) is 7.5 years (range 2–31 years), and a history of pica is unusual. Common signs are failing vision and strabismus. There are three basic lesions: (a) a central granuloma; (b) a peripheral granuloma, which may have elevated retinal folds extending to the disk; and (c) diffuse endophthalmitis or uveitis, sometimes with retinal detachment. The lesions may be mistaken for a retinoblastoma and the eye unnecessarily enucleated. Nematode endophthalmitis was found in 2% of a series of 1,000 eyes removed from children under 15 years old and is believed to cause 10% of the cases of uveitis in children (Table 5–3). (*Rubin and Farber, p. 469*)

421. **(D)** *Balantidium coli* is a ciliated protozoan. Balantidiasis is associated with abdominal pain, severe diarrhea, malaise, abdominal distention, and vomiting. Humans are infected by ingesting water or food contaminated by animal reservoir feces containing the infective cysts. The excysted organisms invade into the bowel wall to produce the symptoms of the disease. Tetracycline or iodoquinol are effective treatments. (*Rubin and Farber, p. 455*)

422. **(B)** Tropical species of mosquitoes in the genera *Culex, Aedes, Anopheles,* and *Mansonia* (family Culicidae, order Diptera, class Insecta, phylum Arthropoda) are the intermediate hosts and vectors of the roundworm (nematode) *W. bancrofti,* a cause of filariasis in humans (the definitive host). When an infected mosquito bites moist skin, the infective larvae in its proboscis creep out, penetrate through the bite, and travel to the lymphatics and lymph nodes, where they mature in a few months into male and female adult worms with tapering ends. The white, threadlike adult worms mate, and the female produces tiny sheathed embryos, microfilariae, that travel from the lymphatic system to the bloodstream, first appearing about a year after the infective bite. The number of microfilariae in the peripheral blood is usually greatest from about 10 PM to 2 AM (nocturnal periodicity), which is the time of peak feeding activity of the mosquito vectors. This is also the optimum time for obtaining blood specimens for diagnostic examination, including centrifuged wet preparations, 5-μm filter preparations, and stained smears. (In the South Pacific, the increase in microfilariae is much smaller and occurs between noon and sunset.) The microfilariae are ingested by mosquitoes taking a blood meal and mature in the mosquito to infective larvae. The larvae are not highly infective, because many fail to penetrate the skin, fail to reach the lymphatics, or are injured by the host immune response. The larvae do not multiply in mosquitoes, nor do the adult worms multiply in people. Thus, thousands of bites per person are required to maintain transmission of the disease in a community. *W. bancrofti* filariasis causes lymphatic inflammation and obstruction, which may progress to elephantiasis, especially in the genitalia and

lower extremities. The vector of filariasis caused by the nematode *O. volvulus* is the black fly or buffalo gnat of the genus *Simulium*. *O. volvulus* causes subcutaneous swellings and sometimes causes blindness. The flagellate species of the genus *Leishmania* cause visceral leishmaniasis (*L. donovani*), cutaneous leishmaniasis (*L. tropica* and *L. mexicana*), and mucocutaneous leishmaniasis (*L. lutzomyia* and *psychodopygus*). The exclusive vector of malaria is the female *Anopheles* mosquito. (*Cotran et al., pp. 397, 398*)

423. **(A)** Mumps is an acute contagious disease caused by a paramyxovirus that is transmitted naturally by respiratory droplets, fomites, or direct contact and enters through the nose or mouth. Although parotitis can be produced in monkeys by injection of mumps virus into the parotid gland or Stenson's duct, the only known natural host is humans. After an incubation period of 2–4 weeks, a prodrome of fever, malaise, headache, and anorexia occurs, followed in a day by parotitis, usually bilateral. Most children become infected with the mumps virus and develop lifelong immunity; 80–90% of adults over 20 years of age are immune to mumps. More than 50% of cases occur in the 5- to 9-year age group, and 90% occur in children under 14 years old. Mumps is uncommon in infants under 1 year old because of placental transfer of maternal mumps antibody. Orchitis is rare before puberty but is the most common extrasalivary manifestation of mumps in postpubertal males, occurring in about 20–30% of patients; it is unilateral in about 80% of these. Therefore, mumps rarely causes sterility in males. Mumps may also involve other salivary glands, ovaries, pancreas, and the central nervous system, but sequelae are rare. Mumps virus can be recovered in routine virologic cell culture and causes cytopathic effects, such as intracytoplasmic eosinophilic inclusions and cell fusion. However, inclusions and syncytia are not seen in vivo in infected tissue. Active immunization of all children with live attenuated mumps virus vaccine at age 15 months is recommended. Vaccination produces a noncommunicable subclinical infection followed

in more than 95% of vaccinees by protective levels of antibody for at least 10 years. Vaccination is recommended also for adolescent and adult males without a history of mumps. (*Cotran et al., pp. 370, 371*)

424. **(D)** *Candida* is by far the most frequent fungus grown from blood cultures. *C. albicans* is the most common isolate, but at least seven other species are known to be pathogenic for humans, including *C. tropicalis, C. pseudotropicalis, C. guilliermondii, C. glabrata, C. krusei, C. paraspilosis*, and *C. stellatoidea*. *C. albicans* is a commensal normally present in the oropharynx, gastrointestinal tract, and vagina. Factors involved in host resistance to *Candida* infection include intact skin and mucosa, neutrophils, circulating and fixed macrophages, eosinophils, lymphocytes, and probably antibodies and complement. *Candida* becomes pathogenic only if the defense mechanisms are compromised. Factors predisposing to *Candida* infection include suppression of inhibitory normal bacterial flora by antibiotic therapy, immunosuppression (human immunodeficiency virus infection, steroid therapy, antineoplastic chemotherapy), intravenous drug abuse, skin or mucosal injury (trauma, surgery, chemotherapy, burns), and foreign bodies (intravenous and Foley catheters, prosthetic cardiac valves, ventricular shunt). Candidiasis may involve skin or mucosa (common in diabetes mellitus) or may be disseminated and involve deeper organs. Although aspergillosis is the second most common disseminated mycosis in the compromised patient and hematogenous seeding occurs, blood cultures from patients with aspergillosis rarely are positive. The *Antinomyces* are gram-positive filamentous bacteria that superficially resemble fungi and cause actinomycosis, a chronic suppurative disease. About half of cases are cervicofacial, and about 20% are pulmonary. Lesions spread contiguously, and hematogenous dissemination is very rare. Blood cultures of patients with actinomycosis are negative. Blood cultures may be positive in patients with cryptococcal meningitis, but *Candida* is isolated far more often. *Mucor* is a saprophytic zygomycete

that may infect immunocompromised patients with diabetic ketoacidosis, but it is rarely cultured from blood specimens. *(Cotran et al., pp. 378–382)*

425. **(E)** Malaria in humans is caused by species of the genus *Plasmodium: P. falciparum, P. vivax, P. ovale,* and *P. malariae.* All are obligate intracellular protozoa with complex life cycles. Sporozoites injected by an infected female *Anopheles* mosquito penetrate hepatocytes and multiply (primary tissue schizogony) to form merozoites. One *P. falciparum* sporozoite forms up to 40,000 merozoites; whereas, sporozoites of the other plasmodia form 2,000–15,000. Asexual development of merozoites in hepatocytes is called the "pre-erythrocytic cycle." Persistent infection in the liver (exoerythrocytic cycle) may cause periodic relapses of malaria due to *P. vivax* and *P. ovale* for several years. Untreated, nonfatal infections with *P. falciparum* terminate within a year, because this organism has no persistent exoerythrocytic cycle. It is very likely that *P. malariae* also has no persistent hepatic infection, but recrudescences may occur for at least 40 years because of latent infection with a small number of circulating parasites (persistent erythrocytic cycle). Because merozoites of *P. falciparum* infect RBCs of all ages, the magnitude of parasitemia (up to 60% of RBCs) is much greater than that of *P. malariae* (which only invades senescent RBCs) and *P. vivax* and *P. ovale* (which only invade reticulocytes and very young RBCs). The level of parasitemia with the last three is usually no more than 1 to 2%. Erythrocytes parasitized by *P. falciparum* develop small electron-dense protrusions (called "knobs") that adhere to vascular endothelium, causing slowed microcirculation with consequent ischemic injury, especially to the cerebrum and kidneys. Although infection with the other plasmodia is rarely fatal, *P. falciparum* malaria is estimated to cause about one million deaths per year in Africa alone. *(Cotran et al., pp. 389–391)*

426. **(A)** Through September 30, 1987, in the United States, 41,770 adult patients with AIDS had been reported to the Centers for Disease Control. No recognized risk factors were reported in only 2,059 of these patients (5%). After additional study of these 2,059 cases, only 1,202 (3%) remain classified as having no identified risk factors. Of these 1,202 patients, 596 currently are under investigation, and it is probable that risk factors will be found in a significant proportion. Information was incomplete or unobtainable in 325 of these 1,202. After additional information became available, risk factors were not identified for 281 of the AIDS patients. Thus, risk factors were not identified in only a small proportion (3% or less) of adult AIDS patients. Because this proportion has not changed over time, it may be inferred that modes of transmission of HIV have not changed. *(Cotran et al., pp. 236–251)*

427. **(E)** When commercially available test kits licensed by the Food and Drug Administration (FDA) are used by reliable laboratories (such as those inspected by the College of American Pathologists and the American Association of Blood Banks), the specificity and sensitivity of the EIA screening test for anti-HIV are both very high, 99% or greater. This has been established by proficiency testing by the CAP and AABB, studies published in the medical literature, and manufacturers of EIA kits, who have submitted data to the FDA for licensure. *(Cotran et al., pp. 236–251)*

428. **(E)** *N. gonorrhoeae,* a nonencapsulated pyogenic gram-negative diplococcus, attaches to columnar and transitional epithelial cells via surface pili. Strains with fewer pili are less virulent than strains having many pili and tend to cause asymptomatic urethritis or cervicitis. *N. gonorrhoeae* does not attach to squamous epithelial cells. *(Cotran et al., p. 362)*

429. **(A)** *V. cholerae* is a facultatively anaerobic, commashaped, gram-negative bacillus with polar flagellation. It does not invade or ulcerate the gut mucosa. It produces a heat-labile protein enterotoxin (choleragen) that has adenosine-diphosphate-ribosyl transferase activity and thus activates the adenylate cyclase of the mucosal cells of the small bowel. This generates increased cyclic adenosine monophosphate (cAMP), causing massive secretion of isotonic fluid in excess of the resorptive capacity of the

colon and resulting in severe diarrhea (Table 5–4). *(Cotran et al., pp. 357, 358)*

430. **(B)** *C. jejuni* is a motile, nonsporing, comma-shaped, slender microaerophilic rod that is best recovered by culture on selective (antibotic-containing) media in 5% O_2 and 8–10% CO_2. Incubation of primary plates should be at 42°C to inhibit other fecal bacteria. The reservoir of infection includes poultry, pigs, rabbits, goats, cattle, and dogs. The infection is acquired orally from food, drink, contact with infected animals, or anal–genital–oral sexual activity. *C. jejuni* causes an estimated 2 million cases of diarrhea or dysentery in the United States per year, including 5–11% of all cases of diarrhea or dysentery in hospitals. The organism produces enterotoxin, but its clinical significance is not well understood. *C. jejuni* invades the epithelium of the jejunum and ileum, causing hyperemia, edema, acute and chronic inflammatory infiltration, and ulceration. Involvement of the colon produces crypt abscesses and ulcerations. Thus, stools may contain exudate and blood. The incidence is higher in children than adults. After an incubation period of 3–5 days, abdominal pain, nausea, headache, and fever occur, along with diarrhea. The disease is usually self-limited, with a 5- to 8-day course, and septicemia and nonenteric infection are uncommon. *C. fetus* (subspecies *fetus* and *intestinalis*) is an opportunistic cause of systemic infection in debilitated patients. *(Cotran et al., pp. 355, 356)*

431. **(C)** *Y. enterocolitica* is a facultatively anaerobic, gram-negative rod that causes enterocolitis and mesenteric lymphadenitis. Although endotoxins are present, these have not been shown to have any pathogenic effect on the gut. An enterotoxin is produced in cultures below 30°C but not at 37°C and thus does not seem to be produced in vivo. The pathogenicity seems to be caused by bacterial invasion of the epithelium of the ileum and colon, causing ulceration and inflammation. Refrigeration of culture specimens for 3 weeks at 4°C in phosphate-buffered isotonic saline (with periodic subculture) to enriched media at 22°–25°C and 37°C increases the yield, because *Y. enterocolitica*

will multiply at this low temperature, and most other fecal organisms are inhibited or killed. The distribution of this pathogen is virtually worldwide, and its reservoirs are extensive, including domestic and wild animals, both sick and healthy, including swine, sheep, cattle, dogs, cats, caged birds, pigeons, deer, rodents, mink, chinchilla, and fish. Transmission to humans is through contaminated food, water, and milk. Person-to-person transmission probably is rare. *(Cotran et al., pp. 356, 357)*

432. **(D)** *B. anthracis,* a large, virulent, aerobic, encapsulated, gram-positive rod, produces endospores that resist boiling and disinfectants and persist in soil for years. Infection causes anthrax, primarily a disease of animals, particularly cattle, sheep, horses, goats, and swine. These ingest the spores in soil contaminating the rough vegetation they eat (Gastrointestinal anthrax is uncommon in humans.) Most human infections result from cutaneous entry of spores from contaminated soil or animal products (hides, carcasses, wool, bone). Within hours to days of entry of spores through a skin scratch, a pruritic red macule appears that soon develops into an edematous papule and then a hemorrhagic vesicle. The vesicle has been called a "malignant pustule," but contains only a few neutrophils, not pus. The vesicle ulcerates, and a small to large black eschar forms. This lesion may heal and no clinical disease results. Alternatively, the ulcer(s) may be followed by severe edema, called "malignant edema," hemorrhagic lymphadenitis, and septicemia. Inhalation of spores, which germinate in the lungs or tracheobronchial lymph nodes, causes hemorrhagic lymphadenitis, mediastinal and pulmonary edema, septicemia, and hemorrhagic bronchopneumonia (wool-sorter's disease). *(Cotran et al., pp. 344, 345)*

433. **(B)** After larvae of the nematode *O. volvulus* are injected into the skin by an infected *Simulium* blackfly, they migrate to the subcutaneous tissue and mature into filiform adult males and females that may live for years, producing huge numbers of tiny microfilariae. The inflammatory reaction to the adult filariae is successively acute, chronic, and fibrous, form-

ing nodules that eventually may calcify. The serious clinical effects are caused by the microfilariae, which cause dermatitis and eye lesions, including punctate keratitis, pannus formation, corneal fibrosis, iridocyclitis, glaucoma, choroiditis, and optic atrophy. Impaired visual acuity and even river blindness may ensue. Diagnosis is made by finding microfilariae in teased snips or in the anterior chamber of the eye (by slit lamp examination) or by finding adult worms in biopsied nodules. About 30 million people in Africa and about 1 million in Central and South America are infected. *(Cotran et al., pp. 398, 399)*

434. **(D)** *Hymenolepis nana* is a tapeworm with humans as both definitive and intermediate hosts. This "dwarf" tapeworm gains entrance to the human intestinal tract when individuals ingest raw foods soiled with infective cysts. Once in the intestine, the worm attaches to the mucosa via a scolex mouthpart. The diagnosis may be confirmed by demonstrating the characteristic proglottids in the feces. *(Rubin and Farber, p. 707)*

435. **(A)** *A. lumbricoides* is the largest roundworm of humans and infects an estimated 1 billion people worldwide. Fertilized *Ascaris* eggs are passed in the stool and mature to the infective stage in 2–3 weeks. When soil contaminated by mature eggs gets on the hands or on raw vegetables and is ingested, larvae hatch in the small intestine, penetrate the mucosa, and migrate in venous blood through the right heart to the lungs. They enter the alveoli, ascend the pulmonary tree, are swallowed, and mature into adult male and female worms in the lumen of the small bowel. In 2–3 months, they begin to produce eggs. Because each female produces up to 200,000 ova per day, ascariasis can be diagnosed by microscopic examination of unconcentrated stool. Because the worm has a short life span of 10–24 months and does not multiply in humans, infection is maintained only by ingestion of fertilized eggs. The eggs are resistant to adverse environments and can survive for years in moist soil. Infection and complications are more common in children. Most

infestations are asymptomatic and are occasionally recognized because of passage of a worm from the anus, mouth, or nose. Loeffler's syndrome may occur during the pulmonary phase. The most serious complications are obstruction of the intestine, pylorus, common bile duct, or pancreatic duct, volvulus, intussusception, and appendicitis. The worms occur in greatest concentration in the jejunum, but obstruction is most common in the terminal ileum. *(Cotran et al., pp. 336, 337)*

436. **(B)** Influenza A virus causes an acute illness characterized by an 18- to 72-hour incubation period, fever, malaise, myalgia, and sometimes nonexudative pharyngitis and (less often) tracheobronchitis. Pneumonia is uncommon, but the disease predisposes to superimposed bacterial pneumonia. Epidemic and pandemic outbreaks occur often in the winter. The pathogen is an orthomyxovirus with a lipid-rich envelope that has surface proteins (influenzal hemagglutinin, HA), enabling the virus to adsorb to receptors on susceptible respiratory mucosal cells. Mucoproteins (which compete for the receptors) and anti-HA antibodies interfere with viral attachment and infection. Once adsorbed, the virions are transferred into endosomes (cytoplasmic vacuoles), and the envelope fuses with endosome membranes to release the nucleocapsid into the cytosol. The segmented, single-stranded RNA genome dissociates from the capsid proteins and viral replication, assemble, and release by budding allow the infection to spread. The host cell nucleus plays no part in influenza virus replication. Influenza A virus undergoes major phenotypic changes (antigenic shift) associated with pandemic spread of influenza at 10- to 14-year intervals. Interpandemic minor changes (antigenic drift) also occur. There are three major (antigenically distinct) types of influenza virus: A, B, and C. Types B and C usually cause less severe cases of influenza and less serious outbreaks than does type A. *(Cotran et al., p. 348)*

437. **(C)** Polyoma virus (*poly*, many; *oma*, tumor) causes murine adenomas, adenocarcinomas, hemangiomas, fibromas, and fibrosarcomas.

In contrast to influenza virus, the polyoma virus is naked (does not have an envelope) and is uncoated (capsid removed) in the host cell nucleus before replication. Polyoma viruses are members of the Papovaviridae family and, thus, have a circular, double-stranded DNA genoma. Members of the Papovaviridae that infect humans are human papillomaviruses, BK virus, which has been isolated from the urine of immunosuppressed renal transplant recipients but does not cause tumors. AS virus, newly described, and JC virus, which causes progressive multifocal leukoencephalopathy (PML), probably by reactivation of a persistent infection. Another polyoma virus, SV40 (simian vacuoloating virus) is probably a rare cause of PML. (*Rubin and Farber, p. 173*)

438. **(D)** HIV, formerly called human T lymphotropic virus III, is a single-stranded RNA retrovirus that has a lipid envelope studded with surface glycoproteins (gp), each of which has two subunits, gp41 (transmembrane gp) and gp120 (surface gp). Human helper T lymphocytes (T4+ cells) and monocytes (macrophages) have a surface antigen called T4 (CD4), which is the receptor for HIV gp120. After HIV gp120 binds specifically to the CD4 receptors, the virion enters the cell. (It has not yet been established whether entry is by direct fusion of the HIV envelope to the cell membrane, by receptor-fusion of the HIV envelope to the cell membrane, or by receptor-mediated endocytosis). Helper T lymphocytes are destroyed by infection with HIV, leading to the severe acquired immunodeficiency syndrome (AIDS). Infected monocytes and macrophages are considerably more refractory to the cytopathic effect of HIV; thus they may serve as a reservoir for persistent HIV infection in the host and also may be the Trojan horse that spreads the infection to the central nervous system, causing encephalopathy. In addition to the CD4 lymphocytes and monocytes, HIV has been found in Langerhans' cells, endothelial cells, astrocytes, oligodendrocytes, microglial cells, and (rarely) neurons. (*Cotran et al., pp. 236–251*)

439. **(A)** The family Paramyxoviridae consists of three genera: *Paramyxovirus* (parainfluenza virus types 1, 2, 3, 4a, 4b, mumps virus, and Newcastle disease virus, and other avian paramycoviruses), *Morbillivirus* (measles, canine distemper, and bovine rinderpest virus), and *Pneumovirus* (respiratory syncytial viruses of humans and cattle and pneumonia virus of mice). Although most other enveloped viruses enter the host cell by receptor-mediated endocytosis, the Paramyxoviridae undergo fusion of the viral envelope with the cell plasma membrane and enter the cytoplasm directly. Adsorption of the virus to the cell surface receptors and envelope–plasma membrane fusion are mediated by viral envelope surface glycoproteins (gp); e.g., parainfluenza and mumps viruses have projecting glycoproteins (HN) responsible for adsorption of these viruses, and glycoproteins (Fo) responsible for fusion. Proteolytic cleavage of Fo into two subunits by a host cell enzyme is necessary for fusion and viral penetration. Thus, only cells with the proteolytic enzyme are penetrated and infected. When the *Paramyxovirus* envelope fuses with the host cell, viral surface proteins become part of the host cell surface, and the cell becomes recognizable as infected and is subject to immune lysis. The Fo gp also is involved in fusion of host cells, spreading by budding of maturing virions from the cell surface. (The lipids of the viral envelope are acquired from the host cell membrane during budding.) The viral HN gp has neuraminidase activity and facilitates release of budding virus. (*Cotran et al., pp. 1225, 1226*)

440–445. **(440-B, 441-D, 442-C, 443-C, 444-D, 445-D)** A large number of mononuclear leukocytes are seen with typhoid fever. Neutrophils predominate in the diarrhea of shigellosis, although (less commonly) some strains of shigella can produce an enterotoxin, resulting in a watery diarrhea without many fecal leukocytes. Salmonellosis and ulcerative colitis cause the appearance of many neutrophils. Ulcerative colitis also may show eosinophils (88% neutrophils, 8% eosinophils). Because little or no inflammatory response is induced by metabolic enterotoxin, inflammatory cells generally are absent in the diarrhea of cholera and infection with enterotoxigenic *E. coli* (Table 5–4). *(Cotran et al., pp. 356, 357; 343, 344)*

446. **(D)** Most patients with AIDS still fall into the categories first observed in 1981. Homosexual and bisexual men constitute the largest group of AIDS patients (73%). *(Cotran et al., pp. 236, 237)*

447. **(B)** A small percentage (1%) of AIDS patients are those with hemophilia who have received multiple units of antihemophilic factor concentrates. *(Cotran et al., pp. 236, 237)*

448. **(A)** Heterosexual men and women who are intravenous drug abusers are the second largest group of people with AIDS (17%) and are becoming an even greater source of new infections. *(Cotran et al., pp. 236, 237)*

449. **(C)** Haitians living in the United States are a small (4%) and decreasing percentage of AIDS patients. Half of these deny homosexual activity and intravenous drug abuse. Thus, a substantial proportion of these could be reclassified as members of the two predominant groups. *(Cotran et al., pp. 236, 237)*

450. **(D)** The anaerobic bacillus, *Clostridium tetani*, is commonly found in the intestinal flora of wild and domesticated animals. The spores produced by these bacteria are deposited out into the environment, especially into the soil, with defecation. Spores enter humans through a traumatic injury. If the wound site becomes anaerobic, the spores germinate and produce a very potent neurologic poison termed "tetanus toxin." This toxin causes uninhibited neural stimulation with resultant tetany, lock-jaw, and rigidity of the facial muscles (risus sardonicus). Prolonged spasms of the laryngeal or respiratory muscles can be fatal. Treatment consists of penicillin, tetanus toxoid, immune serum globulin, and the re-establishment of aerobic conditions in the wound. *(Cotran et al., pp. 368, 369)*

451. **(A)** Scarlet fever is an exanthematous disorder associated with acute pharyngitis or tonsillitis caused by erythrogenic strains of *Streptococcus pyogenes*. While infecting the pharynx or tonsil, the organism produces an erythrogenic toxin. This toxin evokes the systemic rash-like reaction clinically termed "scarlet fever." The erythematous rash is most abundant over the trunk, inner aspect of the arms and legs, and on the face, sparing the mouth. After about a week, the rash subsides, and the skin begins to scale and desquamate. Prompt antibiotic therapy is necessary during the initial pharyngitis stage to avoid later poststreptococcal sequela, such as glomerulonephritis. *(Cotran et al., p. 334)*

452. **(E)** Pseudomembranous colitis is characterized grossly by raised yellowish plaques, measuring between 0.3 and 2.0 cm, cobblestoning the rectosigmoid mucosa. Microscopically, the superficial epithelium is eroded and focally covered by a pseudomembrane comprised of fibrin, necrotic debris, and neutrophils. Most individuals with pseudomembranous colitis have been recently treated with antibiotics. This prior antibiotic therapy may alter the normal bowel flora, allowing the emergence of *Clostridium difficile*. The organism produces a toxin that damages the colonic mucosa with resultant pseudomembrane formation and usually, diarrhea. The toxin may be detected in the stool of affected individuals, serving as a practical way to confirm the diagnosis. Pseudomembranous colitis is treated with vancomycin, fluids, and electrolyte replacement therapy. *(Cotran et al., pp. 368, 369)*

453. **(B)** *Clostridium perfringens* is the bacterial organism that most commonly causes gas gangrene. This ubiquitous organism produces a potent myotoxin when grown in anaerobic conditions, such as those present in certain contaminated wounds. The myotoxin is a lecithinase that lyses cell membranes causing severe myolysis and hemolysis. Prompt debridement of the wound accompanied by hyperbaric oxygen and antibiotic therapy are critical elements of treatment. Clinically, the myolysis is fulminating with accompanying crepitus, dusky necrosis, and a foul odor. The combination of gas bubbles (crepitus) and necrosis give rise to the common clinical

appellation of "gas gangrene." *(Cotran et al., pp. 368, 369)*

454. (C) Botulism is usually caused by ingestion of food contaminated by preformed neurotoxins synthesized by *Clostridium botulinum.* Improper home canning, inadequate refrigeration, inadequate smoking, or insufficient curing of foods provides an environment favorable for the bacteria to proliferate, producing a potent neurotoxin. The subsequent ingestion of these foods without sufficient heating results in a symmetric descending paralysis of cranial nerves, limbs, and trunk. Paralysis of respiratory muscles is fatal. Prompt treatment with antitoxin may prove lifesaving. Botulism can be prevented by fully cooking foods, because moderate heating destroys the preformed neurotoxin. *(Cotran et al., pp. 368, 369)*

455. (E) Epidemic typhus fever is caused by the obligate intracellular organism, *Rickettsia prowazekii.* The organism is transmitted from human to human by body lice (*Pediculus humanus*). After a 1- to 2-week incubation period headache, fever, chills, weakness, and malaise appear. A maculopapular rash soon follows the initial symptoms. Most fatalities in untreated individuals occur in the second or third week after the first symptoms have appeared due to infection of the central nervous system. Microscopically, the organisms can be demonstrated in the endothelial cells of the characteristic typhus nodules. *(Cotran et al., pp. 384, 385)*

456. (B) Rocky Mountain spotted fever is caused by *Rickettsia rickettsii.* The reservoir for this organism is hard-bodied ticks. Ticks transmit the disease to humans when organisms in the ticks' salivary glands are inoculated into bitten individuals. About 1 week after the tick bite, symptoms appear that are characterized by malaise, fever, headache, and myalgia. A rash may then develop as pink macules and later as petechiae. Central nervous system involvement in the second or third week may prove fatal. The organisms may be demonstrated microscopically in infected endothelial cells.

Prompt antibiotic therapy is the treatment of choice. *(Cotran et al., pp. 384, 385)*

457. (D) The chronic suppurative eye disease caused by *C. trachomatis* is one of the leading causes of blindness in the world. The disease is particularly severe in dry sandy regions of the world, where flies and other fomites continually reinfect the conjunctiva. The organism initially evokes a suppurative reaction that later, with further reinfection and lack of antibiotic therapy, will progress to follicular hypertrophy, conjunctival ulceration, scarring, and finally, blindness. Antibiotics, such as the sulfonamides, readily cure the initial infection. The absence of adequate medical care in many of the world's poorer regions accounts for most of the cases that progress to blindness. *(Cotran et al., pp. 1361, 1362)*

458. (A) Human Q fever is caused by the rickettsial organism *Coxiella burnetii.* This Zoonic disease is spread among cattle, sheep, and wild animals by ticks. Humans usually acquire the disease through inhalation of airborne organisms. Slaughterhouse workers, shepherds, cattlemen, and farmhands are most often infected. After a 3-week incubation period, symptoms suddenly develop, characterized by fever, malaise, myalgias, cough, bradycardia, and hepatosplenomegaly. Most people recover without sequela in about 2 weeks after the beginning of symptoms. Antibiotics speed the recovery. *(Cotran et al., p. 384)*

459. (C) Ornithosis, also termed "psittacosis," is caused by *Chlamydia psittaci.* The organism is transmitted to humans during the inhalation of aerosolized bird excreta. The incubation period varies from 1 to 3 weeks and is followed by the sudden onset of fever, chills, malaise, headache, sore throat, and cough. The most characteristic microscopic finding is interstitial pneumonitis. The mortality rate in individuals not promptly treated with antibiotics ranges from 5–40%. *(Cotran et al., pp. 361, 362)*

460. (A) Chagas' disease is caused by hemoflagellate, *Trypanosoma cruzi.* Cardiac involvement is characteristic with this disease, including acute myocarditis, bundle branch block, interstitial fibrosis, and progressive dilatory cardiac failure. Humans acquire the disease from the bite of "kissing bugs" that inhabit cracks in dilapidated buildings and bite sleeping victims at night. The disease is common from Texas to Argentina. Because of this distribution it is sometimes referred to as "American trypanosomiasis." *(Cotran et al., pp. 393, 394)*

461. **(E)** Malaria is a protozoal disease caused by organisms of the *Plasmodium* species. Humans are infected with sporozoites during mosquito bites. The sporozoites travel through the bloodstream to multiply in liver cells. Merozoites are released by the liver and penetrate erythrocytes. Further growth of the parasite in erythrocytes produces both gametocytes and hemolysis. The gametocytes re-enter mosquitoes during a blood meal to complete the infective cycle. *(Cotran et al., pp. 389–391)*

462. **(C)** Lyme disease is a spirochetal disease caused by *Borrelia burgdorferi*. Tick bites transfer the infective agent to humans. Three to four weeks after inoculation, a papule develops at the bite site, shortly followed by a ring-like rash that expands outward and lasts from a month to a year. During this expansion phase, individuals may complain of arthritis, myocarditis, or neurologic symptoms. Antibiotics hasten recovery. *(Cotran et al., pp. 388, 389)*

463. **(B)** Amebiasis is a protozoan disease caused by *Entamoeba histolytica*. Infective cysts are found in contaminated water and pass through the stomach to invade the mucosal tissues of the large bowel, especially the cecum. Symptoms may include abdominal pain, nausea, vomiting, and diarrhea. Infrequent, but life-threatening complications, may include bowel perforation or liver abscess formation. The disease is diagnosed by identifying the characteristic cysts and trophozoites in feces. Treatment is via a number of antiprotozoal agents. *(Cotran et al., pp. 358, 359)*

464. **(D)** Visceral leishmaniasis (kala-azar) is caused by the protozoan organism, *Leishmania donovani*. Blood-sucking flies transfer the infective pro-

mastigotes to humans while biting. The promastigotes invade reticuloendothelial cells, transform into amastigotes, multiply, and are ingested by feeding flies. In the flies, the amastigotes transform back into promastigotes, completing the cycle. The involvement of the reticuloendothelial system explains in large part the pathologic features of kalaazar; namely, lymphadenopathy, hepatomegaly, hyperplastic bone marrow, and splenomegaly. Treatments include preventative measures, parenteral pentavalent antimonials, and meglumine antimoniate. *(Cotran et al., pp. 391–393)*

465. **(A)** Filariasis, a chronic obstructing fibrosis of the lymph vessels, is caused by the organism, *Wuchereria bancrofti*. The infective form of the organism is transmitted to humans during mosquito bites. Once in the human bloodstream, microfilariae come to rest in lymphatics and mature into adult worms. Immunologic reaction to these adult worms is responsible for the gradual obstructive fibrosis of the lymphatics. Extremities or organs drained by these obstructed lymphatics may later develop pronounced swelling and gigantism, also called "elephantiasis." *(Chandrasoma and Taylor, p. 883)*

466. **(E)** Visceral larva migrans is a disease caused by accidental human infection by animal nematodes parasites, such as the dog roundworm *Toxocara canis*. The disease typically affects children living with dogs or cats in crowded conditions. Clinical findings include eosinophilia, pneumonitis, and hypergammaglobulinemia. Ocular involvement can lead to retinal detachment. The disease is usually self-limited, and treatment includes diethylcarbamazine or thiabendazole. *(Chandrasoma and Taylor, p. 498)*

467. **(D)** Hookworm infestation can be caused by either the Old World hookworm *Ancylostoma duodenale*, or by the New World hookworm *Necator americanus*. Both worms live in tropical soils for months as either infective filariform larvae or as free-living rhabdoid larvae and adults. After penetrating the human skin, they circulate into the lungs, migrate to the

epiglottis, are swallowed into the stomach, and come to rest in the small intestine where they propagate while feeding on the mucosal villi. Clinically, there is dermatitis, pneumonitis, and iron deficiency anemia. The diagnosis can be confirmed by observing the characteristic eggs shed out into the feces. Treatment is usually with mebendazole. *(Rubin and Farber, pp. 468–470)*

468. **(C)** The pork tapeworm is *Taenia solium*. Humans acquire the tapeworm infection through the ingestion of raw or undercooked pork. The encysted larvae excyst in the human intestinal tract, mature into adults, and attach to the intestinal wall via scolex mouthparts. The adults discharge eggs into human feces, which may later infect pigs to complete the parasite's life cycle. *(Cotran et al., pp. 395, 396)*

469. **(B)** Pinworm infections are caused by the nematode, *Enterobius vermicularis*. Adult worms live in the lower gastrointestinal tract of infected humans. At night the female worms migrate out to the anal skin to lay eggs, resulting in the classical "night itch" associated with the disease. The eggs are readily infective for other household members who accidentally ingest them. Numerous effective antihelminths are available to treat infections. Reinfection by dormant eggs in clothing and fomites, however, may necessitate multiple courses of therapy. Rarely the worms infect the fallopian tube or appendix producing salpingitis or appendicitis, respectively. *(Cotran et al., p. 332)*

470. **(E)** Rhinoviruses are the most common cause of the "common cold." Spread from person to person by aerosol droplets, over 100 different species exist to confound the human immune system. After a brief incubation period of several days, symptoms of nasal stuffiness, runny nose, itchy eyes, sore throat, and mild fever occur. Treatment is symptomatic. The average duration of illness is about a week. *(Cotran et al., pp. 347, 348)*

471. **(A)** Infectious mononucleosis (IM) is caused by the Epstein–Barr virus. In developed nations, most symptomatic Epstein–Barr infections occur during adolescence. The clinical features of IM include the triad of fever, sore throat, and lymphadenopathy. In the peripheral blood, there is an increased number of circulating atypical lymphocytes. About 2 weeks into the symptomatic phase of the disease, most individuals have developed "heterophile" antibodies that may be detected by laboratory tests to confirm the diagnosis. Over 90% of infected individuals recover without significant sequela. Rarely, splenic rupture, encephalitis, thrombocytopenia, hemolytic anemia, or meningitis complicate the disease. *(Cotran et al., pp. 371–373)*

472. **(D)** Infection with coxsackievirus type A can produce herpangina, a blistering inflammation of the posterior pharynx, tonsils, and soft palate. The lesions begin as macules, progress to tan papules, and then into vesicles that ulcerate. Myalgia, fever, and malaise may accompany the ulcers. The disease is usually self-limited, resolving without significant sequela in about 2 weeks. *(Cotran et al., p. 333)*

473. **(B)** Cervical squamous cell dysplasia is strongly linked to previous infection of the cervix by human papillomavirus. Papillomavirus infection at this site usually produces flat condyloma. A small portion of these condylomas fail to resolve and over time display increasing severe degrees of dysplasia. The viral serotypes of 16 and 18 are most likely to initiate these progressive dysplastic changes. *(Cotran et al., pp. 1208, 1209)*

474. **(C)** Rubella virus, the causative agent of German measles, is a togavirus responsible for the "3-day measles." This mild childhood illness is characterized by rash, fever, malaise, and lymphadenopathy. Adult infections of pregnant females may result in fetal malformations. Hence, the public health officials need to test gravid females for immunity to the rubella virus. *(Cotran et al., p. 467)*

475–479. **(475-D, 476-C, 477-B, 478-E, 479-A)** Many infectious diseases depend on arthropod vectors to carry the transmissible agent to humans.

For example, biting fleas and ixodid ticks spread *Yersinia pestis* (plague) and *Borrelia burgdorferi* (Lyme disease), respectively. The anopheles mosquito is the vector of malaria. Sleeping sickness is transmitted by the tsetse fly. Smallpox, which has been eradicated, had never been spread by insect vectors, only by human-to-human transmission. *(Rubin and Farber, pp. 459, 460; 413, 414; 402, 403; 364; 445–449)*

480. **(D)** *Candida albicans* is a fungal organism. It is an opportunistic infectious agent capable of producing disease in individuals with reduced immunity. Infections are commonly seen in the very young, very old, diabetics, after broad-spectrum antibiotics, with cancer, with severe burns, with indwelling catheters or prosthetic cardiac valves, and with AIDS. Oral infections, as depicted in the scenario, are termed "thrush" and are frequently seen with insulin-dependent diabetics. *(Chandrasoma and Taylor, p. 476)*

481. **(G)** *Toxoplasma gondii* is a protozoan organism. Humans are infected by eating undercooked meat contaminated by cat feces containing transmissible cysts. Congenital toxoplasmosis results in severe consequences including brain damage, mental retardation, seizures, deafness, hydrocephalus, encephalitis, and myocarditis. Toxoplasmosis is also commonly seen with AIDS patients. *(Chandrasoma and Taylor, pp. 438, 439)*

482. **(E)** The scenario depicts an individual with HIV infection, an obligate intracellular virus. The infective agent is a retrovirus with a central core of RNA, an outer antigenic protein coat, and inner reverse transcriptase enzymes capable of manufacturing DNA templates of the viral RNA for replication. The virus preferentially attaches to CD4 membrane sites of lymphocytes. Parenteral, congenital, and sexual routes account for most infections. *(Cotran et al., pp. 239–245)*

483. **(E)** Syphilis is a venereal disease caused by the spirochetal organism *Treponema pallidum*. In primary syphilis, as depicted in the sce-

nario, a chancre usually develops on the glans penis of infected males about a week after exposure. Darkfield microscopic examination of fluid expressed from a chancre will demonstrate diagnostic corkscrew-shaped spirochetes. If the organism is not treated with antibiotics at this stage, the infected individual may go on to develop secondary or tertiary syphilis over time. *(Cotran et al., pp. 239–245)*

484. **(F)** Leprosy, also termed "Hansen's disease," is a slowly progressive mycobacterial infection that affects the cooler portions of the body, especially the skin and peripheral nerves. Clinically, the disease is generally divided into tuberculoid and lepromatous varieties. In the tuberculoid variety, granulomatous inflammation is seen microscopically in facial macular lesions. In the lepromatous variant, a foam cell architecture is seen microscopically in the nodular facial lesions. Both types of leprosy contain diagnostic acid-fast mycobacterial organisms. *(Cotran et al., pp. 385, 386)*

485. **(C)** The scenario portrays infection with herpes simplex II virus. Most herpetic infections of skin or mucous membranes produce vesicles and ulceration. Examination of the vesicle fluid (Tzanck preparations) will usually demonstrate viral-induced cytopathic changes characterized by multinucleate giant cells containing central large acidophilic intranuclear inclusions. These inclusion bodies contain live and dead virion particles. After the initial vesicular outbreak, the virus retreats to neuroganglia, where it slowly reproduces. Repeated attacks of recurrent vesicles in the anatomic distribution of the infected nerve characterize the disease over time. *(Cotran et al., pp. 351–361)*

486. **(B)** The scenario portrays a human infection by the microfilarial organism *Wuchereria bancrofti*. This tropical disease is transmitted from human to human by mosquito bites. Lymphatic filariasis is caused by an inflammatory and fibrous reaction to filarial worms in the lymphatic channels. The gradual development of lymphatic obstruction may produce swelling (elephantiasis) of the scrotum, leg, or arm. *(Cotran et al., pp. 397, 398)*

487. **(C)** AIDS is caused by a nontransforming human retrovirus. Two types of this virus have been found, the HIV-1 and the HIV-2. The HIV-1 is the most common type associated with AIDS in the United States, Europe, and Central Africa. The virus infects the helper/inducer T lymphocytes, markedly impairing the function of the T cells and producing immunosuppression, affecting the cell mediated immunity. *(Cotran et al., pp. 236–251)*

488. **(D)** In addition to the loss of T cells, the monocytes and macrophages are also infected by the AIDS virus. These macrophages are found not in the peripheral blood but rather in tissues. Most likely the macrophages are the reservoir for the human immunodeficiency virus. *(Cotran et al., pp. 236–251)*

489. **(E)** There is experimental evidence that CD4 molecule on the cytoplasmic surface of the lymphocytes is, in fact, a high-affinity receptor for HIV. This explains the selective tropism of the virus for CD4+ T cell and other cells, particularly monocytes/macrophages. The binding of the CD4 is insufficient for infection. The virus must also bind to other surface molecules for entering into the cell. *(Cotran et al., pp. 236–251)*

490. **(A)** In the first stages of this disease, many patients present with peripheral lymphadenopathy. A biopsy of these enlarged lymph nodes show a marked follicular hyperplasia. These follicles contain a pleomorphic amount of cells they are enlarged, irregular, and mitotically active. An attenuation of the mantle zones is seen. These enlarged germinal centers, which are composed of B cells, are showing a hyperplasia of polyclonal type that is activated in patients infected with HIV particles. *(Cotran et al., p. 250)*

491. **(B)** It is believed that the HIV virus is carried into the brain by infected monocytes. The mechanism in which HIV damaged the neurons is not clear. The HIV virus, however, does not affect the neurons. Most researchers believe that the neurological deficit is caused indirectly by viral products and soluble factors produced by macrophages/microglia. *(Cotran et al., p. 242)*

492. **(E)** The epidemiologic studies in the United States have identified groups of adults who are at risk for infection with HIV. Those are homosexual or bisexual men, intravenous drug abusers, homophiliacs, recipients of blood and blood components, heterosexual contact, and in children the transplacental passage from mother to fetus. *(Cotran et al., pp. 236, 237)*

493. **(A)** This is a follow-up to Question 488. *(Cotran et al., pp. 236–251)*

494. **(D)** The most likely cause of respiratory failure in AIDS is infection secondary to pneumonia caused by opportunistic infections. Among these, the most prevalent is pneumocystis carinii pneumonia in which between 20–50% of the AIDS patients present with this infection or develop the infection sometime during their course of their illness. Among other pathogens that can infect the lung, *Candida,* cytomegalovirus, and atypical and typical mycobacteria. *(Cotran et al., pp. 247–249)*

495. **(B)** Many drugs have been used in the fight against AIDS. AZT, which is widely used, acts as an inhibiting the viral reversal transcriptase. A great effort has been made to develop a vaccine, however, up to the present time, none has proved effective. *(Cotran et al., pp. 250, 251)*

496. **(E)** This is a follow-up to Question 487. *(Cotran et al., pp. 236–251)*

REFERENCES

Chandrasoma P, Taylor CR. *Concise Pathology,* 3rd ed. Norwalk, CT: Appleton & Lange, 1998.

Cotran RS, Kumar V, Robbins SL. *Robbins Pathologic Basis of Disease,* 6th ed. Philadelphia: Saunders, 1999.

Rubin E, Farber JL. *Pathology.* Philadelphia: Lippincott, 1999.

CHAPTER 6

Genetic, Metabolic, and Environmental Pathology

Forty-six pieces of DNA and protein, called chromosomes, hold the genetic blueprint from which humans are constructed and maintained. The chromosomes are divided into 22 pairs of autosomes and a pair of sex chromosomes. In males, the sex pair is designated XY. In females, the sex chromosomes are XX. The Lyon hypothesis explains the involution of one X chromosome, which leads to formation of the clinically useful Barr body to determine genetic identity in cases of ambiguous secondary sexual differentiation. Hermaphrodites are those rare individuals who possess both ovarian and testicular tissue, regardless of their karyotype or external sexual genitalia. Pseudohermaphrodites possess only one type of gonadal tissue and usually have the opposite karyotype or secondary sexual characteristics. Common gross abnormalities of chromosome numbers or composition are shown in Table 6–1.

More subtle abnormalities of chromosomes may affect only one base pair or a short strand of pairs. The damage may affect the individual or remain dormant and be expressed in a later generation. Certain of these genetic disorders have well-understood patterns of inheritance and characteristic clinical symptoms (Table 6–2).

The full maturation of an individual is dependent on appropriate environment and nutrition. Lack of certain nutrients, vitamins, or minerals can be characterized into clinical diseases (Table 6–3). Common chemical substances, termed toxins or poison, can be profoundly harmful (Table 6–4), and environmental conditions, such as heat and radiation, can harm or kill people.

Table 6–1. COMMON CHROMOSOMAL ABNORMALITIES

Name	Chromosome Pattern	Clinical Characteristics
Turner's syndrome	45,XO	Webbed neck, short stature, primary amenorrhea, infertility, streak gonads
Klinefelter's syndrome	47,XXY	Eunuchoid habitus with long legs, testicular atrophy, mental retardation, gynecomastia
Down's syndrome	Trisomy 21	Mental retardation, dysplastic ears, epicanthic folds, congenital heart disease
Edward's syndrome	Trisomy 18	Mental retardation, micrognathia, low-set ears, congenital heart disease
Patau's syndrome	Trisomy 13	Mental retardation, microencephaly, microphthalmia, cleft palate, rocker-bottom feet
Cat's cry syndrome	Partial deletion of chromosome 5	Mental retardation, mewing cry, epicanthic folds, microcephaly

Table 6–2. INHERITANCE OF GENETIC DISORDERS

Disorder	Inheritance	Molecular Defect	Clinical Features
Galactosemia	Autosomal recessive	Galactose-1 phosphate uridyl transferase	Jaundice, mental retardation, hepatosplenomegaly, cataracts
Alpha, -antitrypsin deficiency	Autosomal recessive	Alpha, -antitrypsin	Emphysema, cirrhosis
Phenylketonuria	Autosomal recessive	Phenylalanine hydroxylase	Mental retardation
Wilson's disease	Autosomal recessive	Copper excretion	Brain degeneration, cirrhosis
Albinism	Autosomal recessive	Melanin production	Visual impairment, skin cancers
Ochronosis	Autosomal recessive	Homogentisic oxidase	Pigmented cartilage, arthritis
Tay–Sachs disease	Autosomal recessive	Hexosaminidase A	Mental retardation, blindness, cherry red macula
Niemann–Pick disease	Autosomal recessive	Sphingomyelinase	Hepatosplenomegaly, xanthomas, mental retardation, lymphadenopathy
Gauchers' disease	Autosomal recessive	Glucocerebrosidase	Hepatosplenomegaly, bone marrow involvement, mental retardation
Hurler's syndrome (MPS I)	Autosomal recessive	Alpha-L-iduronidase	Hepatosplenomegaly, corneal clouding, dwarfism
Glycogen storage disease (8 types)	Autosomal recessive	Glycogen metabolism	Hepatosplenomegaly, cardiomegaly, skeletal muscle involvement
Glucose-6-phosphate dehydrogenase deficiency	X-linked recessive	Glucose-6-phosphate dehydrogenase	Erythrocyte hemolysis
Fabry's syndrome	X-linked recessive	Trihexosylceramide alpha-galactosidase	Skin, kidney, and neural lesions
Hemophilia	X-linked recessive	Clotting factor VIII or IX	Bleeding
Bruton's agammaglobulinemia	X-linked recessive	Immunoglobulin	Pyogenic infections, autoimmune disorders
Hunter's syndrome	X-linked recessive	L-Iduronosulfate sulfatase	Hepatosplenomegaly, dwarfism, cardiac lesions
Wiskott–Aldrich syndrome	X-linked recessive	Cellular immunity	Loss of cellular immunity, thrombocytopenia, eczema
Duchenne muscular dystrophy	X-linked recessive	Unknown	Muscular weakness, atrophy, and hypertrophy
Achondroplasia	Autosomal dominant	Cartilage cell growth	Short arms and legs
Sickle cell anemia	Autosomal dominant	Hemoglobin	Anemia, autosplenectomy, cirrhosis, gallstones
Huntington's chorea	Autosomal dominant	Unknown	Cortical and thalamic atrophy, dementia
Polycystic kidney disease	Autosomal dominant	Unknown	Renal and other visceral cysts, renal failure
Thalassemia	Autosomal dominant	Rate of hemoglobin synthesis	Anemia

Table 6–3. CLINICAL DEFICIENCY STATES

Substance	Solubility	Deficiency State	Clinical Symptoms
Vitamin A	Lipid	Avitaminosis A	Blindness, xerophthalmia, hyperkeratosis
Vitamin B$_1$ (thiamine)	Water	Beriberi	Heart failure, Wernicke's psychosis
Vitamin B$_2$ (riboflavin)	Water	Ariboflavinosis	Cheilosis, glossitis, keratitis, dermatitis
Niacin	Water	Pellagra	Diarrhea, dementia, dermatitis
Vitamin C	Water	Scurvy	Hyperkeratosis, bleeding
Vitamin D	Lipid	Osteomalacia, rickets	Abnormal bone formation
Vitamin K	Lipid	Hypoprothrombinemia	Bleeding
Iron	—	Iron deficiency	Microcytic hypochromic anemia
Total calories and protein	—	Marasmus, kwashiorkor	Edema, depigmentation, fatty liver

Table 6–4. HARMFUL CHEMICAL SUBSTANCES

Noxious Substance	Site of Action	Clinical Effects
Carbon monoxide	Hemoglobin	Acute: cherry-red blood, coma, death Chronic: degeneration of basal ganglia
Carbon tetrachloride/chloroform	Microsomes	Hepatic fatty change and necrosis, renal tubular necrosis
Cyanide	Cytochrome oxidase	Systemic asphyxiant, cherry-red blood, bitter almond odor
Mercury	Protein	Mucosal ulcers, renal tubular necrosis, cerebral atrophy
Lead	Blood, brain, bone	Mild anemia with basophilic stippling, encephalopathy, intestinal colic, renal tubular acidosis
Arsenic	Sulfhydryl moieties	Diffuse hemorrhages, coagulation necrosis, thromboses

Questions

497. Which best determines the genotype of an organism?

    (A) number of microvilli
    (B) deoxyribonucleic acid (DNA) structure
    (C) pinocytosis
    (D) lysosomal content
    (E) rate of metabolism

498. A father and mother are both clinically well heterozygotes for a genetic disease that is expressed only with homozygous recessive, nonsex-linked inheritance. What percentage of their offspring should be affected?

    (A) 0%
    (B) 25%
    (C) 33%
    (D) 50%
    (E) 100%

499. The father is karyotypically normal. The mother is a clinically well heterozygous carrier for an X-linked trait. What percentage of the female offspring also will be carriers?

    (A) 0%
    (B) 25%
    (C) 33%
    (D) 50%
    (E) 100%

500. A Barr body occurs because of

    (A) ribosomes
    (B) endoplasmic reticulum
    (C) Lyon hypothesis
    (D) cytoplasm
    (E) Golgi apparatus

501. How many Barr bodies usually are seen in each cell with Turner's syndrome?

    (A) none
    (B) one
    (C) two
    (D) three
    (E) five or more

502. How many Barr bodies usually are seen in each cell in classic Klinefelter's syndrome?

    (A) none
    (B) one
    (C) two
    (D) three
    (E) four

503. Giemsa and quinacrine dyes are used in chromosome banding to

    (A) accelerate mitosis
    (B) paralyze the centrioles
    (C) stop the cell in metaphase
    (D) identify the karyotype
    (E) repair damaged chromosomes

504. True hermaphroditism is defined as

(A) ovaries present with male secondary sex characteristics

(B) absence of any gonadal tissue

(C) testis present with female secondary sex characteristics

(D) ambiguous external genitalia

(E) ovarian and testicular tissue in same organism

505. Expected findings in Turner's syndrome include

(A) streak ovaries

(B) neck webbing

(C) primary amenorrhea

(D) 45,XO karyotype

(E) all of the above

506. The 47,XXY karyotype is called

(A) normal male

(B) gonadal dysgenesis

(C) Turner's syndrome

(D) normal female

(E) Klinefelter's syndrome

507. The usual karyotype of Edward's syndrome is

(A) trisomy 13

(B) trisomy 18

(C) trisomy 21

(D) deletion of short arm of chromosome 5

(E) normal karyotype

508. Common findings in Down syndrome include

(A) mental retardation

(B) epicanthic folds

(C) increased incidence of leukemia

(D) increased incidence of congenital heart disease

(E) all of the above

509. A 1-year-old infant has a peculiar catlike mewing cry, mental retardation, and congenital heart disease. The abnormal karyotype is

(A) monosomy 18

(B) trisomy 18

(C) trisomy 21

(D) deletion of short arm of chromosome 5

(E) monosomy 21

510. An X-linked disorder characterized by lysosomal lack of alpha-galactosidase activity with subsequent accumulation of ceramide trihexoside is

(A) galactosemia

(B) Gaucher's disease

(C) metachromic leukodystrophy

(D) Fabry's disease

(E) Wolman's disease

511. Expected findings in Tay-Sachs disease include

(A) macular cherry red spot

(B) death by age 4

(C) neuronal accumulation of GM2 ganglioside

(D) mental retardation

(E) all of the above

512. A 25-year-old man is diagnosed as having an inherited glycogenosis. After heavy exercise, he gets painful cramps, and his urine turns brownish red for a short while. His probable diagnosis is

(A) type I

(B) type II

(C) type IV

(D) type V

(E) Pompe's disease

513. With a short-term dose of 15 rad, what effects would be expected?

(A) death in 2 hours

(B) minor blood changes, at most

(C) nausea, vomiting, and 25% mortality rate

(D) diarrhea, 75% mortality rate

(E) loss of hair, 50% mortality rate

514. An inherited disorder with abnormality in the rate of hemoglobin's globin chain production is

    (A) Huntington's chorea
    (B) hereditary lymphedema
    (C) spherocytosis
    (D) achondroplasia
    (E) thalassemia

515. An autosomal-dominant inherited disorder with disordered connective tissue, aortic cystic medial necrosis, long extremities, and spider fingers is

    (A) von Willebrand's disease
    (B) Milroy's syndrome
    (C) Alport's syndrome
    (D) Marfan's syndrome
    (E) tuberous sclerosis

516. Which of the following statements is correct concerning galactosemia?

    (A) It results from lack of galactose-1-phosphate uridyl transferase activity.
    (B) It is transmitted as autosomal recessive.
    (C) Jaundice, hepatomegaly, and splenomegaly are common.
    (D) Mental retardation and cataracts are common.
    (E) All of the above statements are true.

517. The genetic disease characterized by lack of homogentisic oxidase, black-colored urine, and blue-black pigmentation of cartilage is

    (A) albinism
    (B) hypercholesterolemia
    (C) ochronosis
    (D) neurofibromatosis
    (E) von Recklinghausen's disease

518. Which disease(s) is/are inherited in an X-linked recessive mode?

    (A) hemophilia B
    (B) Bruton's agammaglobulinemia
    (C) hemophilia A
    (D) Wiskott–Aldrich syndrome
    (E) all of the above

519. Identify which statement is correct about sickle cell disease.

    (A) It produces chronic hemolytic anemia.
    (B) It is usually caused by point substitution on globin molecule.
    (C) Homozygotes are most seriously affected.
    (D) It is most common in black populations.
    (E) All of the above statements are correct.

520. What statement is correct about Niemann–Pick disease?

    (A) Enlarged spleen, liver, and lymph nodes are involved.
    (B) It is a lysosomal storage disease.
    (C) Physical and mental retardation are present.
    (D) Lipid-laden macrophages are present.
    (E) All of the above statements are true.

521. The pediatric genetic disease characterized by disordered exocrine gland secretion, pancreatic fibrosis, pulmonary bronchiectasis, and meconium ileus is

    (A) cretinism
    (B) erythroblastosis fetalis
    (C) mucoviscidosis
    (D) anencephaly
    (E) newborn respiratory distress syndrome

522. What statement is/are correct about Duchenne type muscular dystrophy?

    (A) First symptoms appear in early childhood.
    (B) Death is usually by age 20.
    (C) Pseudohypertrophic changes are common in lower extremities.
    (D) Death is commonly caused by respiratory or cardiac difficulties.
    (E) All of the above statements are true.

523. What is the usual mode of inheritance in Wilson's disease?

    (A) sex-linked recessive
    (B) autosomal dominant
    (C) sex-linked dominant

(D) autosomal recessive

(E) not an inherited disease

524. Which of the following are inherited muco-polysaccharidoses?

(A) Hunter's syndrome

(B) Hurler's syndrome

(C) Morquio's syndrome

(D) Sanfilippo's syndrome

(E) all of the above

525. An X-linked disorder characterized by absent hypoxanthine-guanine phosphoribosyltrans-ferase activity, self-mutilation, choroeoatheto-sis, hyperuricemia, and hyperuricosuria is

(A) Lesch–Nyhan syndrome

(B) glucose-6-phosphate dehydrogenase (G6PD) deficiency

(C) pyruvate kinase (PK) deficiency

(D) Milroy's disease

(E) Alport's syndrome

526. Identify common findings in kwashiorkor.

(A) hepatomegaly and diarrhea

(B) changes in hair color or texture

(C) wasting of extremity muscles, with pre-served subcutaneous fat

(D) depigmentation of skin

(E) all of the above

527. The lipid-soluble vitamin important in miner-alization of osteoid is

(A) vitamin A

(B) vitamin B

(C) vitamin C

(D) vitamin D

(E) vitamin E

528. Beriberi results from a lack of which water-soluble vitamin?

(A) vitamin K

(B) pyridoxine

(C) niacin

(D) thiamine

(E) vitamin B_6

529. Indicate functions of vitamin K.

(A) Lack of vitamin K predisposes to bleeding.

(B) Vitamin K is necessary for synthesis of factor II.

(C) Vitamin K is a lipid-soluble vitamin.

(D) Vitamin K may be low in diseases with fat malabsorption.

(E) All of the above are functions of vitamin K.

530. Niacin deficiency is likely to cause

(A) scurvy

(B) pellagra

(C) pernicious anemia

(D) hypoprothrombinemia

(E) ascorbic acid deficiency

531. Iron deficiency usually causes

(A) macrocytic anemia

(B) normochromic, normocytic anemia

(C) megaloblastic anemia

(D) microcytic, hypochromic anemia

(E) anemia rarely occurs

532. An unexpected finding in lead poisoning would be

(A) abdominal pain

(B) renal tubular acidosis

(C) polycythemia

(D) wrist, finger, or foot drop

(E) encephalopathy

533. A 100-kg healthy man ingests 10 g of sodium cyanide on an empty stomach. The expected result is

(A) chronic debilitating arthritis

(B) severe diarrhea

(C) death within an hour or less

(D) ataxia for 1 or 2 hours, then gradual improvement

(E) micronodular cirrhosis

534. Which statement is correct concerning methyl alcohol poisoning?

(A) Poisoning can result from ingestion of 20 mL or more.

(B) Poisoning can result from inhaled fumes.

(C) Poisoning can be caused by ingestion of *Sterno*, paint removers, or solvents.

(D) Poisoning is associated with blindness.

(E) All of the above statements are correct.

535. Which cell is the MOST radiosensitive?

(A) ganglion cell

(B) muscle cell

(C) mature cartilage cell

(D) lymphoid cell

(E) pancreatic epithelial cell

DIRECTIONS (Questions 536 through 587): Each group of items in this section consists of a list of lettered options followed by a set of numbered words or phrases. For each numbered word or phrase, select the ONE lettered option that is most closely associated with it. Each lettered option may be selected once, more than once, or not at all.

Questions 536 through 539

(A) Down syndrome

(B) Edward's syndrome

(C) Patau's syndrome

(D) cat-cry syndrome (cri du chat)

(E) Turner's syndrome

536. Deletion of short arm of chromosome 5

537. Trisomy 18

538. Trisomy 21

539. Trisomy 13

Questions 540 through 543

(A) alpha$_1$-antitrypsin deficiency

(B) hemophilia

(C) achondroplasia

(D) glucose-6-phosphate dehydrogenase (G6PD) deficiency

(E) albinism

540. Bleeding disorder

541. Emphysema and cirrhosis

542. Dwarfism

543. Erythrocyte hemolysis

Questions 544 through 547

(A) niacin deficiency

(B) thiamine deficiency

(C) protein and total calorie deficiency

(D) vitamin D deficiency

(E) iron deficiency

544. Marasmus

545. Beriberi

546. Rickets

547. Pellagra

Questions 548 through 551

(A) lead poisoning

(B) cyanide poisoning

(C) mercury poisoning

(D) carbon tetrachloride poisoning

(E) vitamin A poisoning

548. Anemia with basophilic stippling

549. Binds to sulfhydryl groups of proteins

550. Binds to cytochrome oxidase

551. Fatty liver

Questions 552 through 555

(A) 47,XXY

(B) 45,XO

(C) 46,XY

(D) 46,XX

(E) 45,YO

552. Normal human male karyotype

553. Normal human female karyotype

554. Klinefelter's syndrome karyotype

555. Turner's syndrome karyotype

Questions 556 through 559

(A) Cori's disease
(B) neurofibromatosis
(C) osteogenesis imperfecta
(D) McArdle's disease
(E) Gaucher's disease

556. Autosomal dominant disorder of abnormal collagen synthesis

557. Autosomal dominant disorder with pigmented skin macules and multiple endocrine tumors

558. Hereditary deficiency of glucocerebrosidase

559. Hereditary deficiency of glycogen debrancher enzyme

Questions 560 through 563

(A) Wilson's disease
(B) phenylketonuria
(C) galactosemia
(D) Fabry's syndrome
(E) sickle cell anemia

560. Deficiency of galactose-1-phosphate uridyl transferase

561. Deficiency of phenylalanine hydroxylase

562. Inherited disorder with abnormal hemoglobin molecule

563. Abnormal copper metabolism

Questions 564 through 567

(A) vitamin A
(B) vitamin B_2
(C) vitamin C
(D) vitamin D
(E) vitamin K

564. Lipid-soluble vitamin necessary for the synthesis of clotting factors X and II

565. Deficiency causes scurvy.

566. Deficiency is termed "ariboflavinosis."

567. Deficiency state leads to xerophthalmia, night blindness, and follicular hyperplasia.

Questions 568 through 571

(A) albinism
(B) iron deficiency
(C) folic acid deficiency
(D) cretinism
(E) von Hippel–Lindau disease

568. Macrocytic anemia

569. Microcytic, hypochromic anemia

570. Autosomal recessive inherited disorder with deficiency of melanin production

571. Autosomal dominant inherited disorder

Questions 572 through 575

(A) heat cramps
(B) smoke inhalation
(C) first-degree burn
(D) third-degree burn
(E) malignant hyperthermia

572. Thermal destruction of the epidermis and adnexal structures

573. Most common cause of fire-related deaths

574. Systemic hyperpyrexia on administration of anesthetics

575. Muscle spasms due to depletion of water and salt

Questions 576 through 579

(A) hypocalcemia
(B) hyponatremia
(C) obesity
(D) bulimia
(E) iodine deficiency

576. Goiter

577. Tetany

578. At least 30% over ideal body weight

579. Eating disorder with binge-and-purge episodes

Questions 580 through 583

(A) cystic fibrosis

(B) ochronosis

(C) muscular dystrophy

(D) hemophilia

(E) female pseudohermaphroditism

(F) male pseudohermaphroditism

(G) Turner's syndrome

(H) Klinefelter's syndrome

580. A 4-year-old male has suffered from progressive weakness of his proximal muscle groups for about 6 months. His serum creatine kinase is markedly elevated. His older brother suffers from the same disorder and is now wheelchair-bound at age 10 and has prominent pseudo-hypertrophy of his calf muscles. What is the most likely diagnosis?

581. Shortly after birth, a white infant is noted to have meconium ileus. Over the next several years, the child remains at the lowest tenth percentile for growth and is experiencing mal-absorption and repeated respiratory infections. Examination of this child's sweat reveals an elevated sodium and chloride content. What is the most likely diagnosis?

582. A 20-year-old woman is killed in a motor vehicle accident. At autopsy, normal female external secondary sexual characteristics are present. However, the gonads are found to be testicular and the decedent's karyotype is 46,XY. What is the most likely diagnosis?

583. A 21-year-old female who has never menstruated is examined by her gynecologist. The patient has a small stature, web neck, poorly developed breasts and widely spaced nipples. No Barr bodies are evident on her buccal smear study. What is the most likely diagnosis?

Questions 584 through 587

(A) lead poisoning

(B) carbon monoxide poisoning

(C) pellagra

(D) scurvy

(E) sickle cell anemia

(F) Wilson's disease

(G) Hunter's syndrome

(H) hemophilia

584. A 4-year-old black female with a long history of microcytic anemia since birth presents to the emergency department complaining of severe left-upper quadrant abdominal pain. Her hemoglobin electrophoresis demonstrates 95% hemoglobin S. What genetic disorder is she most likely to have?

585. A 5-year-old male child presents to the emergency department complaining of knee pain. The child denies any recent trauma to the joint. The joint is distended by unclotted blood. The child's factor VIII is found to be less than 5% of normal. The child's sister is well, but his older brother also has episodes of spontaneous bleeding. What genetic disorder is the child most likely to have?

586. A 19-year-old male has been working on his car in an enclosed garage for about 20 minutes. During this time the car's engine has been running. The man begins to develop an intense headache, nausea, and dizziness. What is the most likely diagnosis?

587. A 43-year-old alcoholic with poor nutritional status is admitted to the hospital. His most serious ailments include dermatitis, diarrhea, and dementia. Which vitamin deficiency disease is he most likely to have acquired?

DIRECTIONS (Questions 588 through 591): Each of the numbered items or incomplete statements in this section is followed by answers or by completions of the statement. Select the ONE lettered answer or completion that is BEST in each case.

588. Asbestos exposure may lead to

(A) carcinoma of the lung

(B) fibrocalcific plaques of the pleura

(C) pleural effusion

(D) malignant mesothelioma

(E) all of the above

589. When small particles in the environment are larger than 10 microns in diameter, these particles can be stopped in

(A) the nasopharyngeal filter

(B) pulmonary neutrophils

(C) alveolar macrophages

(D) interstitial lymphates

(E) the mucociliary escalator

590. Currently the most prevalent chronic occupational disease in the world is

(A) asbestosis

(B) silicosis

(C) anthracosis

(D) berylliosis

(E) maple bark disease

591. Name a complication(s) in a person exposed to asbestos.

(A) increased risk of lung carcinoma

(B) increased risk of malignant mesothelioma

(C) symptomatic pulmonary interstitial fibrosis

(D) calcified plaques of the pleura

(E) all of the above

DIRECTIONS (Questions 592 through 594): For each numbered word or phrase, select the ONE lettered option that is most closely associated with it. Each lettered option may be selected once, more than once, or not at all.

(A) silicosis

(B) anthracosis

(C) asbestosis

(D) berylliosis

(E) Caplan syndrome

592. Rheumatoid factor in serum

593. Noncaseating granulomas

594. Most commonly associated with malignant mesothelioma

DIRECTIONS (Questions 595 through 598): Each of the numbered items or incomplete statements in this section is followed by answers or by completions of the statement. Select the ONE lettered answer or completion that is BEST in each case.

595. A 65-year-old male who worked in a shipyard developed a malignant mesothelioma this neoplasm will be related to

(A) coal worker's pneumoconiosis

(B) silicosis

(C) asbestosis

(D) berylliosis

(E) anthracosis

596. A 67-year-old male who worked for many years in a hard rock mine developed chronic cough and shortness of breath. Radiologically it showed extensive pulmonary fibrosis and nodular masses, bilateral on the upper zones of the lung. The most likely diagnosis is

(A) asbestosis

(B) silicosis

(C) anthracosis

(D) berylliosis

(E) coal worker's pneumoconiosis

597. Philadelphia chromosome is characterized by

(A) deletion of the p53 gene from chromosome 17

(B) translocation of the proto-oncogene c-abl from chromosome 9 to chromosome 22

(C) translocation of the proto-oncogene c-myc from chromosome 8 to chromosome 14

(D) translocation of the proto-oncogene bcl-1 from chromosome 11 to chromosome 14

(E) translocation of the proto-oncogene bcl-2 from chromosome 18 to chromosome 14

598. In Burkitt's lymphoma, indicate the oncogene involved in producing this lesion.

(A) BCL-2

(B) BCR

(C) P53

(D) C-MYC

(E) C-ABL

Answers and Explanations

497. **(B)** The genotype (genetic makeup of an organism) is determined by the molecular structure of its DNA contained in chromosomes. Pinocytosis refers to invaginations of the cell membrane, which is useful in fluid measurement. The lysosomal content, number of microvilli, and rate of metabolism of a cell are in part determined by the cell's genotype but do not themselves direct or define the genotype. They are outward expressions (phenotype) of the DNA structure. *(Rubin and Farber, pp. 223–226)*

498. **(B)** Half of the offspring will be identical to the parents, that is, heterozygous for the recessive defect but clinically well. One quarter of the offspring will be homozygous normal and clinically well. The remaining offspring, 25% of the total, will be homozygous for the recessive defect and clinically affected. *(Rubin and Farber, pp. 245, 246)*

499. **(D)** Female offspring receive X chromosomes from the father and mother. The father can contribute only his normal X. The mother can contribute either her normal X or her carrier X. Thus, about one half of the female offspring will be carriers. *(Rubin and Farber, pp. 234–237)*

500. **(C)** According to the Lyon hypothesis, only one X chromatin is genetically active, and the other undergoes heteropyknosis to become the Barr body, inactivation occurs about the 16th day of embryonic life, and inactivation of the same X chromosome persists in all progeny cells. The Barr body is composed mostly of nucleoprotein. *(Rubin and Farber, pp. 284, 285)*

501. **(A)** Turner's syndrome usually has a 45,XO karyotype. According to the Lyon hypothesis, there should be no Barr body (extra X chromosome) in the Turner's cells, because Turner's cells have only one X chromosome. *(Rubin and Farber, p. 236)*

502. **(B)** Classic Klinefelter's syndrome has a 47,XXY karyotype. According to the Lyon hypothesis, all except one X chromosome will involute and become Barr bodies. The expected number of Barr bodies is then one per cell. *(Rubin and Farber, p. 235)*

503. **(D)** Giemsa and quinacrine dyes are used to band the chromosomes, allowing enumeration and identification of the karyotype. After staining, colchicine is used to paralyze the centrioles and microtubules, stopping the cell in metaphase. Giemsa and quinacrine stains do not accelerate mitosis or repair damaged chromosomes. *(Rubin and Farber, p. 210)*

504. **(E)** True hermaphroditism is defined as an organism possessing both ovarian and testicular tissue. An organism with testicular tissue and female external genitalia is a male pseudohermaphrodite. Female pseudohermaphrodites have ovarian tissue and exhibit male external genitalia. *(Cotran et al., p. 176)*

505. **(E)** Turner's syndrome usually has a 45,XO karyotype, although some people are 46,XX/45,XO mosaic. In the fully expressed syndrome, there are streak ovaries (gonadal dysgenesis), webbed neck, short stature, primary amenorrhea, and congenital heart disease. *(Rubin and Farber, p. 236)*

506. **(E)** Klinefelter's syndrome has a male phenotype, sterility, eunochoid body habitus, long legs, and a slight decrease in intelligence. Its karyotype is 47,XXY. Turner's syndrome, also called gonadal dysgenesis, has a karyotype of 45,XO. The normal male and female karyotypes are 46,XY and 46,XX, respectively. *(Rubin and Farber, p. 235)*

507. **(B)** Edward's syndrome has a karyotype of trisomy 18. Clinical features include mental retardation, cardiac defects, micrognathia, and large occiput. Trisomy 13, trisomy 21, and a deletion of the short arm of chromosome 5 are Patau's syndrome, Down syndrome, and cat's cry syndrome, respectively. *(Cotran et al., pp. 170–173)*

508. **(E)** Down syndrome is caused by a trisomy of chromosome 21. Clinical features include mental retardation, epicanthic folds, horizontal palmar crease, flat facial profile, and muscle hypotonia. The incidence of leukemia and congenital heart disease is increased in Down syndrome. *(Cotran et al., pp. 170–171)*

509. **(D)** The clinical picture described characterizes cat's cry syndrome, a genetic disorder with a deletion of the short arm of chromosome 5. Infants with monosomies rarely survive birth. Trisomy 18 and trisomy 21 are Edward's syndrome and Down syndrome, respectively. *(Cotran et al., p. 169)*

510. **(D)** Fabry's disease is an X-linked recessive disorder caused by lack of alpha-galactosidase activity with lysosomal accumulation of ceramide trihexoside. Affected cells contain doubly refractile lipid material that is lamellated in a myelinlike form by ultrastructural examination. Blue–black pruritic skin eruptions are common with the disease. The other listed diseases have autosomal recessive inheritance. *(Cotran et al., p. 155)*

511. **(E)** Tay–Sachs disease is a glycolipid storage disease caused by absent hexosaminidase A activity. Neurons accumulate GM2 ganglioside with resultant mental retardation, deafness, blindness, and death by age 4. The macular cherry red spot is an expected clinical finding. *(Cotran et al., pp. 155, 156)*

512. **(D)** Of the listed choices, only type V, McArdle's disease, is compatible with a normal life span. The defect in McArdle's disease, muscle phosphorylase, causes skeletal muscle damage, with resultant pain and myoglobinuria after heavy exercise. All of the other glycogenoses listed usually are fatal in early childhood. *(Cotran et al., pp. 160, 161)*

513. **(B)** A short-term dose of 15 rad would be expected to produce minor blood changes, if anything. Higher short-term doses, up to about 200 rad, are necessary to produce a mortality rate of about 20%. Over 800 rad, there is a 100% mortality rate. *(Chandrasoma and Taylor, pp. 169–170)*

514. **(E)** Thalassemia is an autosomal dominant inherited disorder characterized by an abnormal rate of globin chain production. All of the other choices are autosomal dominant inherited disorders but have no direct effect on the rate of globin synthesis. *(Cotran et al., pp. 615–618)*

515. **(D)** Marfan's syndrome is a genetic disorder of connective tissue. Aortic cystic medial necrosis is a characteristic lesion and results in a propensity for thoracic dissecting aneurysms. Other features of the disorder include autosomal dominant inheritance, long slender extremities, and long fingers. *(Cotran et al., pp. 148, 149)*

516. **(E)** Galactosemia is a genetic disorder with autosomal recessive inheritance characterized by absent galactose-1-phosphate uridyl transferase activity. This blocked metabolic pathway causes high blood galactose levels and galactosuria. Common findings in the disease are mental retardation, cataracts, jaundice, and hepatosplenomegaly. *(Cotran et al., pp. 476, 477)*

517. **(C)** Ochronosis is an autosomal recessive disorder characterized by the lack of homogenitisic oxidase, black-colored urine, and pigmentation of the cartilage. The pigmented cartilage is more susceptible to osteoarthropathy. The other choices have genetic modes of transmission but lack the clinical findings seen in ochronosis. *(Cotran et al., p. 162)*

518. **(E)** X-linked recessive inheritance has a genetic abnormality carried on the X chromosome. Because of this, the disease usually is apparent only in about half of the male offspring of clinically unaffected heterozygote carrier females. Unaffected males do not transmit the disease. The hemophilias are both X-linked, bleeding disorders. Bruton's agammaglobulinemia and Wiskott–Aldrich syndrome are both X-linked immunodeficiency disorders. *(Cotran et al., p. 173)*

519. **(E)** Sickle cell disease is a genetic disease caused by an inherited abnormal hemoglobin. The most common form in North America, the S form, is caused by a point substitution on the beta-globulin molecule. Normal hemoglobin molecules are termed "A." Sickle hemoglobin is termed "S." Homozygotes are most severely affected with anemia. Vaso-occlusive complications and chronic infections hallmark the disease. The S hemoglobin is most common in black populations. *(Cotran et al., pp. 612–614)*

520. **(E)** Niemann–Pick disease is a lysosomal storage disease caused by reduced or absent sphingomyelinase activity. Sphingomyelin accumulates within lysosomes of the reticuloendothelial cells and macrophages of the spleen, liver, and lymph nodes, causing clinical enlargement as well as physical and mental retardation. An accumulation of galactocerebroside is seen in Krabbe's disease, alternatively called globoid cell leukodystrophy. *(Cotran et al., pp. 156–158)*

521. **(C)** Mucoviscidosis, also called "cystic fibrosis," is characterized by disordered exocrine gland secretion, pancreatic fibrosis, and chronic bronchiectasis. The other disorders, cretinism, newborn respiratory distress syndrome, anencephaly, and erythroblastosis fetalis are pediatric diseases resulting from lack of thyroxine, lack of surfactant, lack of cranial development, and maternal red blood cell alloantibodies, respectively. *(Cotran et al., pp. 477–481)*

522. **(E)** Duchenne type of muscular dystrophy is an X-linked recessive disorder usually limited to males. Pelvifemoral muscle weakness usually first appears in early childhood. Later in the disease, the shoulder, arms, and trunk are involved. Pseudohypertrophic changes are distinctive of this dystrophy. Death by age 20 usually results from respiratory failure, pulmonary infections, or cardiac disorders. *(Cotran et al., pp. 1282–1284)*

523. **(D)** Wilson's disease, also called "hepatolenticular degeneration," is a genetic abnormality of copper metabolism. The usual mode of inheritance is autosomal dominant. The clinical picture is one of cirrhosis, cerebellar and basal ganglia degeneration and a pigmented ring in the cornea (Kayser–Fleischer ring). Treatment with penicillamine has markedly improved the prognosis for this disorder. *(Rubin and Farber, pp. 803–805)*

524. **(E)** The mucopolysaccharidoses are inherited disorders of mucopolysaccharide metabolism. Lack of degradative enzymes results in lysosomal accumulation of mucopolysaccharides. Eventually, the excessive retained mucopolysaccharides result in cell injury and death. *(Rubin and Farber, pp. 249, 253–255)*

525. **(A)** Lesch–Nyhan syndrome has absent hypoxanthine–guanine phosphoribosyltransferase activity with resultant hyperuricemia, hyperuricosuria, and uric acid renal calculi. The major clinical features of the disease are neurologic self-mutilation, mental retardation, spastic movements, and choreoathetosis. Deficiencies of G6PD and PK are X-linked chronic hemolytic anemias. Milroy's disease (hereditary lymphedema) and Alport's syndrome (nephropathy, deafness) are autosomal dominant disorders. *(Cotran et al., pp. 1254, 1255)*

526. **(E)** Kwashiorkor is a nutritional imbalance caused by inadequate protein consumption with adequate or high carbohydrate intake. It usually follows weaning when children are switched to a calorically adequate grain diet with limited quantities of nutritionally poor protein. The clinical picture includes hair

changes, skin depigmentation, hepatomegaly, diarrhea, and muscle wasting. Subcutaneous fat usually is preserved. *(Cotran et al., pp. 437–439)*

527. (D) Vitamin D is important for the proper mineralization of newly made osteoid. Vitamin D is a steroid-based molecule and is lipid-soluble. Other lipid-soluble vitamins include vitamins A, E, and K. All of the B vitamins are water-soluble. *(Cotran et al., pp. 441–446)*

528. (D) Beriberi is caused by a lack of dietary thiamine. The disease consists of high output heart failure, complicating infections, serous effusions, acute pulmonary edema, and hepatic congestion. Niacin deficiency, pellagra, has skin and mucous membrane lesions. Pyridoxine, also called "vitamin B_6," deficiency has a variable clinical appearance. Vitamin K is a fat-soluble vitamin necessary to synthesize certain coagulation proteins. *(Cotran et al., p. 1447)*

529. (E) Vitamin K is a lipid-soluble vitamin necessary for the synthesis of blood clotting factors II, VII, X, and XI. Lack of vitamin K predisposes to bleeding and can be seen in fat malabsorption diseases, such as chronic pancreatitis and obstructive jaundice. *(Cotran et al., pp. 446, 447)*

530. (B) Niacin is an active component in many oxidation–reduction reactions in the body through nicotinamide-adenine dinucleotide (NAD) and NAD phosphate intermediaries. The niacin deficiency state is termed "pellagra" and is associated with dermatitis, dementia, and diarrhea. Scurvy, pernicious anemia, and hypoprothrombinemia are associated with low levels of vitamin C (ascorbic acid), vitamin B_{12}, and vitamin K, respectively. *(Cotran et al., pp. 448, 449)*

531. (D) Iron is an important constituent of hemoglobin, and iron deficiency can lead to anemia. The anemia produces red blood cells that are microcytic and hypochromic. *(Chandrasoma and Taylor, pp. 385–388)*

532. (C) Lead poisoning usually has mild anemia not polycythemia. Accompanying the anemia is basophilic stippling of the erythrocytes. Other common clinical features in lead poisoning include abdominal colic and pain, encephalopathy, gingival lead lines, renal tubular acidosis, and finger, wrist, or foot drop. *(Rubin and Farber, pp. 329, 330)*

533. (C) Ingestion of less than 0.1 g of the inorganic salt of cyanide usually is rapidly fatal. A 10-g dose is massive; death would occur within 10–20 minutes. In acute cyanide poisoning, the cyanide binds to cytochrome oxidase to produce asphyxiation. The blood is cherry red color and has a pungent bitter almond smell. *(Rubin and Farber, p. 328)*

534. (E) Methyl alcohol is found in solvents, *Sterno*, and paint remover. As little as 20 mL of ingested methyl alcohol can be toxic. Poisoning also occurs if fumes are inhaled for a prolonged time, particularly in unventilated rooms. A marked anion gap metabolic acidosis develops. The principal sites of body damage are the brain and retina. Blindness is a common sequela. *(Chandrasoma and Taylor, p. 186)*

535. (D) Cells with high radiosensitivity (the ability to be easily damaged by radiation), include lymphoid cells, hematopoietic cells, germ cells, and intestinal epithelium. In general, the higher the mitotic rate of the tissue, the more likely that the tissue will be damaged by radiation. *(Rubin and Farber, pp. 338–344)*

536–539. (536-D, 537-B, 538-A, 539-C) All of the syndromes have chromosomal aberrations. Down syndrome, Edward's syndrome, and Patau's syndrome are trisomies of chromosomes 21, 18, and 13, respectively. Cat-cry syndrome (cri du chat) has a deletion of the short arm of chromosome 5. *(Cotran et al., pp. 170–173)*

540–543. (540-B, 541-A, 542-C, 543-D) All of the listed conditions are inherited. The mode of inheritance is X-linked recessive in hemophilia and G6PD deficiency. Achondroplasia is an autosomal dominant disorder. The cirrhosis and emphysema seen in $alpha_1$-antitrypsin deficiency is inherited in an autosomal recessive mode. *(Chandrasoma and Taylor, pp. 235–237)*

544–547. (544-C, 545-B, 546-D, 547-A) Deficiencies of the B vitamins, niacin and thiamine, cause pellagra and beriberi, respectively. Lack of protein and total calories is called "marasmus" and is characterized by severe weight loss, edema, depigmentation, and diarrhea. Vitamin D deficiency results in poor mineralization of osteoid and is rickets in infants and children. In adults, the deficient state is osteomalacia. *(Chandrasoma and Taylor, pp. 438–455)*

548–551. (548-A, 549-C, 550-B, 551-D) Lead poisoning is characterized by anemia, erythrocytic basophilic stippling, encephalopathy, renal tubular acidosis, and colic. Cyanide poisons by binding to cytochrome oxidase and asphyxiating all the cells of the body. Mercury damages cells by binding to sulfhydryl protein groups. The kidney is a major site of damage. Carbon tetrachloride poisoning is characterized by hepatic fatty change and necrosis. *(Cotran et al., pp. 419–422)*

552–555. (552-C, 553-D, 554-A, 555-B) The normal human male and female karyotypes are 46,XY and 46,XX, respectively. Klinefelter's syndrome has a 47,XXY karyotype and is characterized by tall eunuchoid habitus, female distribution of hair, small penis, gynecomastia, and infertility. Turner's syndrome has a 45,XO or 45,XO/46,XX mosaic karyotype and is characterized by short stature, web neck, lymphedema, immature nipple development, primary amenorrhea, streak gonads, skeletal abnormalities, and congenital heart disease. *(Cotran et al., pp. 173, 174)*

556–559. (556-C, 557-B, 558-E, 559-A) Osteogenesis imperfecta is a genetic disorder with abnormal collagen production. There is a defect in the synthesis of type I collagen, the major (90%) matrix constituent of bone. The mode of inheritance is autosomal dominant. Affected individuals suffer from extreme bone fragility, multiple fractures, dental imperfections, and blue sclera. Neurofibromatosis is an autosomal dominant disorder characterized by numerous pigmented skin lesions, multiple neural tumors, Lisch nodules, and a tendency for reduced intelligence. Gaucher's disease is an autosomal recessive lysosomal storage disorder in which there is an intracellular accumulation of glucocerebroside due to the genetic lack of glucocerebrosidase enzyme. Clinical features include hepatosplenomegaly, progressive central nervous system degeneration, and skeletal lesions. Cori's disease is an autosomal recessive disorder of glycogen metabolism due to the absence of the debrancher enzyme. There is accumulation of massive quantities of glycogen throughout the body with subsequent death in infancy. *(Cotran et al., pp. 1221, 1222; 1354; 158, 159; 1221, 1222)*

560–563. (560-C, 561-B, 562-E, 563-A) Galactosemia is an autosomal recessive disorder that is most often due to the genetic lack of the enzyme galactose-1-phosphate uridyl transferase. Infants are normal at birth. But, shortly after ingesting galactose containing foods, such as human or bovine milk, there is a marked elevation of galactose levels in serum and urine with subsequent jaundice, vomiting, hepatomegaly, liver failure, neurologic damage, and cataracts unless a galactose-free diet is maintained. Phenylketonuria is an autosomal recessive disease due to an absence of the enzyme phenylalanine hydroxylase. There is hyperphenylalaninemia and increased urinary excretion of its phenylketone metabolites. Clinically, progressive mental retardation is observed unless a phenylalanine-free diet is maintained. Sickle cell disease is an inherited hemoglobinopathy in which there is abnormal beta globin chain production. The abnormal hemoglobin spontaneously deforms the erythrocytes into sickle- and leaf-shaped structures when deoxygenized. These deformed red blood cells hemolyse or clog the smaller blood vessels causing ischemia. Wilson's disease, hepatolenticular degeneration, is an autosomal recessive disorder of copper metabolism characterized by marked accumulation of copper in the brain, liver, and eye. There are usually very low levels of the copper transport protein, ceruloplasmin. *(Cotran et al., pp. 476, 477; 475, 476; 611–615; 875)*

564–567. (564-E, 565-C, 566-B, 567-A) The lipid-soluble vitamin K is necessary for the synthesis of blood clotting factors II, VII, IX, and X in the liver. The resultant abnormality of blood clotting is seen clinically as easy bruising, hematuria, or melena. Scurvy is caused by a deficiency of the water-soluble vitamin C. Scurvy is characterized by abnormal collagen maturation, bleeding gums, abnormal wound healing, and abnormal bone growth. Ariboflavinosis, a lack of vitamin B$_2$, is associated with fissuring of the lips (cheilosis), fissuring at the angles of the mouth (angular stomatitis), tongue atrophy, and corneal vascular opacities. A lack of the lipid-soluble vitamin A can produce night blindness (nyctalopia), conjunctival dryness (xerophthalmia), corneal opacities, corneal ulcerations, and follicular dermatosis. (*Chandrasoma and Taylor, pp. 150–158*)

568–571. (568-C, 569-B, 570-A, 571-E) Macrocytic anemia is usually seen with a deficiency of folic acid. Folic acid is a necessary cofactor for the synthesis of nucleic acids. Folic acid is most plentiful in raw green and yellow vegetables. Iron deficiency produces a microcytic, hypochromic anemia. Chronic blood loss is the most frequent cause of iron deficiency. Albinism is a recessive autosomal disorder due to an inherited lack of effective melanin production. The lack of melanin predisposes these individuals to the early development of actinic-induced skin cancers. Von Hippel–Lindau disease is an autosomal dominant disorder in which there is an increased incidence of hemangioblastomas, angiomas, adenomas, pheochromocytomas, cysts, and carcinomas in various organs throughout the body. A genetic alteration has recently been mapped to chromosome 3. (*Cotran et al., pp. 627–630; 626, 627; 148; 1355*)

572–575. (572-D, 573-B, 574-E, 575-A) Thermal burns are divided into three categories by the depth of tissue destruction. First-degree burns are defined as the thermal loss of only the epidermis. Burns that destroy the epidermis and the superficial dermis, but spare the underlying adnexal structures are termed second-degree. Third-degree burns involve the loss of the epidermis, dermis, and adnexal structures. Smoke inhalation is the most common cause of fire-related deaths. In a house fire, for example, most people die of hypoxia while breathing smokey air with little remaining oxygen and abundant carbon monoxide. Only after

the individual expires of asphyxia does most thermal burning of the body occur. Malignant hyperthermia is a genetic disorder characterized by the development of marked hyperpyrexia during administration of anesthetics. Widespread skeletal muscle necrosis occurs with resultant myoglobinemia, myoglobinuria, and acute renal failure. Exercising in hot, humid weather encourages the loss of water and salt predisposing an individual to develop muscle cramps. These spasms of the voluntary muscles can be prevented and treated by salt and water replacement. (*Chandrasoma and Taylor, pp. 166–168*)

576–579. (576-E, 577-A, 578-C, 579-D) Goiter, a diffuse enlargement of the thyroid gland, is usually seen with iodine deficiency. Iodine is a necessary element in the synthesis of thyroid hormones. One of the body's responses to the lack of this hormone is to encourage hyperplasia of the thyroid gland. Tetany, an involuntary twitching or contracting of muscles, is seen with hypocalcemia. Insufficient parathyroid hormone is the most common cause of hypocalcemia. Obesity is usually defined as a weight at least 30% in excess of ideal body weight. Obese individuals are at increased risk for heart disease, stroke, hypertension, and some forms of cancer. Bulimia is an eating disorder characterized by episodic overeating usually followed by induced vomiting. Bulimics may sustain esophageal tears, aspiration pneumonia, cardiac arrhythmias, acid erosion of their teeth, and occasionally, death. (*Cotran et al., pp. 1138–1140; 1148, 453; 439*)

580. **(C)** Duchenne muscular dystrophy is an X-linked recessive, inherited disorder characterized by progressive muscle weakness. The weakness is usually first detected at age 3 or 4 and begins in the proximal muscle groups, such as the shoulder, trunk, or pelvis. There is a persistent elevation of the serum creatine kinase enzyme throughout the disease. This elevated enzymatic marker is also useful in identifying the heterozygous carrier state. By age 10, most victims are wheelchair-bound. Pseudohypertrophy of the calf muscles due to fatty replacement of diseased muscle is a characteristic finding in the later stages of the disease. Death usually results from muscular respiratory insufficiency. *(Rubin and Farber, pp. 261, 262)*

581.   **(A)** Cystic fibrosis is an inherited disorder affecting exocrine gland secretion throughout the body. The enigmatic genetic alteration is present at the long arm of chromosome 7. Meconium ileus may occur in utero or shortly after birth heralding the onset of the disorder. More commonly, however, the disorder is first diagnosed in 2- or 3-year-old infants who have had repeated pulmonary infections, malabsorption, a retarded growth rate, and poor development. Analysis of sweat reveals the characteristic elevation of both sodium and chloride. Many individuals with cystic fibrosis now live into their mid-20s. Death is usually due to infectious complications. *(Rubin and Farber, pp. 246–249)*

582.   **(F)** The scenario describes male pseudohermaphroditism, a phenotypic female with male karyotype. Unless these individuals are serendipitously studied for karyotype, primary amenorrhea, infertility, or develop tumors in their abdominal testes, most will live their lives as normal, albeit sterile, females. The disorder is usually inherited in an X-linked manner. The corresponding biochemical defect is an inability of cells to respond to androgenic hormones. In utero the lack of androgenic action leads to incomplete descent of the testes and subsequent formation of normal female external genitalia, including a vagina. The uterus, however, is not formed so that primary amenorrhea and sterility result. Chromosomal analysis is diagnostic revealing a male karyotype. The intraabdominal gonads are testes, and this cryptorchidism predisposes to the development of testicular malignancies. *(Chandrasoma and Taylor, p. 1151)*

583.   **(G)** The karyotype of Turner's syndrome is usually 45,XO. A few individuals are 45,XO/ 46,XX mosaics. Turner's syndrome may include the following features: webbed neck, short stature, primary amenorrhea, widely spaced nipples, coarctation of the aorta, wide carrying angle of the arms, poor breast development, rudimentary or streak gonads, lymphedema,

hypoplasia of the nails, abnormal teeth, high arched palate, craniofacial abnormalities, metatarsal and metacarpal deformations, and multiple pigmented nevi. *(Cotran et al., pp. 174–176)*

584.   **(E)** Sickle cell disease is a hereditary hemoglobinopathy in which an aberrant beta hemoglobin chain is made due to an inherited point mutation in the genetic code. This mutation results in the substitution of the amino acid valine for glutamic acid in the sixth position of the beta chain. Upon deoxygenation, this abnormal hemoglobin spontaneously polymerizes in the erythrocyte deforming the cell into a sickle- or leaf-like shape. The sickled erythrocytes hemolyze and occlude small blood vessels. The vascular occlusion may result in ischemic tissue destruction. Most homozygous infants do not develop profound anemia and ischemic sequela until 5 or 6 months after birth due to the protective effect of residual fetal hemoglobin. The common clinical features of sickle cell disease in patients older than 6 months usually include anemia, hyperbilirubinemia, chronic infections, painful vascular occlusive events, and later in the progression of the disease, splenic autoinfarction. Heterozygotes are clinically well and derive a mild protective effect against malarial erythrocytic infection. *(Cotran et al., pp. 611–615)*

585.   **(H)** Hemophilia A is an X-linked disorder in which the activity of blood clotting factor VIII is insufficient for normal hemostasis. These individuals suffer from spontaneous hemorrhages, particularly into the joints. Exsanguination from unexpected trauma or surgical procedures is not unheard of. Replacement therapy with factor VIII concentrates is helpful for temporary correction of the bleeding diathesis in individuals who have not developed inhibitor antibodies. The transfusion of factor VIII concentrates do, however, carry a risk of hepatitis and AIDS transmission. *(Cotran et al., p. 639)*

586.   **(B)** Carbon monoxide poisons by binding irreversibly to hemoglobin with resultant systemic asphyxiation. This colorless, odorless gas is readily formed by incomplete combustion,

such as in automobile engines powered by fossil fuel derivatives. Hypoxia is first noted as headache, nausea, and vomiting with a 20–30% saturation of hemoglobin. Unconsciousness and death are likely at concentrations above 60% saturation. Chronic low-dose poisoning may result in cystic necrosis of the brain. *(Cotran et al., p. 418)*

587. **(C)** The scenario depicts an individual with pellagra, a deficiency of niacin. Pellagra usually has a constellation of symptoms termed "the three Ds"—dermatitis, diarrhea, and dementia. The dermatitis affects the sun-exposed skin, which becomes darker because of increased melanin pigmentation and redder because of increased vascularity. There are atrophic mucous membrane changes throughout the gastrointestinal tract with resultant diarrhea. The dementia occurs due to degeneration of neurons in the cerebral cortex. Niacin is required for the synthesis of nicotinamide adenine dinucleotide, a cofactor active in many oxidation reduction reactions in the cell. *(Cotran et al., pp. 448, 449)*

588. **(E)** Asbestos is a family of crystalline hydrated silicates that form fibers. There is an increased incidence of asbestos-related cancer in asbestos workers. The concentration of particles, the size and the solubility of the different asbestos fibers, is related to the patient developing a disease. The greater pathogenicity of straight and stiff amphiboles is apparently related to their aerodynamic properties and solubility since chrysotiles are more flexible and curled and are more likely to become impacted in the upper respiratory passages. In asbestos-related diseases, it is common to see pleural effusions, fibrous pleural plaques, interstitial fibrosis, bronchogenic carcinomas, and mesotheliomas. *(Cotran et al., p. 732)*

589. **(A)** The nasopharynx is covered by pseudostratified ciliated columnar respiratory epithelium. With age, however, the respiratory epithelium is replaced focally by stratified squamous epithelium over large areas. The mucosa contain numerous mucus glands and abundant lymphoid tissue. One function of

the nasopharyngeal area is to form a filter for inhaled particles. Those larger than 10 microns, in general, are trapped by this filter. The most dangerous particles range from 1–5 microns in diameter, because they escape the nasopharyngeal filter and enter the airways that can be carried all the way to the alveoli of the lungs. *(Cotran et al., pp. 726–728)*

590. **(B)** Silicosis of the lung is caused by inhalation of crystalline silicon dioxide (silica). It is currently the most prevalent chronic occupational disease in the world. Once the particles are inhaled and carried to the lung, they are ingested by the lung macrophages. The toxic effects of the silica over the macrophages cause death of these cells, and the particles are ingested by other macrophages, making the removal of the silica from the lungs impossible. Morphologically, they present as discrete nodules in the upper zones of the lungs. Some of these nodules may undergo central necrosis. In general, they are formed by hard collagenous tissue, which, under polarized light, the silica is birefringent. *(Cotran et al., pp. 730, 731)*

591. **(E)** Same answer as Answer 588. *(Cotran et al., p. 732)*

592. **(E)** Caplan syndrome is defined as a coexistence of rheumatoid arthritis with a pneumoconiosis. The granulomas on Caplan syndrome has a central necrosis and is surrounded by fibroblasts, macrophages, and collagen. This syndrome is not necessarily coexistent with silicosis; it can also occur with another pneumoconiosis. *(Cotran et al., pp. 730–733)*

593. **(D)** Berylliosis is another type of pneumoconiosis that is also manifested by granulomatosis disease in the lung. Characteristically, these granulomas do not undergo caseation necrosis. *(Cotran et al., pp. 730–733)*

594. **(C)** The pneumoconiosis that most likely is related to malignant mesothelioma and bronchogenic carcinoma, as well as pleural effusions is asbestosis. *(Cotran et al., pp. 730–733)*

595. **(C)** Asbestos bodies appear as a golden brown, fusiform or beaded rods in hematoxylin and eosin sections of the lung. If we perform iron stain, it appears to be positive, because the proteinaceous material that covers the asbestos bodies contains iron. These particles present a high risk for developing malignant mesothelioma, as well as bronchogenic carcinoma. In a person exposed to asbestos bodies, there is a 1,000-fold greater increase of contracting malignant mesothelioma. *(Cotran et al., pp. 732–734)*

596. **(B)** This is a follow-up to Question 590. The same answer applies. *(Cotran et al., pp. 730–732)*

597. **(B)** Chronic myelogenous leukemia is affected mostly adults with a peak in incidents in the 30s and 40s. Genetically, CML is distinguished from other chronic myeloproliferative disorders by the presence of a molecular abnormality that involves the BCR gene on chromosome 9 and the ABL gene on chromosome 22. In 90% of the cases of chronic myelogenous leukemia, the karyotyping reveals a Philadelphia chromosome that represents the reciprocate translocation of 9 to 22. In 5–10% of the cases, however, it is more difficult to prove this translocation, and other methods must be used. *(Cotran et al., pp. 680–682)*

598. **(D)** In Burkitt's lymphoma C-MYC proto-oncogene shows an overexpression induced by translocation. In the normal locus, the expression of C-MYC gene is controlled and is only expressed during certain stages of cell cycle. In Burkitt's lymphoma, the translocation of this segment containing C-MYC from chromosome 8 to chromosome 14 produces an overexpression and, therefore, inactivation of C-MYC. The presence of C-MYC gene in Burkitt's lymphoma shows the importance of this oncogene overexpression in the pathogenesis of Burkitt's lymphoma. *(Cotran et al., p. 285)*

REFERENCES

Chandrasoma P, Taylor CR. *Concise Pathology*, 3rd ed. Norwalk, CT: Appleton & Lange, 1998.

Cotran RS, Kumar V, Robbins SL. *Robbins Pathologic Basis of Disease*, 6th ed. Philadelphia: Saunders, 1999.

Rubin E, Farber JL. *Pathology*. Philadelphia: Lippincott, 1999.

CHAPTER 7

Neoplasia and Abnormalities of Growth

Our first priority is to recognize that cancer is only a name given to one part of the collective processes of tissue disorganization, that it has no one external cause, that many external and internal agencies predispose to its development, that it is cell mediated but generally arises without any specific, once-for-all, genetic origin and that, although it may regress or become benign, its tendency is to progress irregularly in several of its growth characteristics.

—Sir David Smithers (1971)

Neoplasia: An abnormal mass of tissue, the growth of which exceeds and is uncoordinated with that of the normal tissues and persists in the same excessive manner after cessation of the stimuli which evolve the change.

—R. A. Willis

The biologic and clinically important subject of neoplasia should be seen in the perspective of abnormal growth and cellular reproduction. This is particularly seen in the concept of the role of genes and gene products—the control of cellular proliferation and growth.

BASIC FACTS AND DEFINITIONS

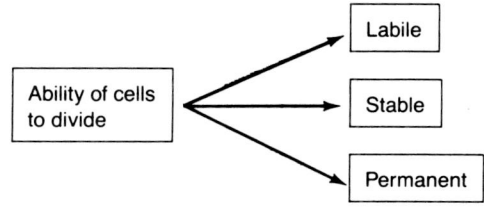

Table 7–1. ABNORMALITIES IN GROWTH

Alteration in Number of Cells	Alteration in Size of Individual Cells	Alteration in Cell Composition and Maturation
Aplasia	Agenesis	Metaplasia
Hypoplasia	Atrophy	Dysplasia
Hyperplasia	Hypertrophy	Neoplasia

The various types of growth abnormalities are summarized in Table 7–1 and further defined in Table 7–2. The normal ability of cells to divide is based on whether they are labile, stable, or permanent.

Two of the most important distinctions in cell proliferation are between hyperplasia and neoplasia (Table 7–3) and benign versus malignant neoplasia (Table 7–4).

Various types of carcinogenic agents identified in human cancer can be seen in Table 7–5. The older concepts of initiation and promotion in chemical carcinogenesis, the multiple hit theory of physical and chemical carcinogenesis, virus oncogenesis, hereditary and acquired carcinogenic chromosomal abnormalities, and their relationship with growth

Table 7–2. DEFINITIONS

Terminology	Definition
Aplasia	Lack of normal cellular proliferation with resultant absence of tissue, e.g., aplastic anemia
Hypoplasia	Decrease in mass of tissue or organ due to decrease in normal cellular proliferation resulting in decrease before tissue or organ reaches normal mature size
Hyperplasia	Increase in mass of tissue or organ because of cellular increase beyond normal range
Agenesis	Congenital lack of tissue or organ owing to total lack of cells concerned
Atrophy	Acquired decrease in mass of tissue or organ because of decrease in size of cellular components after full maturity has been achieved
Hypertrophy	Acquired increase in mass of tissue or organ owing to increase in size of cellular components
Metaplasia	Acquired change of tissue or organ because of change of one adult cell type to a different adult cell type
Dysplasia	Abnormal sequence of changes in maturation or development of cell type in a tissue or organ
Neoplasia	Formation of new growth by abnormal cell proliferation

Table 7–3. ESSENTIAL DIFFERENCE BETWEEN HYPERPLASIA AND NEOPLASIA

Neoplasia	Hyperplasia
Spontaneous or abnormal proliferative response to a stimulus (often unknown type)	A proliferative cellular response to an overstimulation of a normal type
Often not proportional to the stimulus, and proceeds	Proliferation proportional to the stimulus
Unabated in the absence of continuation of stimulus	Ceases on cessation of the stimulus

Note: There are circumstances when the two conditions are superimposed and difficult to separate.

Table 7–4. ESSENTIAL DIFFERENCES BETWEEN BENIGN AND MALIGNANT NEOPLASIAS

Benign	Malignant
Noninvasive by groups of cells or individual cells	Invasive
Encapsulated	Nonencapsulated
Highly differentiated, closely resembling normal cells of origin	Well differentiated or poorly differentiated
Mitoses rare	Mitoses relatively frequent
Slowly growing	More rapidly growing
Nonmetastatic to distant sites	Metastatic to distant sites

factors and control mechanisms are summarized schematically in Figures 7–1 and 7–2. Carcinogenesis can, therefore, be regarded as an interference in the normal gene regulation of growth.

In Table 7–6 some of the mechanisms of increased oncogene activation are summarized. Suppressor genes, often referred to as anti-oncogenes, have been shown in some neoplasms to have a control effect and are related to prognosis. Some examples in human cancer are shown in Table 7–7. It is important to be able to classify the different types of human neoplasms and this is summarized in detail in Table 7–8.

The effects that neoplasms can produce clinically are best understood by the knowledge of their mode of spread (Figure 7–3; Table 7–9) and the various products of tumor expression, which can be exploited diagnostically (Table 7–10). The response of the body to growing neoplasm via the policing immune system is summarized in Table 7–11. The major effects of tumors in terms of their clinical presentation are summarized in Table 7–12. It is important to be aware of the different incidence and death rate for cancer not only in the United States (Table 7–13) but the geographic differences and epidemiology aspect of cancer (Table 7–14).

Table 7–5. SUMMARY OF CARCINOGENIC AGENTS IN HUMAN TUMORS

Chemical	Physical	Viral	Genetic Chromosomal	Hormonal
Polycyclic hydrocarbons	Radiation	HTLV-1	Retinoblastoma (chromosome 13)	Androgen estrogen
Tobacco	Ultraviolet light	HIV	Wilms' tumor (chromosome 11)	D.E.S.
Asbestos		Papilloma viruses	Burkitt's lymphoma (chromosome 14)	? Prolactin
Aflatoxins		Herpes II	Chronic myeloid leukemia (chromosome 22)	
Aromatic amines		E.B. Virus	Acute myeloid leukemia	
Nitrosamines		Hepatitis B	Acute lymphoblastic leukemia	
Heavy metals		Molluscum contagiosum	Neurofibromatosis	
Arsenic		Cytomegalovirus	Multiple endocrine adenomatosis	
Vinyl chloride			Familial polyposis coli	
Chemotherapy drugs			Nevoid basal cell carcinoma syndrome	

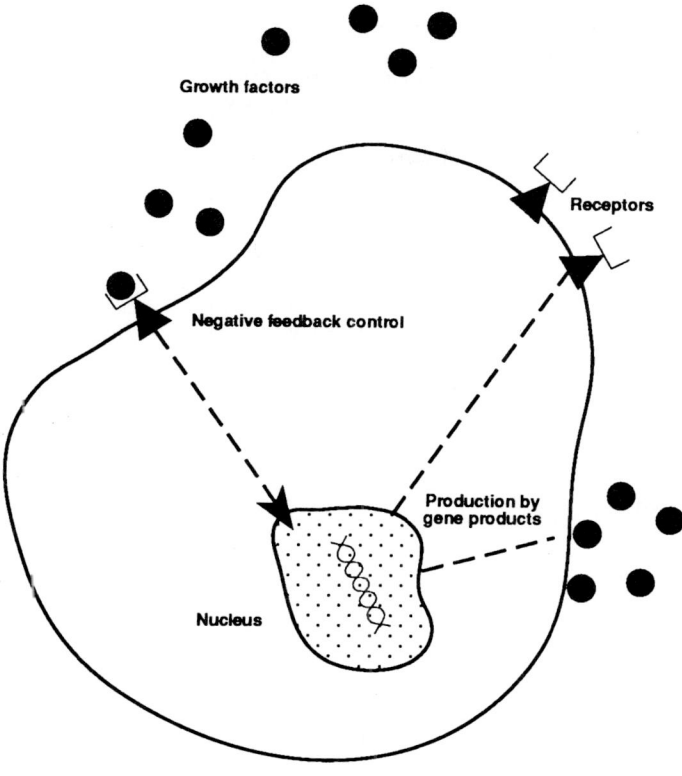

Figure 7–1. Schematic summary of normal cellular growth regulation.

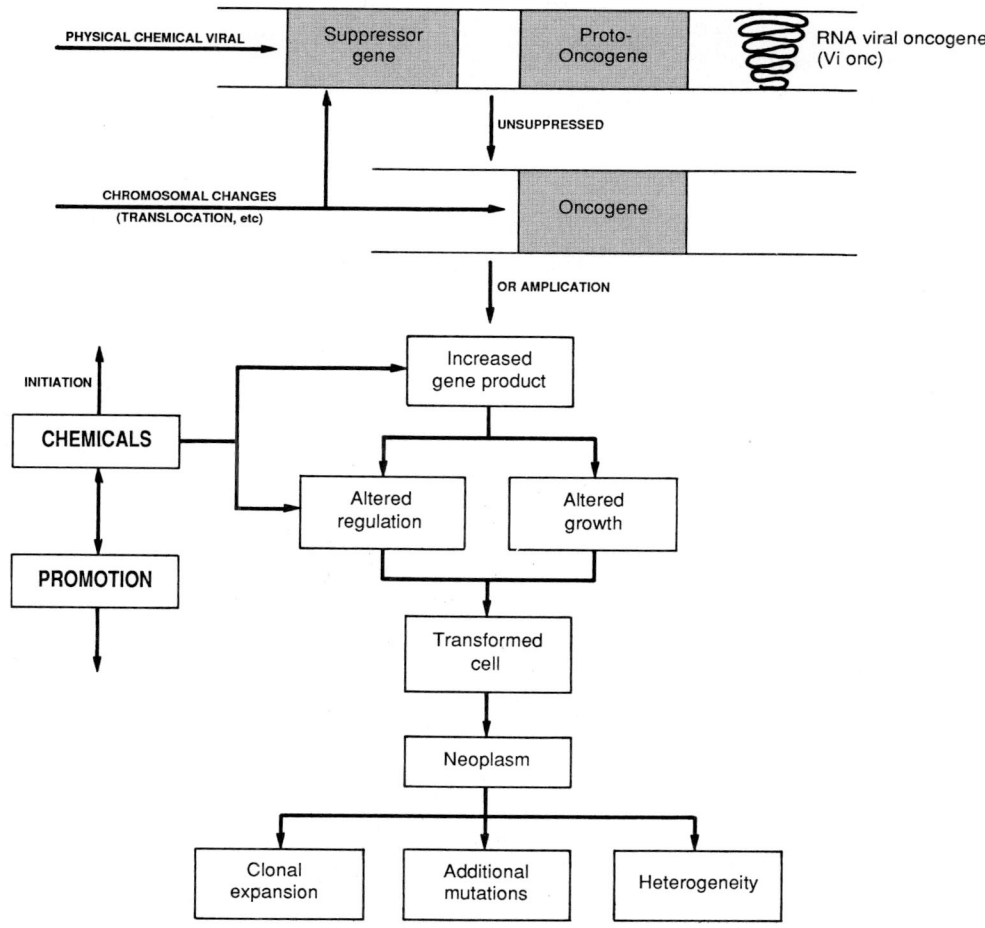

Figure 7–2. Carcinogenesis is a unifying concept.

Table 7–6. EXAMPLES OF POTENTIAL MECHANISMS OF ONCOGENE EXPRESSION

Genetic Alteration	Oncogene Activity	Associated Tumors
Mutation	Recombinant oncogenes	B cell lymphomas
	Insertional activation	Colon carcinoma (K-ras, C-src)
		Myelodysplasic syndromes (K-ras)
Amplification	Increase expression of oncogenes	Neuroblastoma (N-myc)
		Small cell carcinoma of lung (C-myc)
		Breast carcinoma (C-erb)
Decrease	Suppressor genes (anti-oncogenes)	
Deletion	Suppressor genes (anti-oncogenes)	

Table 7–7. EXAMPLES OF HUMAN CANCER IN WHICH SUPPRESSOR GENES (ANTI-ONCOGENES) HAVE BEEN RELATED TO PROGNOSIS

Neuroblastoma
Renal cell carcinoma
Colon carcinoma
Gliomas
Wilms' tumor
Bladder carcinoma
Breast carcinoma
Retinoblastoma
Small cell carcinoma of lung
Osteogenic sarcoma
Meningioma

Table 7–8. CLASSIFICATION OF TUMORS

Tissue or Cell of Origin	Benign	Malignant
Epithelial ectodermal endodermal		
Squamous	Squamous papilloma	Squamous cell carcinoma (epidermoid carcinoma)
Transitional	Transitional cell papilloma	Transitional cell carcinoma
Glandular	Adenoma	Adenocarcinoma (columnar cell mucous secretion, etc.)
	Adenomatous polyp	
	Cystadenoma	
Basal cell	Basal cell papilloma	Basal cell carcinoma (locally malignant)
Melanocyte[a]	Nevus junctional compound intradermal	Malignant melanoma
Connective tissue mesodermal		
Fibrous tissue	Fibroma	Fibrosarcoma
	Dermatofibroma	Dermatofibrosarcoma
	Myxofibroma	Myxofibrosarcoma
Nerve sheath	Neurofibroma	Neurofibrosarcoma
Adipose tissue	Lipoma	Liposarcoma
Smooth muscle	Leiomyoma	Leiomyosarcoma
Skeletal muscle	Rhabdomyoma	Rhabdomyosarcoma
Cartilage	Chondroma	Chondrosarcoma
Bone	Osteoma	Osteogenic sarcoma
Blood vessel	Hemangioma	Hemangiosarcoma
Embryonic cells		
Retinoblasts		Retinoblastoma
Neuroblasts (ganglion)		Neuroblastoma
Kidney		Nephroblastoma (Wilms' tumor)
Liver		Hepatoblastoma

(continued)

Table 7–8. CLASSIFICATION OF TUMORS (continued)

Tissue or Cell of Origin	Benign	Malignant
Pancreas		Pancreatic blastoma
Notochord		Chordoma
Enamel organ		Ameloblastoma (adamantinoma)
Rathke's pouch		Craniopharyngioma
Medulloblast (cerebellum)		Medulloblastoma
Mixed cell type miscellaneous	Benign teratoma	Malignant teratoma
Kidney	Renal cell adenoma	Renal cell carcinoma (hypernephroma)
Liver parenchyma		Hepatocellular carcinoma (hepatoma)
Placenta (trophoblasts)	Hydatidiform mole	Choriocarcinoma
Lymphatics	Lymphangioma	Lymphangiosarcoma
Mesothelium	Mesothelioma (benign) (?)	Malignant mesothelioma (Wilms' tumor)
Hematopoietic and reticuloendothelial		
Lymphatic tissue	Lymphoma (?)	Malignant lymphoma
Lymphocytes		Lymphatic leukemia
Granulocytes		Myeloid leukemia
Monocytes		Monocytic leukemia
Platelets		Megarkaryocytic leukemia
Plasma cells	Plasmacytoma	Multiple myeloma
Red cell precursors	Some forms of polycythemia rubro vera	Erythroderma (DiGuglielmo's disease)
Nervous system		
Glial cells (astrocytes)		Glioblastoma multiforme
Ependymal cells		Ependymoma
Meduloblasts		Medulloblastoma
Choroid plexus		Papilloma of choroid plexus
Pineal gland		Pinealoma
Schwann cells		Schwannoma (neuroadenoma)
Testis		Seminoma
		Teratoma
Ovary		Dysgerminoma
	Granulosa/thecoma	
	Serous cystadenoma	Serous cystadenocarcinoma
	Mucinous cystadenoma	Mucinous cystadenocarcinoma
		Papillary cystadenocarcinoma
		Solid undifferentiated carcinoma
	Brenner tumor	
		Arrhenoblastoma
		Endodermal sinus tumor
	Benign cystic teratoma	Solid malignant teratoma (choriocarcinoma)

[a] Often considered under a separate heading. Because the melanocyte is derived from neural crest and resides in an epithelial location, it is included in this classification as part of epithelial tumors.

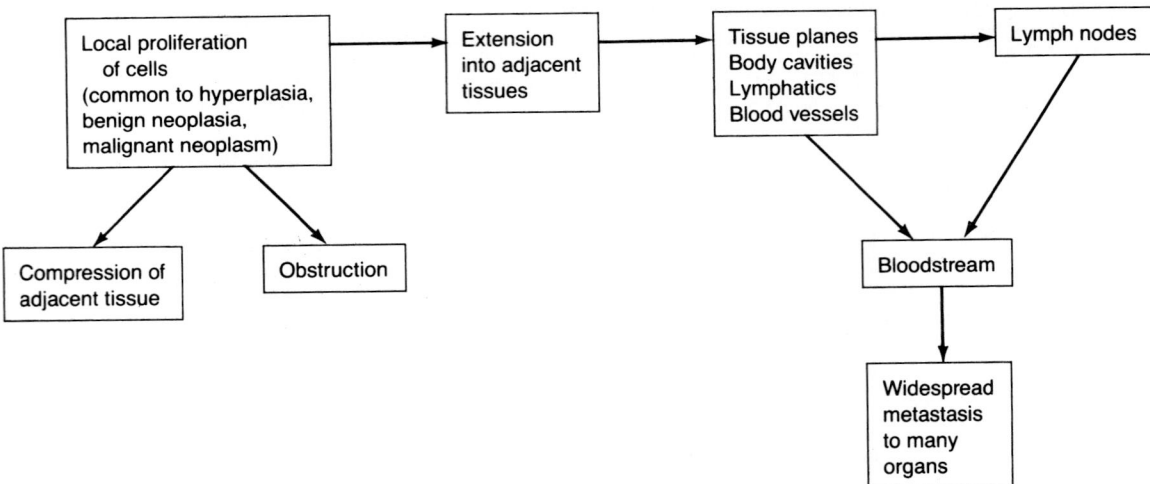

Figure 7–3. Sequential pathways in tumor growth or spread.

Table 7–9. IMPORTANT MODES OF TUMOR SPREAD WITH COMMON EXAMPLES

Mode of Spread	Example
Local spread or invasion	Most common malignant tumors Basal cell carcinoma almost exclusively
Coelomic cavities	Many types of primary epithelial tumors, such as carcinoma of stomach, ovary, and lung Many secondary (metastatic) tumors, such as carcinoma of breast
Cerebrospinal fluid	Primary brain tumors involve the meninges Metastatic carcinomas and malignant melanoma
Lymphatic spread to lymph nodes	Particular epithelial tumors (carcinomas), very occasional mesodermal tumors (sarcomas)
Bloodstream spread	Particularly mesodermal tumors—sarcomas and, in later stages of spread, carcinomas

Table 7–10. SOME EXAMPLES OF TUMOR PRODUCTS AND MARKERS OF IDENTIFICATION

Carcinoembryonic antigen (CEA)	Carcinomas and breast, colon, stomach, pancreas, and lung
Alphafetoprotein (AFP)	Hepatocellular carcinoma, some germ cell neoplasms
Human chorionic gonadotrophin (HCG)	Trophoblastic tumors and some germ cell tumors
Prostatic specific antigen (PSA)	Prostatic carcinoma
Prostatic acid phosphatase	Prostatic carcinoma
Catecholamines	Pheochromocytoma or neuroblastoma
Calcitonin	Medullar carcinoma (C-cell) of thyroid
Serotonin on 5HIAA	Carcinoid tumors
Neurone-specific Enolase	Small cell carcinoma of lung neuroblastoma
Glycoprotein complex	
CA-125	Ovarian carcinoma
CA 19-9	Colonic and pancreatic carcinoma
CA 15-3	Breast carcinoma

Table 7–11. EXPRESSION OF IMMUNOLOGICAL REACTION IN PATIENTS WITH CANCER

Immune surveillance and spontaneous regression

Lymphocytic/monocyte and plasma cell influence in early cancer

Antitumor antibodies   < against live tumor cells
                          < against tumor products

Immune complexes contact tumor antigens   < serum tissue

In-vitro cell mediator immune reaction   < cytotoxic B and T cells
                                            T-cell–surveillance
                                            NKCL–NK cells
                                            –macrophages

Response to various forms of immunotherapy (*often limited*)

Table 7–13. RELATIVE INCIDENCE OF SELECTED CANCERS IN THE UNITED STATES

Rank	Male	Female
1.	Prostate	Breast
2.	Lung	Colorectal
3.	Colorectal	Lung
4.	Urinary	Uterus
5.	Leukemia/lymphoma	Leukemia/lymphoma
6.	Oral	Ovary
7.	Skin (excluding melanoma)	Skin (excluding melanoma)
8.	Pancreas	Pancreas

Table 7–12. EXAMPLES OF MAJOR EFFECTS OF TUMORS

Obstruction or compression	Hyperplasia of prostate with urinary obstruction Benign neoplasia of bronchus, bowel, or base of brain Malignant tumors of bronchus, bowel, etc.
Ulceration	Skin tumors, benign or malignant, especially basal cell rodent ulcer, carcinoma of stomach, colon carcinoma
Infection	Any tumor of skin with surface ulceration or tumor of bronchial tree of gastrointestinal tract or bladder Lymphomas and leukemias in which immune suppression may occur
Anemia	Effect of blood loss from ulcerated tumor, effects of bone marrow replacement by tumor cells Unknown mechanisms
Cachexia	Extremely variable and complex, seen in a variety of metastatic tumors or obstructive tumors, such as esophageal carcinoma
Effects of products of tumors	Hormones: thyroid, adrenal, catecholamine, protein by appropriate neoplasms of these tissues Inappropriate hormone production, ie, antidiuretic hormone by bronchogenic carcinoma

Table 7–14. AGE-ADJUSTED CANCER DEATH RATES IN 50 COUNTRIES

	Highest Ranks		Lowest Ranks		USA (Rank)	
	Male	*Female*	*Male*	*Female*	*Male*	*Female*
All cancers	Hungary Czechoslovakia Belgium	Denmark Scotland Hungary	Peru (50th)	Peru (50th)	26th	20th
Lung	Scotland Belgium Holland	Scotland Hong Kong United States	Peru (50th)	Peru (50th)	12th	3rd
Colorectal	Czechoslovakia Denmark Austria	New Zealand Denmark Hungary	Peru (50th)	Peru (50th)	22nd	20th
Prostate	Martinique Switzerland Norway		Hong Kong (50th)		23rd	
Breast		England Malta Denmark		Peru (50th)		16th
Leukemia	Luxemburg Iceland Hungary	Kuwait Luxemburg Denmark	Surinam (50th)	Surinam (50th)	6th	11th
Stomach	Costa Rica Japan Former Soviet Union	Former Soviet Union Costa Rica Ecuador	United States (50th)	United States (50th)	50th	50th

Questions

DIRECTIONS (Questions 599 through 648): Each of the numbered items or incomplete statements in this section is followed by answers or by completions of the statement. Select the ONE lettered answer or completion that is BEST in each case.

599. Which of the following is/are neoplasms of epithelial origin?

    (A) carcinoma of the esophagus
    (B) carcinoma of the stomach
    (C) laryngeal papilloma
    (D) basal cell carcinoma
    (E) all of the above

600. A needle biopsy of the liver shows a mucinous-secreting adenocarcinoma. The most likely site of origin is

    (A) bladder
    (B) cerebellum
    (C) anal canal
    (D) colon
    (E) prostate

601. Which of the following characteristics is typical of a sarcoma?

    (A) pleomorphism
    (B) blood vessel invasion
    (C) metastases to distant sites
    (D) mesodermal origin
    (E) all of the above

602. Angiogenesis in a neoplasm is better characterized as

    (A) blood-borne spread of tumor cells
    (B) invasion of blood vessels by tumor cells
    (C) a tumor arising from primitive blood-forming tissue
    (D) the ingrowth of new blood vessels into a growing tumor
    (E) central necrosis seen in rapidly growing tumors due to outgrowing of the blood supply

603. Which of the following tumors is/are associated with hormone dependence?

    (A) carcinoma of the prostate
    (B) carcinoma of the breast in females
    (C) carcinoma of the thyroid
    (D) carcinoma of the endometrium
    (E) all of the above

604. On gross examination, a keloid is characterized as

    (A) a protruding tumor-like scar
    (B) a form of early granulation tissue
    (C) a benign tumor of melanocytic origin
    (D) the outcome of most infected wounds
    (E) a granuloma in response to mycobacteria

605. A tumor composed of tissues representing all three embryologic germ layers is called

    (A) adenocarcinoma
    (B) carcinosarcoma
    (C) mixed mesodermal tumor
    (D) teratoma
    (E) papillary adenocarcinoma

606. A benign neoplasm characterized by an abnormal amount of tissue indigenous to the area is best described as

(A) carcinosarcoma
(B) embryonal tumor
(C) hamartoma
(D) mixed tumor
(E) teratoma

607. Which of the following best describes the phenomenon of epithelial dysplasia?

(A) an increase in thickness of the epithelium because of increased number of cells
(B) a decrease in thickness of the epithelium because of decrease in number of dividing cells
(C) an irregular proliferation and maturation of cells throughout the layers of the epithelium
(D) an increase in thickness of the epithelium because of enlargement of the component cells
(E) absence of epithelium because of lack of cell proliferation

608. Which of the following statement(s) is/are correct?

(A) The incidence of malignancy tends to increase with age.
(B) Carcinoma of the breast is more frequent in females than in males.
(C) Hormones may inhibit or promote tumor growth.
(D) Certain tumors characteristically appear in certain age groups.
(E) All of the above statements are correct.

609. Which of the following is/are a neoplasm of mesenchymal origin?

(A) leiomyoma
(B) hemangioma
(C) lipoma
(D) rhabdomyoma
(E) all of the above

610. The pathologic condition in which one type of adult tissue is replaced by another is termed

(A) dysplasia
(B) anaplasia
(C) metaplasia
(D) aplasia
(E) hypoplasia

611. A unequivocal feature of malignancy is

(A) cellular pleomorphism
(B) lymphocytic infiltration at the edges of the tumor
(C) metastases
(D) numerous mitotic figures
(E) plasma cell infiltration at the edges of the tumor

612. Decrease in size of a previously normal-sized and normally developed organ is called

(A) aplasia
(B) hypoplasia
(C) atrophy
(D) metaplasia
(E) agenesis

613. An epithelial neoplasm, forming glandular structures, and invading the surrounding tissue is better described as

(A) adenocarcinoma
(B) adenomatous hyperplasia
(C) adenomatous polyp
(D) adenomyosis
(E) carcinosarcoma

614. Endoscopic findings of the gastric mucosa and duodenum show a submucosal discrete nodules. They are composed of pleomorphic cells in nests with fine fine granules of brownish pigment in the cytoplasm. The most likely diagnosis is

(A) adrenal cell carcinoma
(B) small intestinal adenocarcinoma
(C) hepatocellular carcinoma
(D) metastatic malignant melanoma
(E) gastric carcinoma

615. The most common cause of death from cancer in women in the United States is

(A) carcinoma of the urinary bladder
(B) carcinoma of the liver
(C) carcinoma of the cervix of uterus
(D) carcinoma of the breast
(E) carcinoma of the ovary

616. The most common form of cancer seen in most black African countries is

(A) carcinoma of the colon
(B) carcinoma of the cervix and uterus
(C) carcinoma of the breast
(D) carcinoma of the lung
(E) carcinoma of the pancreas

617. Which of the following tumors has been associated most strongly with a possible viral etiology?

(A) leiomyoma of the uterus
(B) carcinoma of the lung
(C) carcinoma of the esophagus
(D) Burkitt's lymphoma
(E) histiocytic lymphoma

618. Indicate the tumor which is most commonly associated with the overproduction of carcino-embryonic antigen

(A) carcinoma of the esophagus
(B) testicular seminoma
(C) carcinoma of the colon
(D) malignant lymphoma
(E) testicular teratoma

619. Which of the following characteristics is/are typical of benign neoplasms?

(A) encapsulation
(B) low mitotic index
(C) well differentiated
(D) slow growth
(E) all of the above

620. An increase in the number of cells in an organ or tissue is known as

(A) agenesis
(B) aplasia
(C) metaplasia
(D) hyperplasia
(E) hypertrophy

621. The etiology of bronchogenic carcinoma is most clearly associated with

(A) genetic abnormalities in patients
(B) familial tendency
(C) cigarette smoking
(D) respiratory viruses
(E) emphysema

622. Workers in the aniline dye industry are most prone to which of the following tumors?

(A) carcinoma of the lung
(B) carcinoma of the stomach
(C) squamous cell carcinoma of the skin
(D) basal cell carcinoma of the skin
(E) carcinoma of the urinary bladder

623. Exposure to sunlight (although does not seem to be the only predisposing factor) is most closely associated with

(A) squamous cell carcinoma of the skin
(B) carcinoma of the lung
(C) carcinoma of the stomach
(D) malignant melanoma
(E) carcinoma of the urinary bladder

624. Which term is most likely to fit the description of the uterus during pregnancy?

(A) hyperplasia
(B) hypertrophy
(C) aplasia
(D) agenesis
(E) dysplasia

625. Which of the following best describes post-menopausal small uterus?

(A) hyperplasia
(B) hypertrophy
(C) aplasia
(D) agenesis
(E) atrophy

626. Which term most closely describes lack of development in a lobe of the lung in a new-born infant?

(A) hyperplasia
(B) hypertrophy
(C) aplasia
(D) agenesis
(E) atrophy

627. A localized thickness of the buccal mucosa resulting from an increase in the number of epithelial cells is

(A) hyperplasia
(B) hypertrophy
(C) aplasia
(D) agenesis
(E) dysplasia

628. Which of the following tumors is most associated with ingestion of aflatoxins?

(A) carcinoma of the cervix
(B) carcinoma of the endometrium
(C) carcinoma of the urinary bladder
(D) hepatocellular carcinoma (hepatoma)
(E) carcinoma of the stomach

629. Which of the following is most associated with industrial exposure to naphthalenes and related products?

(A) carcinoma of the cervix
(B) carcinoma of the stomach
(C) carcinoma of the endometrium
(D) carcinoma of the urinary bladder
(E) hepatocellular carcinoma (hepatoma)

Questions 630 through 633. (Refer to Figures 7–4 and 7–5.)

630. The gross appearance (Figure 7–4) is best described as

(A) an ulcer
(B) an adenoma
(C) an inflamed polyp
(D) a papilloma
(E) a sarcoma

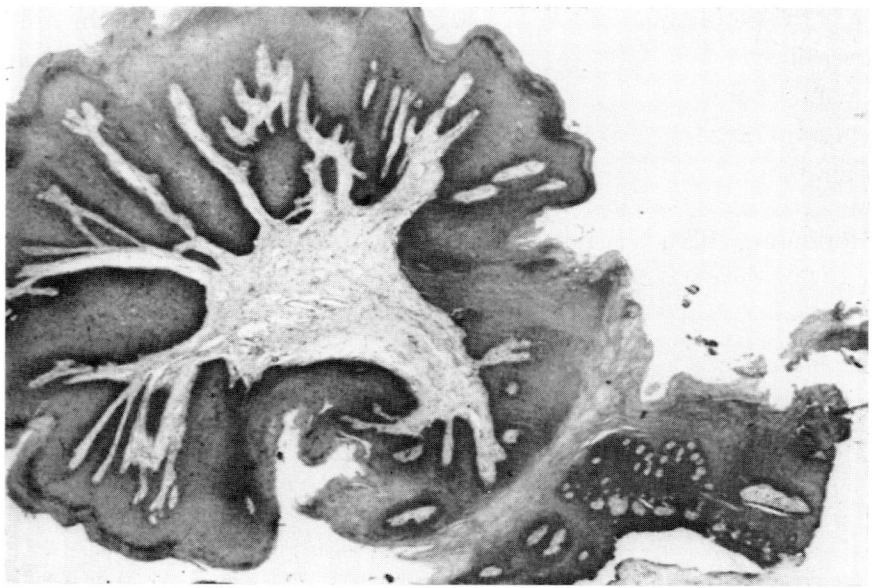

Figure 7–4. Low-power photomicrograph of a skin lesion removed from the shoulder of a 40-year-old white male.

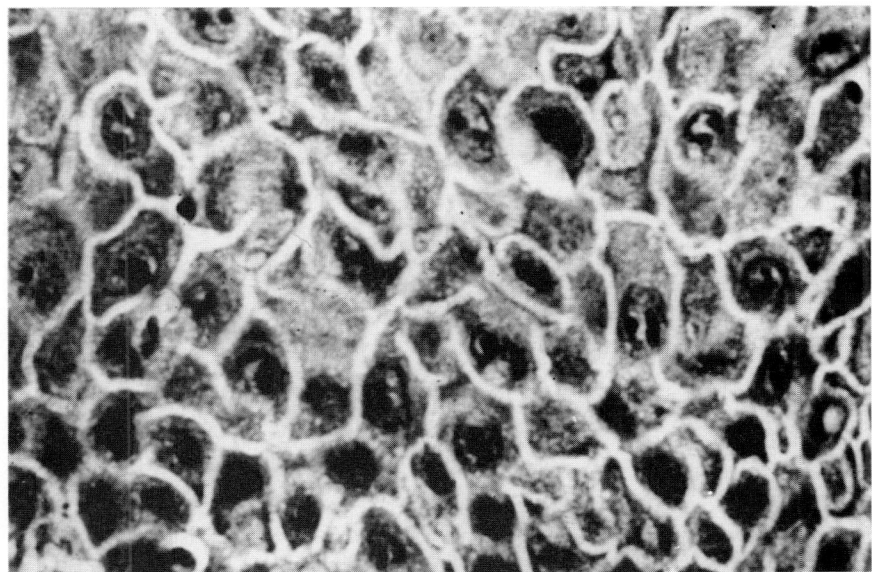

Figure 7–5. High-power photomicrograph of a section taken from the lesion depicted in Figure 7–4.

631. The high-power view (Figure 7–5) enables the epithelium to be recognized as

(A) columnar epithelium
(B) stratified squamous epithelium
(C) transitional cell epithelium
(D) mesothelium
(E) smooth muscle

632. On the basis of the appearance, the lesion is best classified as

(A) sweat gland adenoma
(B) transitional cell carcinoma
(C) squamous papilloma
(D) squamous cell carcinoma (poorly differentiated)
(E) leiomyosarcoma

633. After complete excision of the lesion, the most likely sequela would be

(A) metastatic spread to regional lymph nodes
(B) metastatic spread to lungs via the bloodstream

(C) recurrence of the lesion locally
(D) none of the above
(E) all of the above

Questions 634 through 636. (Refer to Figure 7–6.)

634. The photomicrograph demonstrates

(A) malignant spindle cells
(B) malignant epithelial cells
(C) ferruginous (asbestos) bodies
(D) acid-fast bacilli
(E) Curschmann's spirals

635. Additional history useful in assessing this patient includes

(A) excessive smoking
(B) asthma
(C) exposure to tuberculosis
(D) occupation
(E) none of the above

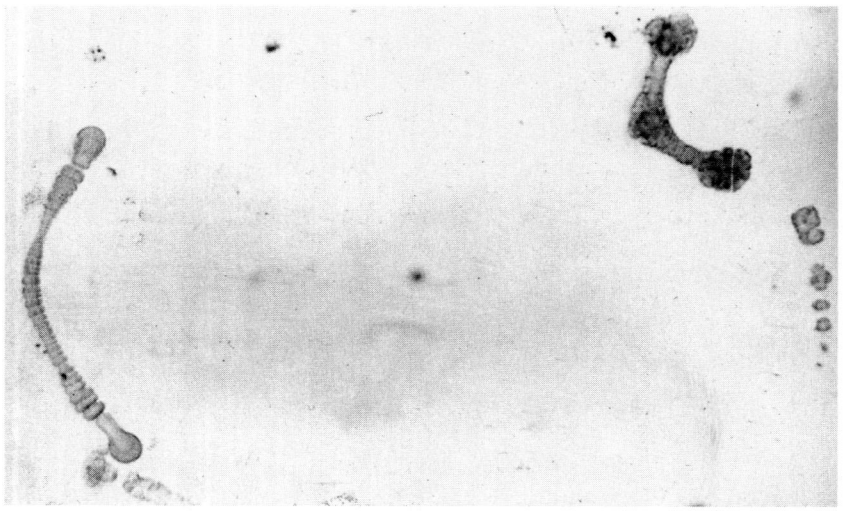

Figure 7–6. A 60-year-old male has dyspnea and bilateral pulmonary infiltrates. Sputum examination shows features seen in the photomicrograph.

636. The patient also is more likely to have or develop

(A) mesothelioma of pleura
(B) history of other allergies
(C) metastatic tumor deposits in lymphatics of the lung
(D) tuberculous pneumonia
(E) status asthmaticus

Questions 637 and 638. (Refer to Figure 7–7.)

637. The photomicrograph shows

(A) normal cervical squamous epithelium
(B) transitional epithelium
(C) chronic cervicitis
(D) squamous carcinoma in situ (intraepithelial carcinoma)
(E) invasive squamous carcinoma

638. The chance that this patient has metastatic carcinoma in the inguinal lymph nodes is

(A) 0%
(B) 10%
(C) 30%
(D) 50%
(E) 100%

Questions 639 and 640. (Refer to Figure 7–8.)

639. The photomicrograph demonstrates

(A) normal squamous epithelium to the right and squamous epithelium showing dysplasia to the left
(B) normal squamous epithelium to the left and squamous epithelium showing dysplasia to the right
(C) variants of cervical squamous epithelium
(D) normal squamous epithelium to the left and metaplastic epithelium to the right
(E) squamous metaplasia of epithelium at left and malignant squamous epithelium at right

640. The lesion depicted may

(A) regress
(B) remain unchanged
(C) develop into carcinoma
(D) all of the above
(E) none of the above

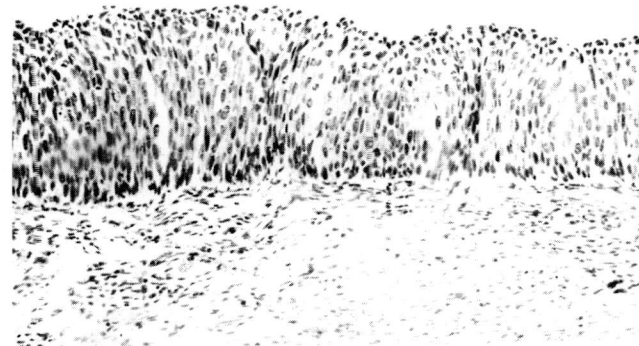

Figure 7–7. Photomicrograph from a section of a LEEP (loop electrocautery excisional procedure) biopsy in a 25-year-old female with an abnormal pap smear.

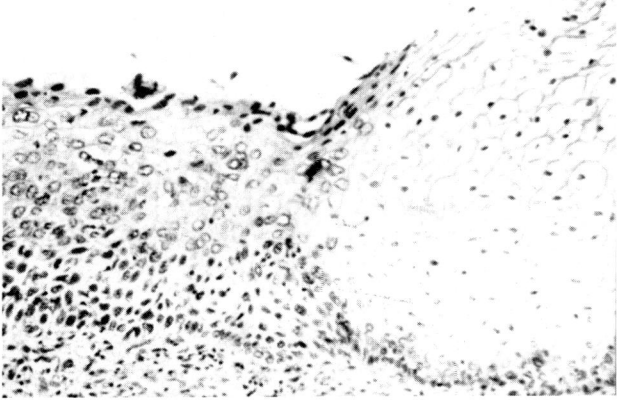

Figure 7–8. Photomicrograph of a section taken from a biopsy of the cervix performed after a Papanicolaou smear that contained abnormal cells.

Questions 641 through 644. (Refer to Figures 7–9 and 7–10.)

641. The low-power appearance (Figure 7–9) is best described as

   (A) diverticulum

   (B) pseudopolyposis

   (C) sessile polyp

   (D) pedunculated polyp

   (E) annular constriction

642. The high-power appearance (Figure 7–10) is best described as

   (A) well-differentiated adenocarcinoma

   (B) poorly differentiated adenocarcinoma

   (C) inflammatory polyp

   (D) adenomatous polyp

   (E) metaplasia

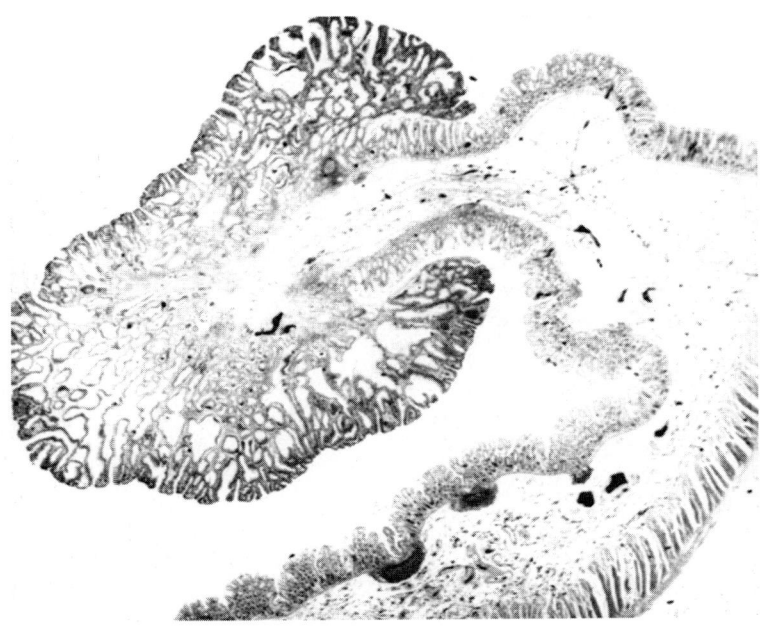

Figure 7–9. Low-power photomicrograph of a segment of large intestine.

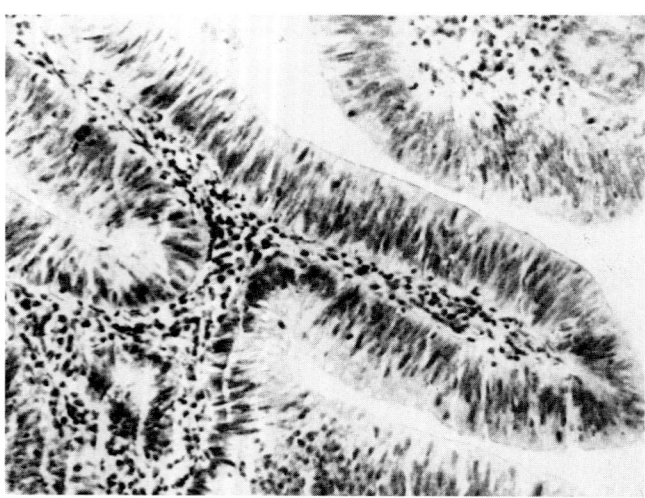

Figure 7–10. High-power view of the lesion shown in Figure 7–9.

643. The ultimate outcome of the lesion is

(A) metastasis via the lymphatics
(B) blood-borne tumor spread to the liver
(C) both of the above
(D) neither of the above
(E) no further growth after removal

644. The best assessment of prognosis based on these findings alone is

(A) poor
(B) moderate
(C) excellent
(D) impossible to determine
(E) dependent on patient's age

Questions 645 through 648. (Refer to Figure 7–11.)

645. The lesion is most likely

(A) inflammatory
(B) ischemic
(C) infectious
(D) neoplastic
(E) immunologic

646. The lesion is most likely

(A) tuberculous pneumonia
(B) healing pulmonary infarction
(C) Wegener's granulomatosis
(D) bronchogenic carcinoma
(E) centrilobular emphysema

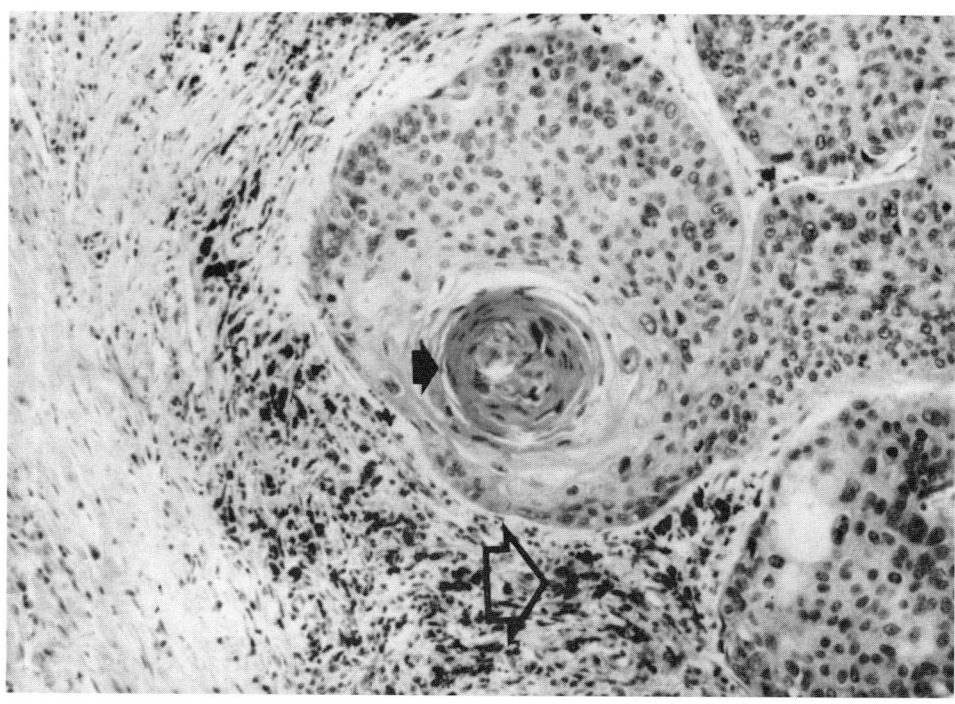

Figure 7–11. Histologic section of a lesion removed from a 60-year-old male.

647. The small solid arrow points to

  (A) a Langhans' giant cell
  (B) coagulated bronchial epithelium
  (C) fibrinoid necrosis of a pulmonary artery
  (D) a squamous pearl
  (E) a psammoma body, or calcospherite

648. The large open arrow points to

  (A) degenerating elastic fibers
  (B) epithelioid cells
  (C) polymorphonuclear leukocytes
  (D) anthrocotic pigment
  (E) pores of Kohn

DIRECTIONS (Questions 649 through 712): Each group of items in this section consists of a list of lettered options followed by a set of numbered words or phrases. For each numbered word or phrase, select the ONE lettered option that is most closely associated with it. Each lettered option may be selected once, more than once, or not at all.

Questions 649 through 651

  (A) malignant neoplasm
  (B) benign neoplasm
  (C) hyperplasia
  (D) aplasia
  (E) teratoma

649. Adenoma

650. Lack of red cell precursors in bone marrow

651. Liposarcoma

Questions 652 and 653

  (A) carcinoma
  (B) sarcoma
  (C) adenoma
  (D) papilloma
  (E) teratoma

652. A benign tumor of epithelial origin attached to the normal epithelium by a stalk

653. A malignant tumor of mesodermal origin

Questions 654 through 659

  (A) a tumor that predominantly metastasizes via the bloodstream
  (B) a lymph node filled with tumor composed of abnormal epidermoid cells
  (C) a Krukenberg tumor
  (D) a tumor that produces alpha-fetoprotein (AFP)
  (E) cells that produce human chorionic gonadotropin (HCG)

654. Choriocarcinoma

655. Secondary carcinoma of the stomach in ovaries

656. Hepatocellular carcinoma

657. Osteogenic sarcoma

658. Bronchogenic carcinoma

659. Fibrosarcoma

Questions 660 through 662

  (A) neuroblastoma
  (B) malignant fibrous histiocytoma
  (C) bronchogenic carcinoma
  (D) squamous cell carcinoma
  (E) adenocarcinoma

660. Cells of origin thought to be derived from fetal neural crest

661. More common in childhood than in adult life

662. The adrenal is the most common site.

Questions 663 and 664

  (A) stage I
  (B) stage II
  (C) stage III
  (D) stage IV
  (E) insufficient data to stage completely

663. Breast carcinoma, T1, N0, M0

664. Colon carcinoma, T3, N2, M1

Questions 665 and 666

(A) papillary thyroid carcinoma
(B) mammary fibroadenoma
(C) pleural mesothelioma
(D) gastric adenocarcinoma
(E) liver cell carcinoma

665. A tumor associated with asbestos exposure in a nonsmoker

666. A tumor associated with hepatitis B virus carrier state

Questions 667 through 670

(A) hyperplasia
(B) dysplasia
(C) atrophy
(D) aplasia
(E) metaplasia

667. Increase in the thickness of the cardiac left ventricle with essential hypertension

668. Cellular change seen with cervical intracellular neoplasia (CIN), grade II

669. Congenital absence of a pulmonary lobe or segment

670. Squamous epithelium found in the bronchial mucosal of a smoker

Questions 671 and 672

(A) prostate specific antigen
(B) calcitonin
(C) catecholamines
(D) CA 19-9
(E) CA 15-3

671. Most likely product of a medullary carcinoma of thyroid

672. Most likely product of a pheochromocytoma

Questions 673 through 676

(A) lipoma
(B) osteogenic sarcoma
(C) rhabdomyosarcoma

(D) renal cell carcinoma
(E) liposarcoma

673. Malignant tumor of adipocytes

674. Benign tumor of adipocytes

675. Production of osteoid by malignant cells

676. Myosin may be detected with monoclonal antibodies

Questions 677 through 680

(A) adenoma
(B) adenocarcinoma
(C) chondroma
(D) chondrosarcoma
(E) leiomyoma

677. Benign neoplasm of smooth muscle cells

678. Malignant neoplasm arising from glandular cells

679. Benign neoplasm arising from glandular cells

680. Benign neoplasm arising from cartilage cells

Questions 681 through 684

(A) gastric adenocarcinoma
(B) cervical squamous cell carcinoma
(C) colonic adenocarcinoma
(D) cutaneous basal cell carcinoma
(E) appendiceal adenocarcinoma

681. More frequently seen in Western populations with high-fat, low-fiber diets

682. More frequently seen in African women

683. More frequently seen in whites who have extensive actinic dermatitis

684. More frequently seen in Japanese and Russian populations

Questions 685 through 688

(A) Epstein–Barr virus
(B) hepatitis B virus
(C) mumps virus
(D) human immunodeficiency virus
(E) human papilloma virus

685. Carcinoma of the cervix

686. Hepatocellular carcinoma

687. Burkitt's lymphoma

688. Kaposi's sarcoma

Questions 689 through 692

(A) undescended testicle
(B) tuberous sclerosis
(C) ulcerative colitis
(D) Paget's disease of the bone
(E) xeroderma pigmentosum

689. Increased incidence of cutaneous neoplasms

690. Increased incidence of colonic adenocarcinoma

691. Increased incidence of seminoma

692. Increased incidence of osteosarcoma

Questions 693 through 696

(A) hepatic angiosarcoma
(B) liver cell carcinoma
(C) vaginal adenosis
(D) mammary phylloides tumor
(E) oral carcinoma

693. Ingestion of aflatoxins

694. Chewing betel nuts and leaves

695. Maternal antepartum administration of diethylstilbesterol

696. Vinyl chloride exposure

Questions 697 through 700

(A) neuron stimulating factor
(B) monoclonal immunoglobulin
(C) corticosteroids
(D) prostate-specific antigen
(E) erythropoietin

697. Renal cell carcinoma

698. Prostatic adenocarcinoma

699. Multiple myeloma

700. Adrenal cortical adenoma

Questions 701 through 704

(A) malignant melanoma
(B) malignant mesothelioma
(C) adenocarcinoma
(D) squamous cell carcinoma
(E) transitional cell carcinoma
(F) lymphoblastic leukemia
(G) Hodgkin's disease
(H) fibrosarcoma

701. A 62-year-old man who has been smoking two packs of cigarettes a day for the past 35 years is found to have a 2.5-cm solitary nodule in the left upper lobe of his lung. A fine needle aspiration biopsy reveals abundant malignant cells with intercellular bridges, intracellular keratin production, and keratin pearl formation. No glandular structures are evident. What is the most likely diagnosis?

702. A 32-year-old woman is seen by her family physician because of an enlarging pigmented skin lesion on her back that now measures about 2 × 1.5 cm. It is variegated by hues of brown, black, and pink. The central portion of the lesion is raised and beginning to ulcerate. A biopsy shows nests of atypical melanocytes scattered up through the epidermis and invading down into the dermis. What is the most likely diagnosis?

703. A 6-year-old child with Down syndrome is noted to have recent onset of bleeding gums and pallor. At the doctor's office the child's white blood cell count is found to be markedly elevated due to a monomorphic population of immature lymphoid cells. A bone marrow biopsy reveals almost complete replacement of the medullary space by similar appearing blast cells. What is the most likely diagnosis?

704. A 67-year-old postmenopausal woman has been feeling excessively tired for about 2 months. Her lab work is remarkable for a microcytic anemia and an elevated CEA. A barium enema x-ray study reveals an "apple-core" mass lesion in the right colon. A biopsy of this area demonstrates malignant gland-forming epithelial cells. What is the most likely diagnosis?

Questions 705 through 708

(A) adenocarcinoma
(B) lymphoma
(C) adenoma
(D) hemangioma
(E) transitional cell carcinoma
(F) insulinoma
(G) malignant astrocytoma
(H) chronic myelogeneous leukemia

705. A 45-year-old male has had a slowly growing reddish nodule on his forearm for about 2 years. He finally decides to have a surgeon remove it. Microscopically the nodule is composed of benign varying sized blood vessels. What is the most likely diagnosis?

706. A 51-year-old female is found to have an elevated white blood cell count on her annual physical. The elevated count is due to an increased number of myelocytes, metamyelocytes, and band neutrophils. A chromosomal analysis of these myeloid cells reveals the presence of a Philadelphia chromosome. What is the most likely diagnosis?

707. A retired rubber worker notices that his urine is occasionally brownish or reddish in color. At the doctor's office this tinctorial abnormality is found to be hematuria. His bladder is examined via cystoscopy and a biopsy of a large ulcerating tumor is obtained. The lesion is composed of malignant transitional cells. What is the most likely diagnosis?

708. A 41-year-old woman has a seizure while at work and is taken to the hospital. On examination she denies ever having had seizures before. A CT scan of the brain demonstrates a large poorly circumscribed, focally necrotic tumor in the frontal and parietal lobes. A biopsy of this area contains malignant astrocytes. What is the most likely diagnosis?

Questions 709 through 712

(A) metaplasia
(B) dysplasia
(C) hypertrophy
(D) atrophy
(E) hyperplasia

709. Replacement of one differentiated cell type by another mature cell

710. Disordered growth accompanied by nonuniformity of cellular appearance

711. Increase in cell number

712. Increase in cell size

DIRECTIONS (Questions 713 through 722): Each of the numbered items or incomplete statements in this section is followed by answers or by completions of the statement. Select the ONE lettered answer or completion that is BEST in each case.

713. During pregnancy there is an increase in the uterine smooth muscle cells of the myometrium. This is known as

(A) physiologic hypertrophy
(B) physiologic hyperplasia
(C) physiologic metaplasia
(D) pathologic hyperplasia
(E) pathologic metaplasia

714. The increase in size of a neoplasm depends on the doubling time which

(A) is related to the growth fraction and rate of cell loss
(B) is related to its clonality
(C) is the same as the cell cycle time
(D) is related to the age of the patient
(E) is related to the length of the cell cycle time

715. Routinely in cancers of the breast the estrogen and progesterone receptors are measured to

(A) confirm the histologic diagnosis
(B) determine the necessity for further diagnostic evaluation
(C) prove that the neoplasm is monoclonal
(D) predict the response to anti-estrogen therapy
(E) predict the likelihood of metastases

716. In non-neoplastic cells, the tumor suppressor gene p53 is a

(A) cell surface protein that is a growth factor receptor

(B) cellular matrix protein that binds growth factors

(C) nuclear protein that can inhibit cell growth

(D) secreted peptide growth factor

(E) nuclear protein that is a receptor for growth inhibiting steroids

717. What is the role of laminin in a malignant neoplasm in invasion and production of metastasis?

(A) It is an autocrine growth factor.

(B) It is a collagenase that degrades the extracellular matrix.

(C) It promotes adhesion of neoplastic cells to the extracellular matrix.

(D) It promotes movement of neoplastic cells through the degraded extracellular matrix.

(E) It inhibits neoplastic cell binding to fibronectin.

718. In what organ has cytologic screening produced a marked reduction in mortality?

(A) breast

(B) lung

(C) uterine cervix

(D) pancreas

(E) prostate

719. In carcinoma of the breast, the first area to develop metastases via lymphatic or blood-stream is

(A) the axillary lymph nodes

(B) the arterial system to the brain

(C) the portal circulation to the liver

(D) the systemic venous system to the heart

(E) the lungs through the pulmonary artery

720. In a malignant tumor, it is important to evaluate the existence of metastasis to determine

(A) grade

(B) stage

(C) histologic type

(D) response to chemotherapy

(E) clonality

721. What is the most common skin cancer?

(A) sweat gland carcinoma

(B) basal cell carcinoma

(C) squamous cell carcinoma

(D) Merkel cell carcinoma

(E) metastatic carcinoma

722. The wild type of p53 can be best characterized as

(A) an oncogene

(B) mitogen

(C) a tumor suppressor gene

(D) a metastases inhibitory gene

(E) a proto-oncogene

Answers and Explanations

599. **(E)** This is a question of terminology (Table 7–8). The terms "carcinoma" and "papilloma" are used to denote neoplasms that are of epithelial origin. *(Cotran et al., pp. 261–264)*

600. **(D)** This is a practical problem often faced by pathologists and clinicians when patients have symptoms of metastasis before the primary site is discovered. All primary tumors can produce metastasis to the liver, but the colon is by far the most common site and often produces a mucus-secreting adenocarcinoma arising from the glandular epithelium. *(Cotran et al., pp. 827–833)*

601. **(E)** Sarcomas tend to remain locally invasive or to spread by the bloodstream. This probably is related to the fact that they are of mesodermal origin (Tables 7–8 and 7–9) and often have large vascular spaces that readily connect with the vasculature of normal surrounding tissues, hence, their ability to spread more rapidly by that route. Pleomorphism or a variation in size and shape and appearance of the nuclei and the cell in general is relatively characteristic of these neoplasms. *(Rubin and Farber, pp. 164–167)*

602. **(D)** As the name implies, angioneogenesis is the formation of new blood vessels. It has been shown that these often are of host origin, growing into the tumor and stimulated by the release from the tumor of substances designated angiogenesis factors. *(Cotran et al., pp. 301–302)*

603. **(E)** All of the tumors listed may be altered by hormonal treatment or manipulation, such as ablation of estrogen-producing tissues in carcinoma of the breast or castration and administration of estrogen in carcinoma of the prostate. In the thyroid, the cancer actually may produce thyroid hormone and be destroyed by uptake of radiolabeled iodine by the functioning tumor cells. Not all of the cancer cells in prostate, breast, or thyroid, however, are hormone dependent. This depends on the presence of estrogen or progesterone receptors in breast cancer, the production of hormone receptors in prostate cancer, and the actual production of a functioning hormone in carcinoma of the thyroid. *(Chandrasoma and Taylor, p. 297)*

604. **(A)** Keloid is an overexuberant production of collagen bundles, usually following a wound that may be trivial. It often is a tumorlike mass but is not neoplastic in the true sense of the word in that the phenomenon is self-limiting and does not progress or spread or metastasize as do other forms of neoplastic growth. The formation of keloid often is a racially determined condition, and blacks have a high propensity for producing such scarring, with gross distortion, particularly in response to burns. *(Rubin and Farber, p. 99)*

605. **(D)** Teratoma, which may be benign or malignant, is the only tumor type in which all three germ cell layers are represented. All the others contain one or two cell types. Teratomas typically are seen in the ovaries or testis but also occur in other sites, such as the mediastinum and retroperitoneum. *(Cotran et al., pp. 262–263)*

606. **(C)** Hamartoma is a conglomeration of tissues that are normal to the area but haphazardly arranged in an abnormal fashion. All of the neoplasias listed contain a mixture of different cell types, but only in the hamartoma are the cells normal to that particular area. These are best regarded as developmental anomalies rather than true neoplasms, and they are never malignant and, therefore, do not metastasize. *(Cotran et al., p. 263)*

607. **(C)** This is a question of definition of the different types of cell growth (Tables 7–1 and 7–2). As described, dysplasia is an abnormal sequence of changes in maturation or development of cell types in a tissue or organ. It is best seen in the cervix of the uterus, where normally an ordered regular maturation of basal cells results in flattened squamous epithelium at the surface. In dysplasia, nucleated cells appear throughout the layers even at the surface and can be shared and thus recognized in cytologic preparations. Dysplasia can, therefore, occur in any epithelium where maturation produces a series of layers. Dysplasia, in company with dyscrasia and dystrophy, is often used in describing tissues with other perversions of cell growth. All are self-limiting and distinct from neoplasia. *(Rubin and Farber, p. 217)*

608. **(E)** It is true that incidence of malignancy tends to increase with age. It also is true that hormones may inhibit or promote tumor growth. Certain tumors characteristically appear in certain age groups. Carcinoma of the breast is more frequent in females than in males. *(Chandrasoma and Taylor, pp. 269–271)*

609. **(E)** Hemangioma, lipoma, rhabdomyoma, and leiomyoma are tumors of mesenchymal mesodermal origin (Table 7–8). *(Chandrasoma and Taylor, pp. 267–268)*

610. **(C)** Metaplasia is defined as an acquired change of tissue or organ resulting from change in one adult cell type to a different adult cell type (Table 7–2). All of the other terms describe various forms of cellular proliferation or lack of proliferation, but only metaplasia implies a change from one established adult type to another. An example is squamous metaplasia of the bronchus, in which the normal stratified squamous epithelium replaces the nor-

mal columnar cell epithelium. Similar changes are seen in the uterine cervix, in which columnar epithelium sometimes replaces the squamous epithelium at the squamocolumnar junction. *(Chandrasoma and Taylor, p. 254)*

611. **(C)** Cellular pleomorphism, numerous mitotic figures, lymphocyte infiltration at the edge of the tumor, and plasma cell infiltration at the edge of the tumor are features common to all forms of malignancy and may even be seen in some benign tumors. However, as shown in Table 7–4, metastasis, ie, spread of the tumor beyond the normal site widely in the body, is a feature characteristic of only truly malignant tumors. *(Chandrasoma and Taylor, pp. 263, 264)*

612. **(C)** The definitions of the various types of cellular proliferations or abnormalities of cell proliferation and development are shown in Table 7–2. A decrease in the size of a previously normal-sized and developed organ is defined as atrophy. It is an acquired decrease in the size of cellular components after full maturation has been achieved. This is in contradistinction to agenesis, where the tissue or organ may never reach the normal adult size because of lack of tissue components. Examples are disuse atrophy of muscles that have become denervated or atrophy of the uterus in the postmenopausal period. *(Chandrasoma and Taylor, pp. 250, 251)*

613. **(A)** The term or prefix *adeno* implies a tumor of glandular epithelial origin. However, adenomatous polyp simply implies growth that is limited and does not exhibit the changes described here of invasion into the adjacent tissue (Table 7–8). Adenomyosis is the appearance of glandular elements in the myometrium, and a carcinosarcoma, although containing invasive and glandular components, also has a sarcomatous element, as its name suggests. The best example, therefore, is an adenocarcinoma in which all of the features described are present. *(Chandrasoma and Taylor, pp. 266, 267)*

614. **(D)** A malignant tumor that produces multiple nodules and, therefore, metastatic spread in a structure, such as the gastric mucosa and small

intestine, is a relatively rare phenomenon. Added to this, the presence of fine granules of brownish pigment would fit the description of melanin, and, therefore, malignant melanoma, a malignant tumor rising from the melanocytes of the skin, fits this description best. Malignant melanoma is one of the few tumors to metastasize to the stomach and small intestine. It is often pigmented because of the production of melanin, although sometimes the tumor is so undifferentiated as to no longer produce melanin (so-called amelanotic melanoma). *(Rubin and Farber, p. 1284)*

615.   **(D)** It is estimated that in 1991, 44,000 women in the United States died of breast carcinoma, and the age-corrected death rate per 100,000 of the population was 27.4 for breast cancer. *(Chandrasoma and Taylor, pp. 822, 823)*

616.   **(B)** The incidence of cancer differs considerably both in its crude incident rate and in its death rate in underdeveloped countries, particularly in black African countries as compared to white races in the United States and Europe. Carcinoma of the lung, colon, breast, and pancreas tend to be major neoplasms in Western developed countries and are relatively uncommon in Africa. Carcinoma of the uterine cervix, however, is one of the most frequent malignancies in African countries. It has been suggested that this is associated with early and frequent sexual activity. Recent data related this antecedent to herpes virus infections. *(Rubin and Farber, pp. 980–983)*

617.   **(D)** There has been a great deal of investigation of the possible etiologic role of viruses, which has established the oncogene and oncovirus theories. A number of tumors have come under suspicion, including some forms of cancer of the uterine cervix and possibly some lymphomas. Burkitt's lymphoma is associated with the Epstein–Barr virus and was described first in young African children. There is no direct evidence that leiomyoma of the uterus, carcinoma of the lung, and carcinoma of the esophagus have viral etiologies. This is another example of the fact that malignancy may occur morphologically in different forms and may

have different pathways of etiology and that chemical carcinogenesis, hereditary factors, viruses, and other factors may interact at different levels and have more or less strong associations in a specific type of tumor. *(Chandrasoma and Taylor, pp. 288–289)*

618.   **(C)** CEA is a form of glycoprotein. It usually is expressed by cells of the fetal intestine. Although it is produced in some form by a variety of tumors and some non-neoplastic conditions, it is most typically seen in carcinoma of the colon. Its very consistent appearance in carcinoma of the colon has led to its use not only diagnostically but in following up patients after surgery to determine if recurrence or metastasis has occurred. Some of the other tumors listed, particularly testicular teratomas and seminomas, may produce similar by-products that are unrelated to CEA. *(Chandrasoma and Taylor, pp. 295–296)*

619.   **(E)** As seen in Table 7–4, benign tumors tend to be encapsulated and slowly growing. Therefore, they have a low mitotic index; i.e., at any time, particularly when sections are taken of the fixed tissue at death of the tumor, few mitoses are seen. In this respect, they appear closely similar to their normal tissue counterparts and tend to be well differentiated. All of these factors, however, are variable. The inability to invade in single cells or groups of cells and not to produce metastasis via the blood vessels and lymphatics is a particularly important distinction between benign and malignant. *(Cotran et al., pp. 261–266)*

620.   **(D)** The term "hyperplasia" (Tables 7–2 and 7–3) is an increase in mass of tissue or organ because of cellular increase beyond the normal range. The terms "aplasia," "agenesis," "hypertrophy," and "metaplasia" clearly are different and usually are easily distinguishable. *(Cotran et al., pp. 32–35)*

621.   **(C)** The relationship between cigarette smoking and lung cancer is probably one of the most convincing associations between a social habit and a prevalent form of neoplasia. Although there may be other factors, including

the role of such substances as asbestos and even viruses, cigarette smoking is clearly and unequivocally shown to be a major carcinogenic event in this very important tumor. *(Cotran et al., p. 409)*

622. **(E)** The increased incidence of bladder cancer among aniline dye workers was one of the earliest industrial cancers recognized before the turn of the century and was thought to be caused by naphthylamines and related amines, including benzene. There is a complex relationship between the enzyme beta-glucuronidase and the release of 2-amino-l-naphthol in the bladder. This is further exaggerated by cigarette smoking, which increases the carcinogenic effect by interfering with betaglucuronidase production. *(Cotran et al., p. 1007)*

623. **(D)** Production of malignant melanoma of the skin in the white races, particularly those of Celtic origin, in such countries as Australia and New Zealand and parts of the United States; e.g., Texas, Arizona, and New Mexico, has a clear, direct relationship with ultraviolet light. Carcinoma of the lung has no such relationship with sunlight, and the skin of blacks is particularly immune to the effect of ultraviolet light in production of both basal cell and squamous cell carcinoma. Intraocular malignant melanoma is an extremely rare tumor in blacks and is unrelated to sunlight as far as can be determined. *(Cotran et al., pp. 1177, 1178)*

624. **(B)** Table 7–2 shows that hyperplasia is an increase in the size of an organ or tissue resulting from increase in cell proliferation; whereas, hypertrophy is an increase in size of an organ resulting from increase in size of the cells. This is what happens in the uterus during pregnancy. Dysplasia may occur in the uterine cervix but is unrelated to pregnancy per se. *(Cotran et al., pp. 32–35)*

625. **(E)** The postmenopausal small uterus results from a decrease in the size of the component cells (atrophy) (Table 7–2). It is the opposite of the answer to Question 26. *(Cotran et al., pp. 132–135)*

626. **(D)** Lack of development of the lobe of the lung in a newborn fits the term "agenesis," which is a congenital lack of tissue or organ resulting from total lack of cells. Although aplasia may share certain features, it is often an acquired rather than a congenital lack of development and is seen also in adults. *(Cotran et al., p. 466)*

627. **(A)** Hyperplasia is an increase in mature tissue or organs resulting from increase in cell number beyond the normal range (Tables 7–2 and 7–3). A localized thickness of the buccal mucosa resulting from increased numbers of epithelial cells fits this description. This is not hypertrophy, because the cells do not necessarily increase in size, and there are more cells than normal. Dysplasia may often accompany hyperplasia in some situations, but the two may be separate entities, as in this case. *(Rubin and Farber, p. 9)*

628. **(D)** Aflatoxins produced by certain fungi may contaminate food and have been shown to produce changes in the liver in humans and in other animals, including the turkey. It is closely associated with hepatocellular carcinoma, particularly in parts of Africa. *(Rubin and Farber, p. 825)*

629. **(D)** Industrial exposure to naphthalene, as seen in aniline dye workers (see Question 24), is associated with an increased incidence of urinary bladder carcinoma caused by by-products of naphthalene and their concentration in the urine. It is another form of chemical carcinogenesis that has been well established and prove. *(Cotran et al., p. 309)*

630. **(D)** The low-power photomicrograph (Figure 7–4) shows a papillary tumor on a stalk that is well circumscribed with what appears to be a central core of connective tissue and an epithelial covering. The high-power photomicrograph (Figure 7–5) shows the cells to be of squamous type with intercellular bridges and the pavement type epithelium characteristic of squamous epithelium. The tumor is, therefore, a papilloma (Table 7–8). Because the cells of origin are clearly squamous in type, and it is well differentiated, the tumor is referred to as a well-

differentiated benign squamous cell papilloma. *(Rubin and Farber, pp. 157, 158)*

631. **(B)** *(Rubin and Farber, p. 157)*

632. **(C)** After complete excision of this lesion, the most likely predictable sequence would be that nothing further would occur, because the benign tumor has been completely excised. Therefore, by definition, it would not spread to regional lymph nodes or to the bloodstream and should not occur locally unless tissue was left behind. The prognosis is good with such a lesion if it is adequately treated. *(Rubin and Farber, pp. 156, 157)*

633. **(D)** *(Rubin and Farber, pp. 156, 157)*

634–636. **(634-C, 635-D, 636-A)** The association between mesothelioma, which is a malignant tumor of the pleura, and asbestos exposure over many years has now been well established. It is reasonably well established that there is an increased incidence of cancer arising from the bronchial epithelium, so-called bronchogenic carcinoma. The characteristic asbestos bodies are demonstrated clearly (Figure 7–6) in the photomicrograph, and the other features are clearly distinguishable. Although excessive smoking may add to the problem, this is not particularly the case in mesothelioma, although it would be in lung cancer. *(Cotran et al., pp. 732–742)*

637 and 638. **(637-D, 638-A)** The photomicrograph (Figure 7–7) shows epithelium from the ectocervix in which there is total disorganization of the cells, with nucleated cells appearing throughout the layers and with the cells showing marked pleomorphism and irregularity in the size and shape of the nuclei. This is the picture of carcinoma in situ or a malignant process still confined to the epithelial layer, with no evidence of invasion of the underlying tissue. If the area of the cervix is completely removed at this stage, there is no further likelihood of malignant spread. *(Cotran et al., pp. 1051–1053)*

639 and 640. **(639-A, 640-D)** The photomicrograph from the cervix (Figure 7–8) shows normal squamous epithelium to the right and squamous epithelium showing severe dysplasia to the left. The distinction between the severe dysplasia seen in this photomicrograph and that in Figure 7–7 may be difficult to determine in some instances, but there is still an attempt at regular layering of the cells although there are nucleated cells shedding at the surface. If this is the situation, the lesion may under some circumstances regress, may remain unchanged for periods of time, or may develop into a true in situ or even invasive malignancy. It is for this reason that such severe dysplasia is regarded as potentially malignant. *(Cotran et al., pp. 1051–1053)*

641–644. **(641-D, 642-D, 643-D, 644-C)** The low-power photomicrograph (Figure 7–9) shows a pedunculated structure composed of glandular spaces on a stalk that is connected to epithelium characteristic of the large intestine. The high-power photomicrograph (Figure 7–10) shows the epithelium to be well differentiated, similar to that seen in the normal bowel but disorganized in the fashion of a glandular tumor. There is no evidence of invasion of the stalk by groups or clumps of cells; therefore, this represents a benign tumor of glandular type; i.e., an adenoma (Table 7–8). Because of its pedunculated nature, it is described as an adenomatous polyp. These lesions are extremely common throughout the large bowel and can produce malignant change with subsequent invasion. In this instance, there is no such evidence, and, therefore, the prognosis is excellent. This is similar to that seen in Questions 630 through 633, where the pedunculated lesion of the skin was removed completely with no residual area of tumor, resulting in cure. *(Cotran et al., pp. 827–833)*

645–648. **(645-D, 646-D, 647-D, 648-D)** The photomicrograph (Figure 7–11) clearly shows a neoplastic process. There are sheets and clumps of cells that do not have a normal appearance of any tissue. The tumor is composed of cells of an epithelial type, and the center shows an area of keratohyalin, which is characteristic of squamous cell carcinoma or a carcinoma arising from squamous cell epithelium. There is, adjacent to the tumor, black pigment characteristic of anthracotic pigment, which often is seen in the lungs of city dwellers and in those who smoke cigarettes. Although the anthracotic pigment is not related directly to cigarette smoking, it is a clue to the site of the tumor. The tumor is, therefore, a squamous cell carcinoma arising in the lung and is a characteristic of bronchogenic carcinoma. *(Cotran et al., pp. 743–744)*

649–651. (649-B, 650-D, 651-A) These definitions are described in Table 7–8. An adenoma is defined as a benign neoplasm that is growing locally and is well circumscribed and very similar in appearance to the cells from which it arose. The term "adenoma" usually applies to a particular benign neoplasm of glandular origin. The lack of production of red cell precursors in bone marrow is a description of aplasia; often this results in a disease known as "aplastic anemia," in which the red cells are no longer replenished from the stem cell pool and severe anemia results. There are many other reasons why red cells are not replaced or are actually destroyed, but in this situation, it is a lack of production of the precursors. A liposarcoma is a sarcoma or malignant neoplasm of mesodermal or mesenchymal origin, the prefix *lipo* meaning "of fat cells." This is a particularly rare form of malignant tumor arising from the adipose tissue. *(Chandrasoma and Taylor, pp. 260–263)*

652 and 653. (652-D, 653-B) The benign tumor of epithelial origin attached to the normal epithelium by a stalk is a papilloma (Table 7–8). If the epithelium is of glandular type, it can be referred to as a "papillary adenoma," which is a combination of these descriptions. A malignant tumor of mesodermal origin, by definition, is a sarcoma. The prefix determines the cell of origin; (e.g., *lipo*sarcoma, *fibro*sarcoma, and *osteo*sarcoma). *(Chandrasoma and Taylor, pp. 260–263)*

654–659. (654-E, 655-C, 656-D, 657-A, 658-B, 659-A) A choriocarcinoma is a malignant neoplasm of trophoblastic origin that, although it may pre-

dominantly metastasize via the bloodstream, most characteristically produces HCG, as does the normal trophoblast. A secondary carcinoma of the stomach in the ovaries, the Krukenberg tumor, is a metastatic tumor that originates in other sites than the stomach, although that is the most classic, and metastasizes to the ovaries either via the bloodstream or via the peritoneal cavity or both. A hepatocellular carcinoma is one of the tumors that secretes AFP, a substance normally seen only in fetal life and the fetal equivalent of albumin. Other tumors, such as teratomas and testicular tumors, may also produce AFP. Osteogenic sarcoma is a malignant neoplasm of mesodermal origin (Table 7–8) and arises from cells of the osteoblast type in bone. It is a highly malignant tumor, usually seen in young people, with a second peak at an older age. It characteristically metastasizes via the bloodstream, although there have been rarer occasions when lymph nodes have been involved in some forms of osteogenic sarcoma. Bronchogenic carcinoma; however, a tumor of epithelial origin arising in the lungs and characteristic of epithelial tumors, tends to go via the lymphatic rather than the bloodstream, although it can eventually be widely disseminated through the bloodstream after traversing the lymphatics and the lymph nodes. A fibrosarcoma is a malignant neoplasm of mesodermal origin from fibroblastic tissue and is characteristically metastasized via the bloodstream through thin-walled blood vessels often closely associated with the tumor. Very occasionally, a fibrosarcoma may metastasize primarily via the lymphatics (Table 7–9). *(Chandrasoma and Taylor, pp. 813–814; 776; 659–661; 970–971; 547–553)*

660–662. (660-A, 661-A, 662-A) Neuroblastoma is a malignant neoplasm thought to arise from primitive neural crest cells. It is a tumor of infancy and early childhood, most commonly occurring in the adrenal gland. Most patients have an enlarging abdominal mass. Examination of the urine reveals elevated levels of the neuroendocrine metabolites, metanephrine, and vanillylmandelic acid. Hematogenous metastases occur early in the disease. The karyotypic abnormalities associated with neuroblastoma include partial deletion of the short arm of chromosome 1 and amplification of the oncogene N-myc. Treatment is a combination of surgery, chemotherapy, and radiation. The prognosis depends on the age of the patient, stage of disease, histology of the tumor cells, and oncogene status. *(Cotran et al., pp. 485–487)*

663 and 664. (663-A, 664-D) The TNM staging system is a useful method to enumerate the extent of malignant disease quickly, categorize patients for therapy, and predict prognosis. The T icon represents the size of the primary tumor, with T1 being the smallest sized tumor, and T2 through T4 designating increasingly larger tumor sizes. The N icon is for the nodal status. N0 indicates no known nodal metastases. N1 through N3 indicate increasing, more distant lymph node involvement. The absence or presence of distant non-nodal metastases is designated by M0 or M1, respectively. The stage of disease is determined by plugging the appropriate T, N, and M numbers into a site- or organ-specific staging formula. For example, a stage I breast carcinoma is T1, N0, M0. Whereas, a stage II breast carcinoma is T1, N1, M0; or T2, N0, M0; or T2, N1, M0; or T3, N0, M0. The prognosis decreases with each increasing stage. The 5-year survival for stages I, II, II, and IV breast cancers are 85, 66, 41, and 10%, respectively. *(Rubin and Farber, p. 171)*

665 and 666. (665-C, 666-E) Asbestos is strongly associated with an increased risk of subsequently developing malignant mesothelioma. Asbestos is a fiber-shaped silicate found in nature occurring in crocidolite, chrysotile, and amosite forms. Inhaled fibers are deposited in the alveolar spaces and phagocytized by macrophages. Eventually interstitial pulmonary fibrosis may result. Ferruginous bodies are iron-coated asbestos fibers and may be seen microscopically. Pleural thickening and mesothelioma occur not only in individuals who work with asbestos, such as shipbuilders, but also in their family members who are exposed to the worker's asbestos-soiled clothes. The hepatitis B viral carrier state is associated with an increased risk of developing hepatoma (liver cell carcinoma). Preceding the emergence of the cancer there is antecedent cirrhosis and liver cell dysplasia. Hepatoma is most common in Africa and the Far East in geographic areas with a high prevalence of the hepatitis B carrier individuals. *(Cotran et al., pp. 733; 888, 889)*

667–670. (667-A, 668-B, 669-D, 670-E) A number of terms exist (Tables 7–1 and 7–2) to define alterations either in the number of cells, the size of individual cells, the composition of cells, or the maturation of cells. Hyperplasia is the increase in size of individual cells. Left ventricular hypertrophy due to essential hypertension is a common physiologic example. Dysplasia is a preneoplasic abnormality of maturation associated with nuclear hyperchromatism and enlargement. Aplasia is the absence of normal cellular proliferation or populations. It can involve a few cells, a complete developmental line of cells, a portion of an organ, or an entire organ. Metaplasia is the acquired change of one adult cell type into another adult cell type. Usually metaplasia is a protective alteration because the metaplastic cells are frequently more resistant to the inciting physiologic or environmental stresses. *(Cotran et al., pp. 32–35; 776; 778; 466)*

671 and 672. (671-B, 672-C) The products synthesized by certain benign and malignant tumors can be used as markers of identification for diagnosis and as an aid in detecting tumors at an earlier stage (Table 7–10). Medullary carcinoma arises from the parafollicular C cells of the thyroid. These cells manufacture and secrete the hormone calcitonin. Medullary carcinomas either secrete increased serum levels of calcitonin, or calcitonin molecules can be demonstrated in these tumor cells with special techniques. Pheochromocytomas are neoplasms of the adrenal medulla. They characteristically produce increased levels of catecholamines and their metabolites. *(Cotran et al., pp. 1131; 1165, 1166)*

673–676. (673-E, 674-A, 675-B, 676-C) Liposarcoma is a malignant tumor composed of fat-forming cells. These malignant tumors of adipocytes occur most commonly in the retroperitoneum, mesentery, and soft tissues of middle-aged and elderly individuals. A lipoma is a benign tumor of adipocytes. It is seen most often in the hypodermis of middle-aged and elderly individuals. Osteogenic sarcoma is a malignant tumor of bone-forming cells. Osteoid production is a characteristic feature. Rhabdomyosarcoma is a malignant tumor of skeletal muscle cells. Myosin can be demonstrated immunohistochemically in most of these tumors. Osteogenic sarcoma and rhabdomyosarcoma are most commonly encountered in children and young adults. The nomenclature for tumors is detailed in Table 7–8. *(Cotran et al., pp. 1260–1262; 1236–1237; 1265)*

677–680. (677-E, 678-B, 679-A, 680-C) The nomenclature of tumors can be complex (Table 7–8). In general, benign tumors are named by combining the cell type with the suffix *oma*. For example, a benign tumor of chondrocytes (cartilage cells) is called a chondroma," and a benign tumor of leiomyocytes (smooth muscle cells) is called a "leiomyoma." Malignant epithelial tumors are generally named by adding the cell type to the suffix *carcinoma*. For example, a malignant tumor of glandular cells (adenocytes) is called an "adenocarcinoma." Malignant tumors of mesenchymal cells are usually named by adding the suffix *sarcoma* to the cell type. For example, a malignant tumor of chondrocytes is termed a "chondrosarcoma." *(Cotran et al., pp. 261–273)*

681–684. (681-C, 682-B, 683-D, 684-A) Colonic carcinoma occurs most commonly in Western populations with high-fat, low-fiber diets. A low residual diet slows colonic transit times perhaps exposing the bowel epithelium to carcinogenic fatty substances for prolonged periods of time. African female populations have a high incidence of cervical squamous cell carcinoma for a number of reasons: lack of pap smear screening, high prevalence of viral promoters, and early age of first sexual activity. Basal cell carcinomas of the skin occur much more frequently in individuals with extensive actinic dermatitis. Gastric adenocarcinoma is most common in Japan and the former Soviet Union, and relatively rare in North American populations (Table 7–14). The reason for this disparity is not known. *(Chandrasoma and Taylor, pp. 662, 663; 790–794; 889, 890; 580–584)*

685–688. (685-E, 686-B, 687-A, 688-D) Close viral associations are seen with several types of human cancers. Dysplasias and carcinoma of the cervix are strongly associated with genital infection of the human papilloma virus, particularly subtypes 16, 18, 31, and 33. Hepatocellular carcinoma is seen with hepatitis B virus carrier states. Dysplasia and cirrhosis may precede the development of liver cell carcinoma. Burkitt's lymphoma of the African type is strongly associated with Epstein–Barr viral infections. Epstein–Barr virus infection is also related to the subsequent development of nasopharyngeal carcinomas. Kaposi's sarcoma is seen most frequently in individuals with AIDS due to human immunodeficiency virus infection. *(Chandrasoma and Taylor, pp. 268; 334; 559–561; 790–794)*

689–692. (689-E, 690-C, 691-A, 692-D) A number of clinical conditions and disorders predispose to the later emergence of neoplasms. Xeroderma pigmentosum, for example, is a genetic disorder that lacks the usual DNA cellular repair mechanisms for mitigating against actinic damage. As a result these individuals develop multiple skin cancers at an early age. Ulcerative colitis is another disorder associated with subsequent neoplastic transformation. In this disease, there is chronic ulcerative inflammation of the large intestine, epithelial dysplasia, and a significantly increased risk of colonic adenocarcinoma. Undescended testes are associated with sterility and an increased risk of such germ-cell tumors as seminoma. Individuals with Paget's disease of the bone have an increased incidence of subsequent osteosarcoma. *(Cotran et al., pp. 296; 820; 263–264; 1225–1227)*

693–696. (693-B, 694-E, 695-C, 696-A) A number of chemical substances are related to tumorous development. Aflatoxin, a fungal metabolite, can contaminate improperly stored food, particularly grains and peanuts. The ingested aflatoxin is oxidized in the liver and exerts its carcinogenic effect by binding to guanine. Chewing betel leaves and nuts is likely to produce oral carcinomas. This practice correlates with Sri Lanka's and parts of India's high incidence of oral tumors. The maternal antepartum administration of diethylstilbestrol produces an increased risk of subsequent vaginal adenosis and vaginal clear cell carcinoma in their female offspring. These tumors usually do not make their appearance until the daughters are at least age 20. Vinyl chloride workers are at increased risk to develop angiosarcomas of the liver. (*Chandrasoma and Taylor, pp. 283–286*)

697–700. (697-E, 698-D, 699-B, 700-C) Renal cell carcinoma may secrete erythropoietin, a hormonal red cell growth factor. Erythrocytosis and polycythemia may occur. Prostate adenocarcinoma may secrete prostate-specific antigen and prostatic acid phosphatase. Early detection of localized disease may be achieved by measuring the serum levels of these markers. Multiple myeloma is a malignancy of plasma cells. The malignant plasma cells may secrete intact whole immunoglobulin molecules, free light chains, or rarely, free heavy chains. The immunoglobulins may be observed in the serum, urine, or both serum and urine. Adrenal cortical carcinomas may retain their native cell's ability to secrete corticosteroid products. These products may be measured in the serum or the metabolites may be detected in the urine. (*Chandrasoma and Taylor, pp. 289–292*)

701.   (D) Squamous cell carcinoma of the lung is seen most commonly in cigarette smokers. Squamous metaplasia and squamous cell dysplasia usually precede the development of an overt malignancy. The microscopic appearance of the tumor is varied, depending on the grade of the tumor. Usually multicell keratin pearl formation, intercellular bridges (prickles), or intracellular keratin production must be observed histologically to definitively diagnose the squamous cell type. Other associated features include sheetlike architecture, enlarged hyperchromic nuclei, and eosinophilic cytoplasm. Early lesions may be cured by surgery. However, the overall prognosis of lung carci-

noma is dismal, because the 5-year survival is only 8%. (*Chandrasoma and Taylor, p. 548*)

702.   (A) Melanoma is a malignant neoplasm of melanocytes. Most melanomas arise in basal layers of the epidermis and remain confined to the epidermis in a radial growth phase for some time. Later in the tumor's development, it will grow down into the dermis (vertical growth phase) and gain access to the lymphatics. Clinically, most melanomas display a variegated brown, tan, pink, or black appearance. Irregular edges, enlargement, and central nodular ulceration may also be noticed. The microscopic appearance is characterized by nests of cells and single cells with eccentric nuclei, prominent macronucleoli, and cytoplasmic melanin pigment. The prognosis of melanoma is related to its depth of invasion measured by either the Clark's level or Breslow's thickness. Deeply invading tumors and thicker tumors are associated with a poor prognosis. (*Chandrasoma and Taylor, pp. 892, 893*)

703.   (F) Down syndrome is caused by a trisomy of chromosome 21. Prominent epicanthal folds, mental retardation, congenital cardiovascular abnormalities, oblique palpebral fissures, increased susceptibility to infections, hyperflexibility, muscle hypotonia, dysplastic ears, and infertility characterize the syndrome. Individuals with Down's syndrome have a 20-fold increased risk of developing lymphoblastic leukemia during childhood. (*Cotran et al., pp. 129–132*)

704.   (C) Adenocarcinoma is the most common type of malignancy arising in the large intestine. Iron deficiency microcytic, hypochromic anemia, may be the presenting symptom due to bleeding from tumorous ulceration. Alternatively, the tumor may be suspected by detection of occult fecal blood tests, bowel obstruction, or through the development of hepatic enlargement due to metastases. The gross appearance of the tumors is usually polypoid or ulcerating. Many ulcerating tumors involve the full circumference of the bowel and appear radiographically as an "applecore" lesion. The microscopic appearance is that of gland-forming malignant cells. Usually mucin production is prominent. The prognosis is related to the stage of the disease. TMN and modified Duke's staging protocols are clinically useful to predict an individual's prognosis. *(Chandrasoma and Taylor, pp. 622–626)*

705. **(D)** Hemangiomas are benign tumors composed of blood vessels. They occur in the dermis of all age groups, although they are most common in infancy and childhood. Those tumors forming large vessels may be termed "cavernous hemangiomas." Those formed by small blood vessels are called "capillary hemangiomas." Most hemangiomas are removed for diagnostic or cosmetic reasons. Rarely, rupture of an intravisceral hemangioma can be fatal. The malignant counterpart, angiosarcoma, is distinguished by the anaplasia its endothelial cells demonstrate, invasiveness, and ability to metastasize. *(Cotran et al., pp. 532, 533)*

706. **(H)** Chronic myelogenous leukemia is a myeloproliferative disease of middle age with a slight male predominance. Common clinical features include splenomegaly, hepatomegaly, anemia, fatigability, easy bruising, and bleeding. Examination of the peripheral blood reveals an increased number of myeloid white blood cells, mostly segmented neutrophils, band neutrophils, metamyelocytes, and myelocytes. The bone marrow displays trilineage hyperplasia. The Philadelphia chromosome is present in about 90% of cases. This karyotypic abnormality consists of a translocation of a portion of the long arm from chromosome 22 to chromosome 9. *(Rubin and Farber, pp. 1112–1114)*

707. **(E)** Malignant tumors composed of bladder transitional epithelium are termed "transitional cell carcinomas." They are commonly associated with employment in the dye, rubber, paint, and chemical industries due to exposure to occupational carcinogens. The most frequent initial complaint is that of gross hematuria. The tumors are divided histologically into three grades, with grade I tumors being the most (well) differentiated and grade III tumors being the least (poorly) differentiated. The prognosis and treatment is determined by the stage of disease at initial presentation. *(Rubin and Farber, p. 929)*

708. **(G)** Malignant tumors composed of astrocytes are called "malignant astrocytomas." These tumors occur most frequently in middle-aged and elderly adults. The heralding clinical event may be a seizure. Malignant astrocytomas are characterized microscopically by proliferations of atypical astrocytes with anaplasia and increased mitoses. Those tumors that, in addition, demonstrate glomeruloid endothelial hyperplasia, extreme astrocytic pleomorphism, and palisading of tumor cells next to necrotic foci are termed "glioblastoma multiforme." Malignant astrocytoma and glioblastoma multiforme have a dismal prognosis, with most affected individuals dying within a year of diagnosis. *(Rubin and Farber, pp. 1513–1516)*

709–712. (709-A, 710-B, 711-E, 712-C) By definition, hyperplasia constitutes an increase in the number of cells in an organ or tissue, which may then have a subsequent increase in volume. The hyperplasia could be divided into physiologic and pathologic hyperplasia. Examples of physiological hyperplasia such as that which occurs in pregnant uterus is secondary to hormonal changes. In addition, have compensatory hyperplasia in cases when a portion of the liver is removed, and the cells divide to compensate for the deficit. Pathologic hyperplasia is exemplified by hormonal stimulation of the endometrium (estrogen), which is unopposed and leads to glandular hyperplasia. This change in turn, could lead to cancerous proliferation. Hypertrophy is defined as increasing size of the cells that eventually also leads to increase of the size of the organ. Hypertrophy could also be physiologic or pathologic. These changes occur mostly in the organs that cannot adapt to an increase in demand of function by mitotic division. Good examples are the myocardium, as well as the skeletal muscle. Atrophy is defined as shrinkage of the size of the cells, by loss of cell substance. The atrophy can be secondary to decreased workload, loss of innervation, diminished blood supply, inadequate nutrition, loss of endocrine stimulation and aging. Dysplasia means disorderly growth and is encountered principally in the epithelial lining of different organs and is characterized by a constellation of changes that include loss of polarity and uniformity of the individual cells, as well as hyperchromatia and increase in mitotic activity. *(Cotran et al., pp. 32–37)*

713.   **(A)** Hypertrophy in the pregnant uterus is secondary to hormonal stimulation. The massive physiologic growth of the uterus during pregnancy is a good example of hormone-induced hypertrophy involving both hypertrophy and hyperplasia. The cells are stimulated by hormones, through the receptors, which interact with the nuclear DNA, resulting in an increase in synthesis of smooth muscle proteins and increase in cell size. *(Cotran et al., pp. 33, 34)*

714.   **(A)** The growth of the tumor is related to the amount of cells dividing versus the rate of cell loss. Thus, a tumor in which the cell production is excessive, with low cell loss they grow more rapidly than in the tumors in which there is an equilibrium between the cell loss and the cell division, or a tumor in which the cell loss exceeds the amount of cell production. *(Cotran et al., pp. 299–301)*

715.   **(D)** Many breast cancers contain receptors for estrogen and progesterone. Recently, more markers have been used to predict the response to treatment as well as patient survival. When these tumors are positive for estrogen and progesterone receptors, hormonal manipulation can be used as part of the arsenal in treatment of breast cancer. *(Cotran et al., p. 1106)*

716.   **(C)** P53 is a tumor-suppressor gene located on chromosome 17. Frequently, this gene is altered in human tumors. In normal cells, however, p53 is a nuclear protein that can inhibit cell growth. *(Cotran et al., pp. 290, 291)*

717.   **(D)** Laminin is one of the most abundant glycoproteins in basement membrane. It binds not only with the basement membrane but with specific receptors of the surface of the cell and with such matrix components as collagen type IV. It is also known to mediate the cell attachment to connective tissue substrates. With these functions, it will also promote adhesion of neoplastic cells to the extracellular matrix. *(Cotran et al., p. 100)*

718.   **(C)** Mortality from cervical carcinoma has been consistently falling through the years, and that is secondary to multiple factors, such as cytologic screening (PAP smears), early detection and treatment of dysplasia, as well as carcinoma in situ before they become invasive lesions. *(Chandrasoma and Taylor, pp. 790, 791)*

719.   **(A)** Different ways of spreading breast cancer, either local, or systemic can occur. The local extension is throughout the ductal system or invasion directly through the breast stroma. The systemic invasion is done by lymphatic spread or bloodstream spread. The lymphatic spread is the most likely route to metastasize to the lymphatics and to the axillary lymph nodes. The axillary nodes are the primary group that is affected, and occasionally the internal mammary, supraclavicular and, cervical nodes could also contain metastasis. *(Chandrasoma and Taylor, pp. 826, 827)*

720.   **(B)** A malignant neoplasm is graded according to the degree of differentiation of the tumor cells, as well as the number of mitoses per high power field. Although this is not an absolute criteria, most neoplasms that contain a high number of mitoses and the cells are undifferentiated; they behave in an aggressive fashion. Staging of a malignant tumor is based on different parameters, such as size, local extension, or metastatic spread. Staging has assumed a great importance in the selection of the therapy for the patient. Staging has proven to be of greater clinical value than grading. *(Cotran et al., pp. 321, 322)*

721.   **(B)** Basal cell carcinoma is the most common malignant tumor of the skin. This tumor is characterized mainly by being locally aggressive. They originate in the basal layer of the epidermis. Basal cell carcinomas will rarely metastasize; many histological varieties have been described. In general, they originate in sun-exposed areas and in the face. *(Rubin and Farber, pp. 1291, 1292)*

722. **(C)** The p53 product can be detected in essentially all normal cells, although it is present at extremely low levels and seems to have a much shorter half-life, as compared with the mutated p53 in transformed cells. The lifespan of wild (normal) p53 is only about 30 minutes. Inactivation of p53 is generally associated with the loss of the wild-type allele. The generation of a mutated, transforming one, is present in a number of malignant tumors. Many studies show a role for p53 in cell cycle regulation. Last, introduction of wild-type p53 into cell growing in culture usually blocks self proliferation at the G1-S transition point in the cell cycle. *(Cotran et al., pp. 290, 291)*

REFERENCES

Chandrasoma P, Taylor CR. *Concise Pathology,* 3rd ed. Norwalk, CT: Appleton & Lange, 1998.

Cotran RS, Kumar V, Robbins SL. *Robbins Pathologic Basis of Disease,* 6th ed. Philadelphia: Saunders, 1999.

Rubin E, Farber JL. *Pathology.* Philadelphia: Lippincott, 1999.

CHAPTER 8

Photographic Exercises
Questions

DIRECTIONS: Each of the numbered items or incomplete statements in this chapter is followed by answers or by completions of the statement. Select the ONE lettered answer or completion that is BEST in each case.

Questions 723 through 727. (Refer to Figure 8–1.)

723. Which of the following best describes Figure 8–1?

(A) hyperplasia of the epithelial lining
(B) loss of continuity of the epithelial surface
(C) neoplastic transformation of the epithelium
(D) metaplastic transformation of the epithelium
(E) atrophic changes of the epithelium

724. Which of the following is the most appropriate diagnostic term for the illustrated condition?

(A) hypertrophic gastritis
(B) peptic ulcer
(C) gastric carcinoma
(D) intestinal metaplasia of gastric mucosa
(E) congenital gastric atrophy

725. The most likely etiology is

(A) ingestion of carcinogens in the diet
(B) the result of megaloblastic anemia
(C) associated with overproduction of acid and pepsin
(D) an inherited enzyme deficiency
(E) a viral organism

726. Which type of tissue alteration does this condition illustrate?

(A) gummatous inflammation
(B) tuberculous inflammation
(C) ulcerative inflammation
(D) fat necrosis
(E) granulomatous inflammation

727. What is the most likely complication of the illustrated condition?

(A) gastric leiomyomatosis
(B) hypertension
(C) atrophic gastritis
(D) pernicious anemia
(E) hemorrhage

Questions 728 through 731. (Refer to Figures 8–2 and 8–3.)

728. Which of the following processes best describes the pathologic changes illustrated in Figures 8–2 and 8–3?

(A) chronic nongranulomatous inflammation
(B) chronic granulomatous inflammation
(C) acute suppurative inflammation
(D) peptic ulceration
(E) hyperplasia

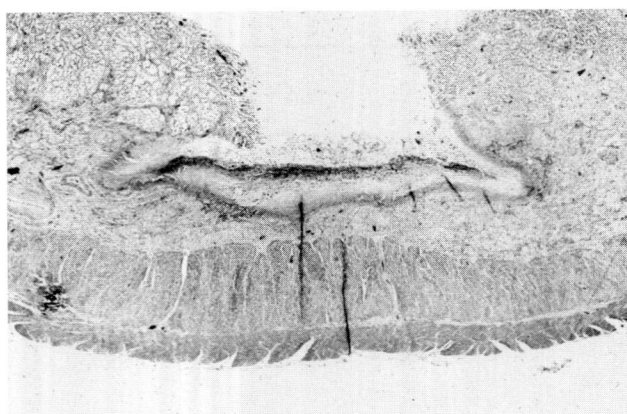

Figure 8–1. Low-power photomicrograph of a lesion in the stomach.

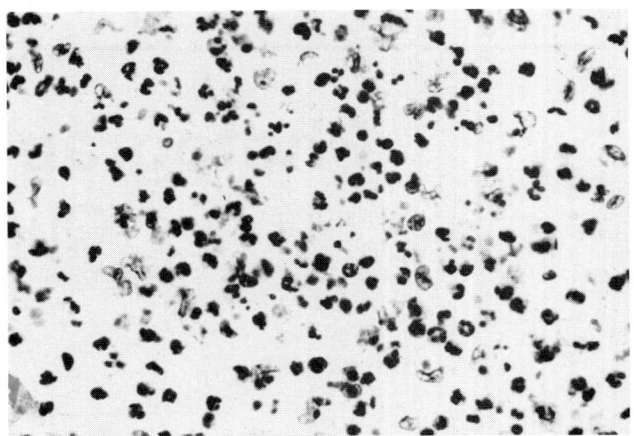

Figure 8–3. High-power photomicrograph of a transverse section of appendix.

729. Which is the most probable outcome if untreated?

(A) malignant transformation
(B) complete resolution
(C) ischemic necrosis with perforation
(D) spontaneous healing and repair
(E) atrophy

730. Characteristic morphologic findings include

(A) neutrophils
(B) luminal suppurative debris
(C) edema and vascular congestion
(D) acute inflammation
(E) all of the above

731. Which statement about this pathologic process is true?

(A) It usually resolves without treatment.
(B) It always is associated with a carcinoid tumor.
(C) It may be associated with obstruction by a fecalith.
(D) It is more frequently seen in underdeveloped rather than developed societies.
(E) It is never seen in elderly individuals.

Questions 732 through 735. (Refer to Figures 8–4 and 8–5.)

732. Which of the following is the most appropriate description?

(A) diffuse interstitial pneumonia
(B) lobar pneumonia
(C) lobular (broncho) pneumonia
(D) chronic granulomatous disease
(E) pulmonary fibrosis

733. Which of the following is the most likely cause?

(A) adenovirus
(B) *Streptococcus pneumoniae* (pneumococcus)
(C) *Escherichia coli*
(D) *Mycobacterium tuberculosis* (tubercle bacillus)
(E) asbestos particles

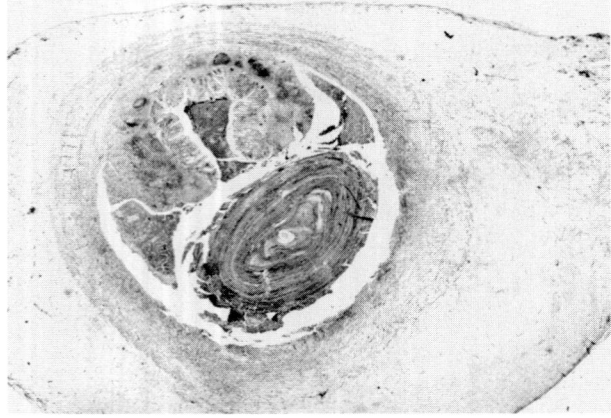

Figure 8–2. Low-power photomicrograph of a transverse section of appendix.

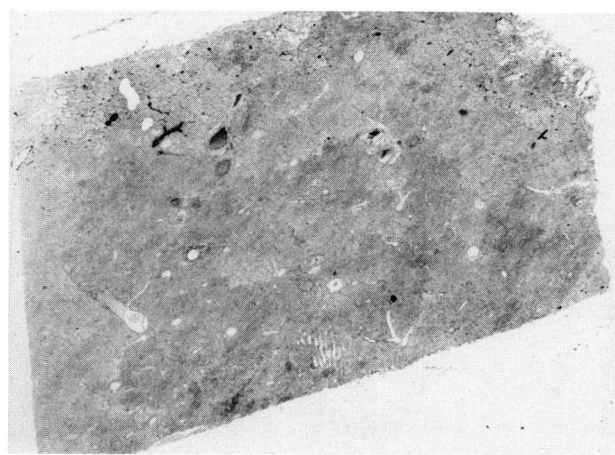

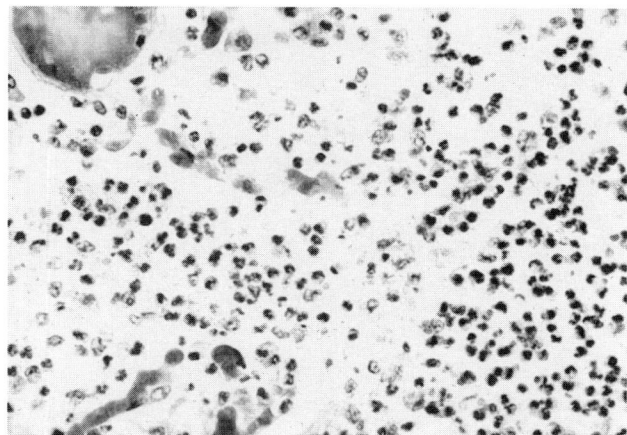

Figures 8–4 (*top*) and 8–5 (*bottom*). Low-power and high-power photomicrographs of an inflammatory process in the lung.

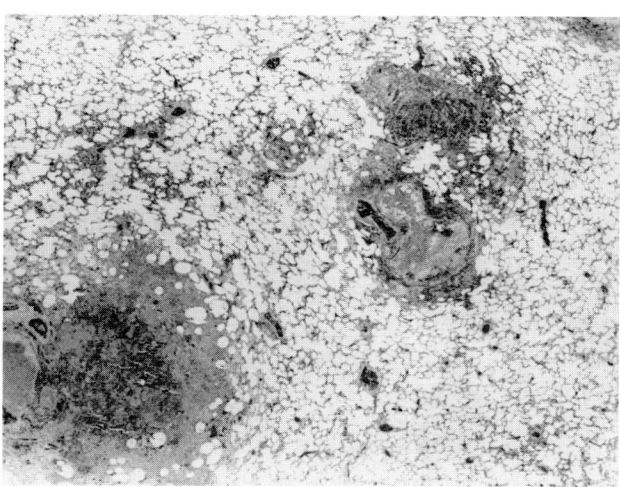

Figure 8–6. Photomicrograph of the lung.

Questions 736 through 739. (Refer to Figures 8–6 and 8–7.)

736. Which of the following is the most appropriate description?

(A) diffuse interstitial pneumonia
(B) lobar pneumonia
(C) lobular (broncho) pneumonia
(D) chronic granulomatous disease
(E) pulmonary fibrosis

734. The characteristic microscopic feature seen in the acute phase of this process is

(A) multinucleate giant cells
(B) fibrin and neutrophils in the alveoli
(C) lymphocytic inflammation
(D) fibrocytes and granulation tissue
(E) granulomatous inflammation

735. The most likely sequela is

(A) malignant nodal metastasis
(B) calcification
(C) gangrene
(D) complete resolution
(E) dense fibrosis and scar formation

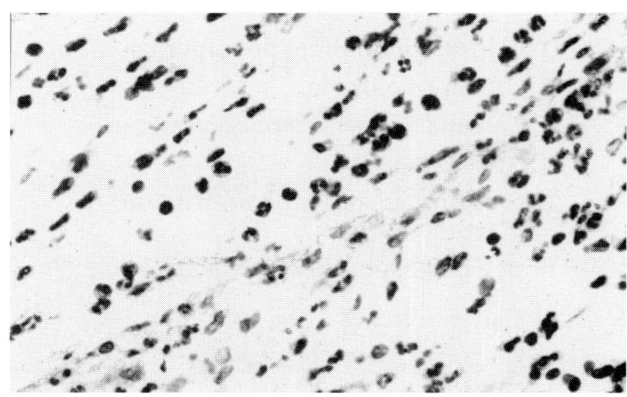

Figure 8–7. Photomicrograph of the lung.

737.   Which of the following is the most likely cause?

(A) adenovirus
(B) pneumococcus *Streptococcus pneumoniae* (pneumococcus)
(C) *Escherichia coli*
(D) *Mycobacterium tuberculosis* (tubercle bacillus)
(E) asbestos particles

738.   The characteristic microscopic feature of this process is

(A) malignant gland-forming cells
(B) ferruginous bodies
(C) peribronchial and bronchial neutrophilic inflammation
(D) giant cell granulomas
(E) malignant squamous cells

739.   Which is most likely outcome of the process?

(A) pancreatitis
(B) complete resolution with no residual abnormalities
(C) widespread calcification
(D) partial resolution with some permanent damage to bronchi and bronchioles
(E) gangrene

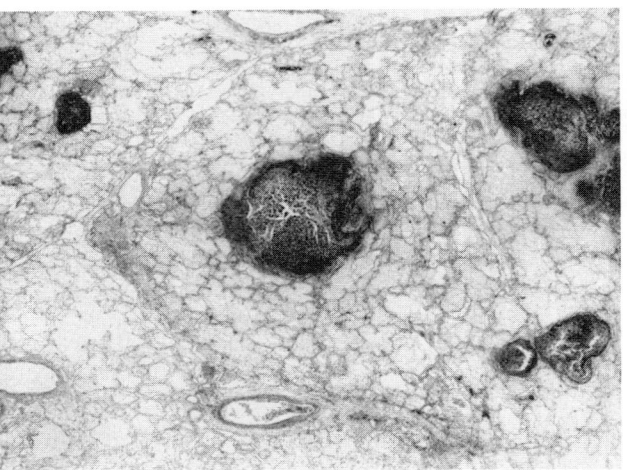

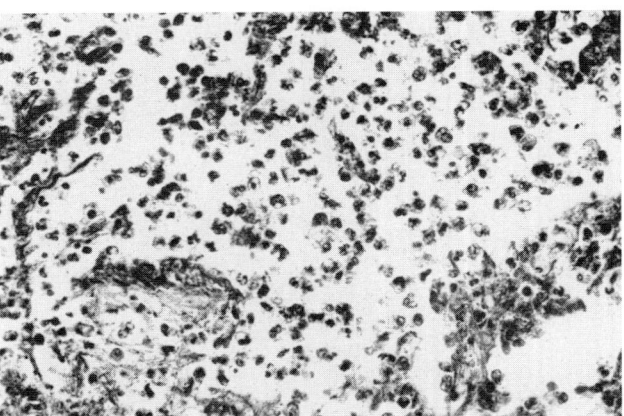

Figures 8–8 (*top*) and 8–9 (*bottom*). Low-power and high-power photomicrographs of lung tissue with several discrete solid areas.

Questions 740 through 743. (Refer to Figures 8–8 and 8–9.)

740.   Which is the most appropriate description of Figures 8–8 and 8–9?

(A) diffuse interstitial pneumonia
(B) lobar pneumonia
(C) lobular (broncho) pneumonia
(D) abscesses
(E) chronic granulomatous disease

741.   Which is the most likely causative agent?

(A) adenoviruses
(B) *Mycobacterium tuberculosis* (tubercle bacillus)
(C) mixed aerobic and anaerobic pyogenic bacteria
(D) asbestos particles
(E) *Mycoplasma pneumoniae*

742.   What is the most likely predisposing event?

(A) inhalation of asbestos material
(B) aspiration of infected material into the respiratory tract or septicemia
(C) opportunistic infection with *Mycoplasma pneumoniae*
(D) pneumoconiosis
(E) idiopathic pulmonary fibrosis

743.   Which of the following events is/are likely to occur?

(A) abscess formation in the pleural cavity
(B) brain abscess
(C) empyema
(D) focal scar formation
(E) all of the above

Questions 744 through 747. (Refer to Figures 8–10 and 8–11.)

744. The process demonstrated is

(A) postmortem blood clot

(B) thrombotic occlusion

(C) acute inflammation

(D) chronic inflammation

(E) tumor embolus

745. The most probable outcome of this process is

(A) acute suppurative inflammation

(B) chronic granulomatous inflammation

(C) metastatic spread of tumor cells

(D) infarction of tissue distal to the obstruction

(E) dissolution and disappearance of the blood clot

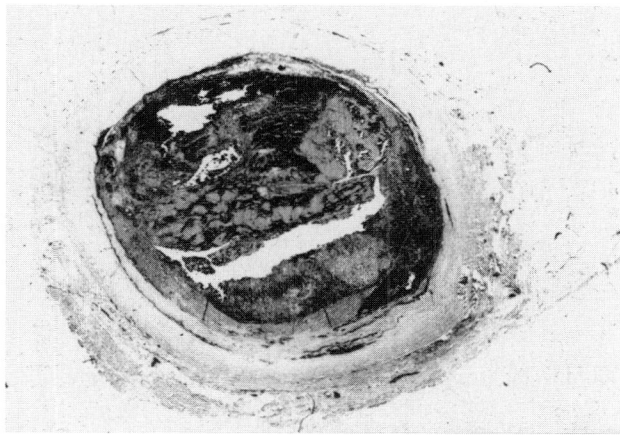

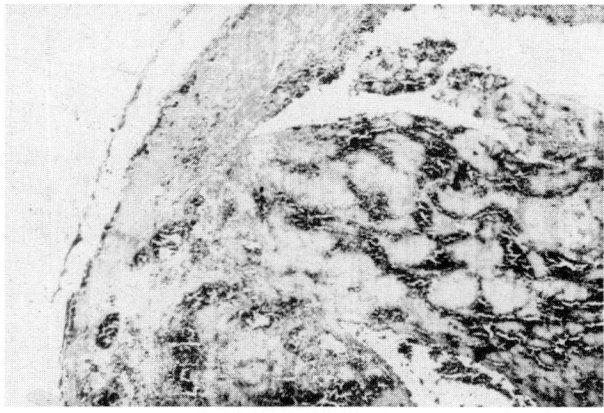

Figures 8–10 (*top*) and 8–11 (*bottom*). The low-power photomicrograph shows blood vessels with filled lumen. The high-power photomicrograph focuses on the occluded material and the adjacent vessel wall.

746. The extent and final outcome of this process depends on

(A) the degree of occlusion

(B) the state of collateral circulation

(C) the state of tissue oxygenation before occlusion

(D) whether the vessel is an end-artery type

(E) all of the above

747. Predisposing factors include

(A) alterations of blood flow

(B) damage to intima of vessel wall

(C) hypercoagulable state

(D) stasis of blood

(E) all of the above

Questions 748 through 751. (Refer to Figures 8–12 and 8–13.)

748. The pathologic process is best described as

(A) hyperplasia of the epithelium

(B) granulomatous inflammation

(C) malignant neoplasm

(D) benign neoplasm

(E) acute suppurative inflammation

749. The microscopic picture would suggest

(A) ulcerative colitis

(B) Crohn's disease of the colon

(C) adenocarcinoma of the colon

(D) adenomatous polyp of the colon

(E) amebic dysentery

750. Which is likely to occur if this process is left untreated?

(A) hemorrhage

(B) metastases

(C) obstruction

(D) ulceration

(E) all of the above

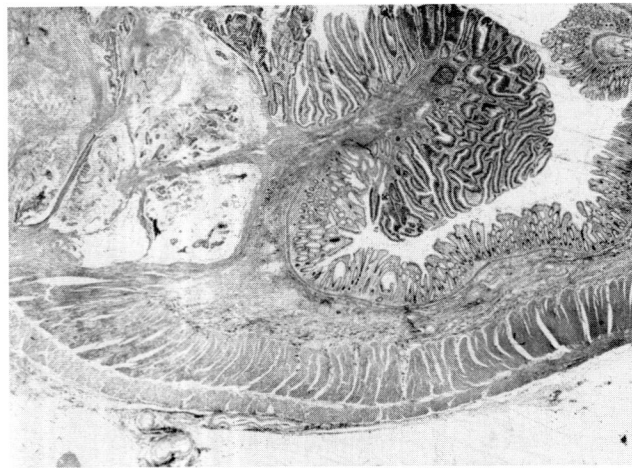

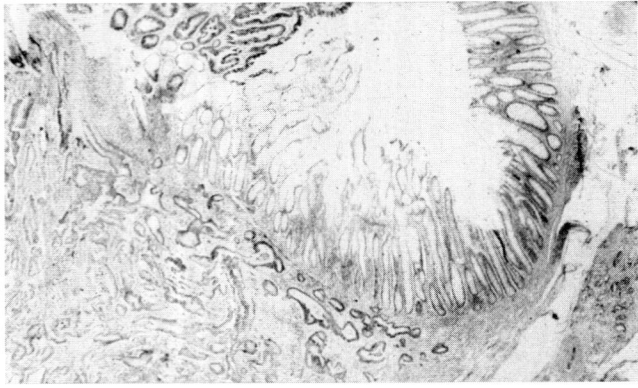

Figures 8–12 (top) and 8–13 (bottom). The gross specimen is a colon that has been opened. The photomicrograph is a representative section of the lesion.

751. Which statement(s) concerning this process is/are accurate?

(A) It arises from gland-forming epithelium.

(B) It is associated with relatively low-fiber diets.

(C) It is more common in developed countries.

(D) It is more often seen in patients over 45 years of age.

(E) All of the above statements are correct.

Questions 752 through 755. (Refer to Figures 8–14 and 8–15.)

752. Which of the following best describes the condition illustrated?

(A) pulmonary infarct

(B) lung abscess

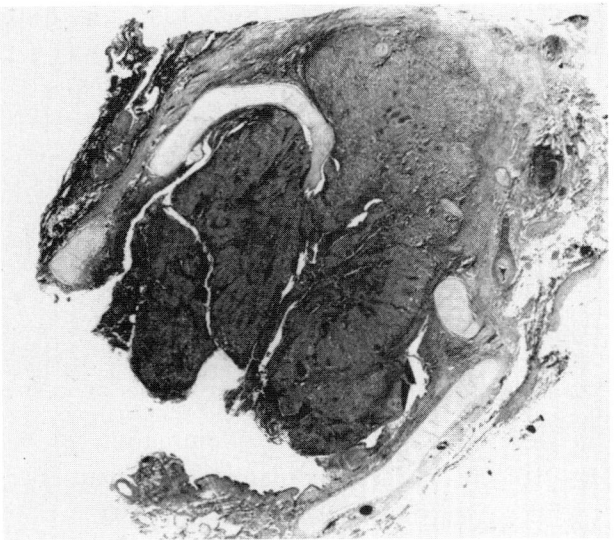

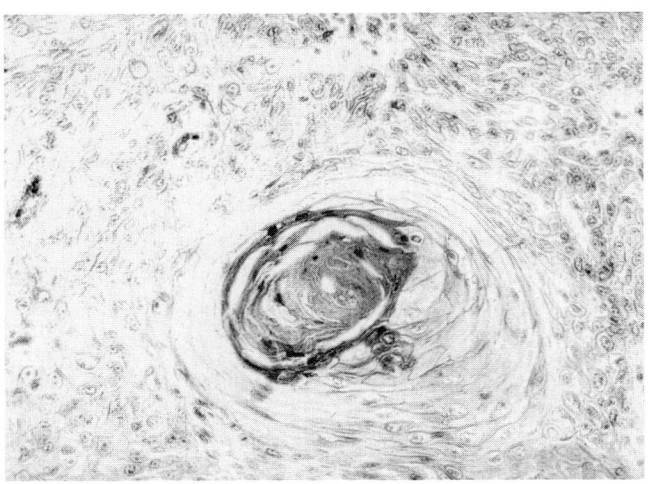

Figures 8–14 (top) and 8–15 (bottom). The low-power photomicrograph is of a lung, and the high-power photomicrograph is of a section of the abnormality demonstrated.

(C) malignant tumor

(D) benign tumor

(E) granuloma

753. The microscopic appearance most suggests

(A) pulmonary infarct

(B) lung abscess

(C) epidermoid carcinoma

(D) adenoma of the bronchus

(E) tuberculosis

754. Complications of this condition include

(A) hemorrhage

(B) metastases

(C) pneumonia distal to obstruction

(D) ulceration

(E) all of the above

755. Which is the most likely etiologic factor?

(A) low-fiber diet

(B) hypercoagulate state

(C) sickle cell anemia

(D) cigarette smoking

(E) bacterial infection

Questions 756 through 759. (Refer to Figures 8–16 and 8–17.)

756. Which of the following best describes the lesion depicted?

(A) malignant tumor of the breast

(B) fat necrosis

(C) benign tumor of the breast

(D) abscess of the breast

(E) granuloma

757. The microscopic appearance is most characteristic of

(A) adenocarcinoma of the breast

(B) fibroadenoma of the breast

(C) fat necrosis

(D) duct obstruction with abscess formation

(E) tuberculous mastitis

758. Which of the following is the single most important prognostic variable for the depicted process?

(A) status of progesterone receptors

(B) status of estrogen receptors

(C) overexpression of oncogene C-erb

(D) stage of disease

(E) high proliferative index

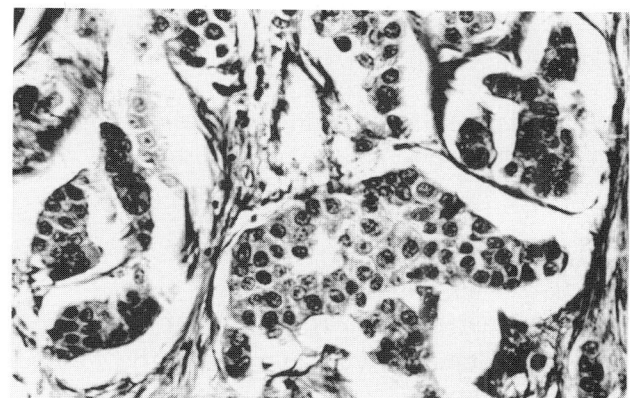

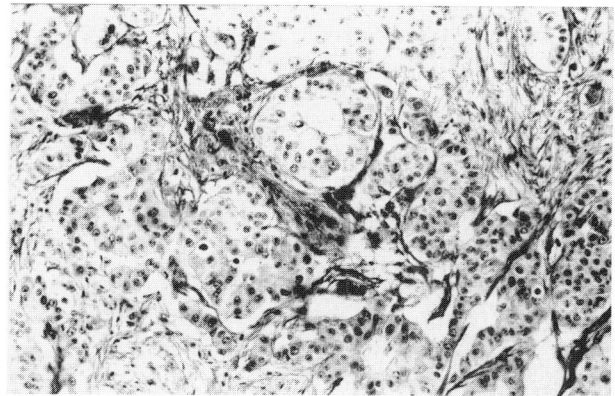

Figures 8–16 (*top*) and 8–17 (*bottom*). The specimen is from a female breast removed surgically for the condition shown. The photomicrograph shows the histologic features of the lesion.

759. Which item is most likely to be associated with this condition?

(A) low-fat diet

(B) male sex

(C) similar condition in older female relatives

(D) oriental ancestry

(E) multiparity, late menarche, and early menopause

Questions 760 through 762. (Refer to Figures 8–18 and 8–19.)

760. Which of the following is the most appropriate description of the condition?

    (A) ectopic pregnancy
    (B) benign tumors of the uterus
    (C) malignant primary tumor of the uterus
    (D) metastatic malignant tumors
    (E) congenital muscular deformity of the uterus

761. Which is the best diagnostic term to describe these lesions?

    (A) benign leiomyomas
    (B) leiomyosarcomas

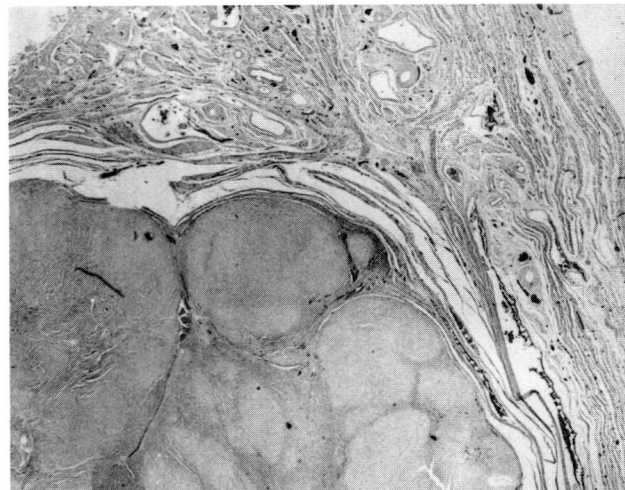

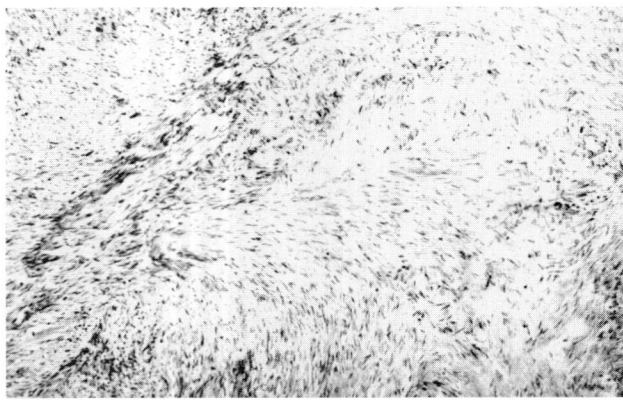

Figures 8–18 (top) and 8–19 (bottom). A uterus contains multiple, discrete, firm, white nodules. The photomicrograph shows the histologic picture of the lesion.

    (C) adenocarcinoma of endometrium
    (D) squamous cell carcinoma of the cervix
    (E) teratoma of the uterus

762. Which statement(s) concerning this condition is/are correct?

    (A) The tumors are benign.
    (B) The tumors are composed of smooth muscle cells from the uterine myometrium.
    (C) The tumors are the most common neoplasm of the female genital tract.
    (D) The tumors are frequently multiple.
    (E) All of the above statements are correct.

Questions 763 through 766. (Refer to Figure 8–20.)

763. The floccular, darkly staining material represents

    (A) apoptosis
    (B) karyolysis
    (C) swollen damaged mitochondria
    (D) viral inclusions
    (E) karyorrhexis

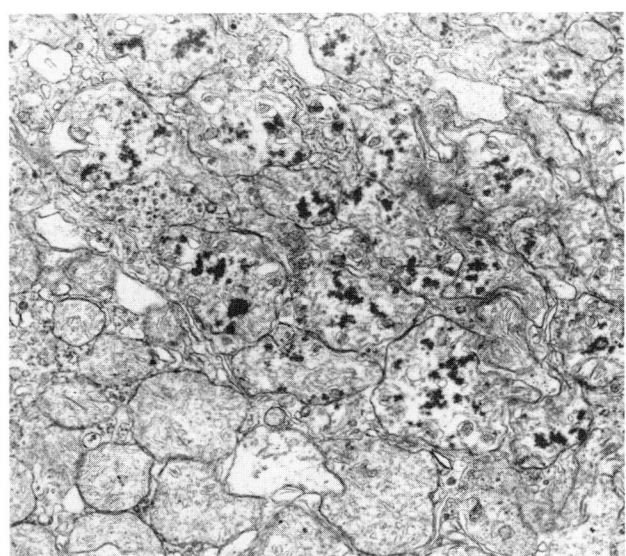

Figure 8–20. Electron micrograph of the cytoplasm of part of a proximal tubule cell of the kidney.

764. Which of the following best describes the condition depicted?

(A) lipid peroxidation with cell membrane damage

(B) damage to lysosomes, with cell swelling

(C) decreased respiration of mitochondria with flocculation

(D) clumping of chromatin

(E) damage to endoplasmic reticulum

765. The features are consistent with

(A) cytoplasmic cloudy swelling

(B) early ischemic damage or poisoning with mercuric chloride

(C) cytomegalovirus infection

(D) saponification

(E) no alterations present

766. Which of the following best represents the mechanism involved?

(A) toxic poisoning of the lysosomal system of the cell

(B) viral transformation of cellular DNA

(C) abnormality of lipid storage

(D) disruption of oxidative phosphorylation in the mitochondria

(E) failure of organogenesis

Questions 767 through 770. (Refer to Figure 8–21.)

767. The egg pictured is from which parasite?

(A) *Trichinella spiralis*

(B) *Trichuris trichiura*

(C) *Schistosoma mansoni*

(D) *Ancylostoma duodenale*

(E) *Ascaris lumbricoides*

768. Which of the following is the most frequent host for the adult forms?

(A) snail

(B) fish

(C) human

(D) mosquito

(E) dog

769. The intermediate host in the parasite life cycle is a

(A) tick

(B) cow

(C) fly

(D) snail

(E) mosquito

770. Which statement(s) concerning this disorder is (are) correct?

(A) Adult male and female worms copulate in the human host.

(B) Cercarial larvae found in contaminated water infects human hosts by penetration of the skin.

(C) This is a common disease infecting millions of people worldwide.

(D) Depending on the species, the large intestine or the bladder is the site of lodgment of eggs.

(E) All of the above statements are correct.

Questions 771 through 773. (Refer to Figure 8–22.)

771. The organisms shown are

(A) bacteria

(B) rickettsiae

(C) fungi

(D) viruses

(E) protozoa

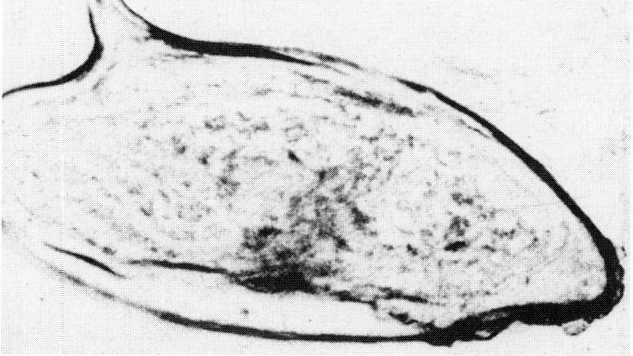

Figure 8–21. Egg seen by microscopy in stool sample.

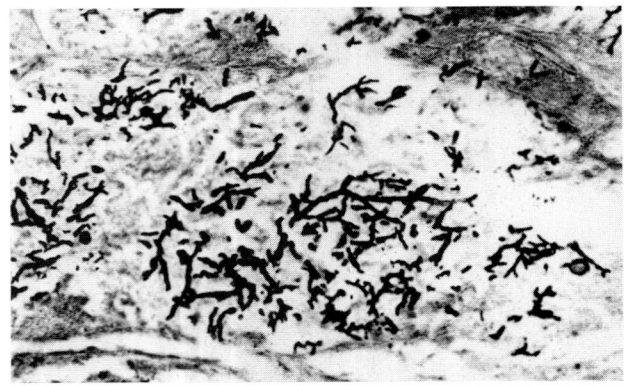

Figure 8–22. Photomicrograph of an area of consolidation in the lung.

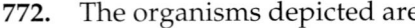

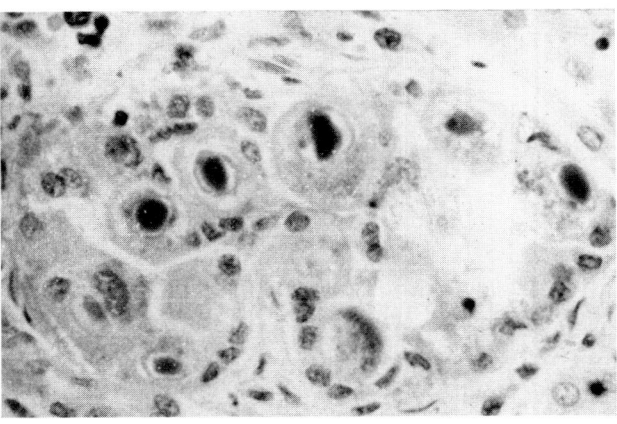

Figure 8–23. Young adult male with acquired immune deficiency syndrome (AIDS). An autopsy showed the changes in the renal tubules shown in the photomicrograph.

772. The organisms depicted are

    (A) Staphylococci

    (B) *Rickettsia burnettii*

    (C) *Aspergillus*

    (D) Epstein–Barr virus

    (E) *Entamoeba histolytica*

773. Which of the following most appropriately describes this condition?

    (A) skin is usual portal of entry

    (B) viral organism of high virulence

    (C) rarely involves lungs or blood vessels

    (D) opportunistic infection seen most commonly in immunocompromised hosts

    (E) only occurs in black males

Questions 774 through 777. (Refer to Figure 8–23.)

774. Figure 8–23 shows

    (A) storage material

    (B) viral inclusion bodies

    (C) fungal infection

    (D) amyloidosis

    (E) fatty infiltration

775. The most likely cause of the disease is

    (A) chemical poisons

    (B) heredity

    (C) malnutrition

    (D) immune deficiency

    (E) hyperimmune state

776. The clinical and pathologic features best fit

    (A) ganglioside storage disease

    (B) glycogen storage disease

    (C) cytomegalovirus infection

    (D) systemic candidiasis

    (E) thiamine deficiency

777. Which statement concerning this disorder is correct?

    (A) The epidemic form is most common.

    (B) It is seen only in the tropics.

    (C) It is never seen in renal transplantation or AIDS.

    (D) It is most commonly seen in immunologically compromised hosts.

    (E) A bacterial organism is the etiologic agent.

Questions 778 through 781. (Refer to Figure 8–24.)

778. The photomicrograph shows a

    (A) group of malignant cells

    (B) colony of bacteria

    (C) portion of a tapeworm

    (D) distorted bile duct

    (E) nidus of future calculus

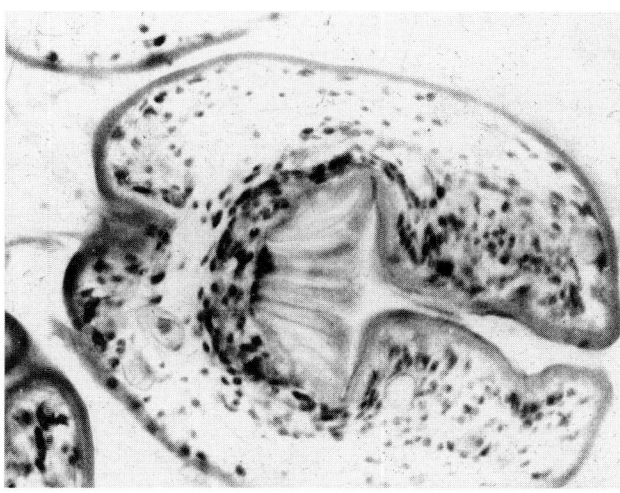

Figure 8–24. A 50-year-old male had a hepatic lobe resected because of a large cyst. The photomicrograph depicts part of the content of the cyst diagnostic of this condition.

779. The most likely cause of the cyst is

(A) hydatid disease
(B) pyogenic abscess from portal pyemia
(C) bile duct dilatation
(D) stasis
(E) necrosis within the center of a tumor

780. The disease is usually caused by

(A) congenital abnormalities
(B) transmission via infected feces
(C) gallstones
(D) bacteremia or appendicitis
(E) unknown etiology

781. Which is a correct statement about the depicted disorder?

(A) Disease is always congenital.
(B) Sheep are never a secondary host.
(C) Humans are the most frequent primary host.
(D) Dogs are the most frequent primary host.
(E) Ova in dog feces are never infective for humans.

Questions 782 through 784. (Refer to Figure 8–25.)

782. The photomicrograph demonstrates

(A) gram-positive cocci
(B) gram-negative bacilli
(C) *Actinomyces*
(D) spirochetes
(E) Donovan bodies

783. The most likely diagnosis is

(A) chancroid
(B) granuloma inguinale
(C) lymphogranuloma venereum
(D) gonorrhea
(E) syphilis

784. Which statement is most accurate concerning this disease?

(A) The organism thrives outside the human body.
(B) The disease is usually transmitted venereally.
(C) The disease is usually transmitted by food contamination.
(D) The organism survives for prolonged periods on dust and debris.
(E) The disease is not seen in sexually active populations.

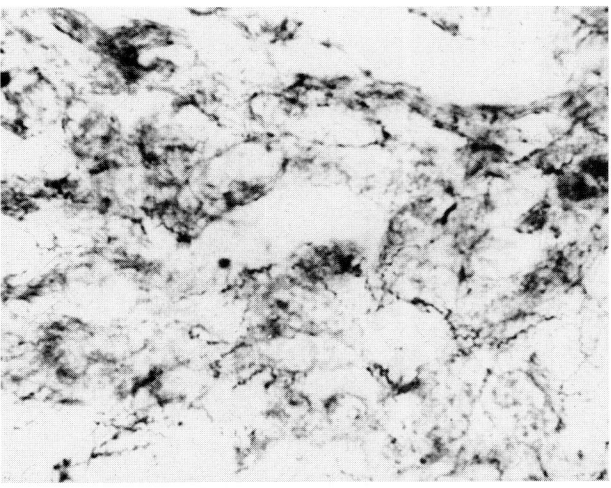

Figure 8–25. Photomicrograph depicting a special stain on a section of a penile ulcer.

Questions 785 and 786. (Refer to Figure 8–26.)

785. The photograph demonstrates

 (A) tuberculous pneumonia
 (B) metastatic carcinoma
 (C) disseminated intravascular coagulation
 (D) lung abscess
 (E) pulmonary infarct

786. The source of entry into the lung is

 (A) aspiration of infected material
 (B) infection of contaminated material into the bloodstream
 (C) spread from primary tumor
 (D) penetration injury of lung
 (E) embolism from the deep calf veins

Questions 787 through 790. (Refer to Figure 8–27.)

787. The process illustrated is best described as

 (A) benign neoplasia
 (B) malignant neoplasia
 (C) healing
 (D) acute suppurative inflammation
 (E) chronic granulomatous inflammation

788. A more precise diagnostic term is

 (A) an osteoid tumor
 (B) osteogenic sarcoma

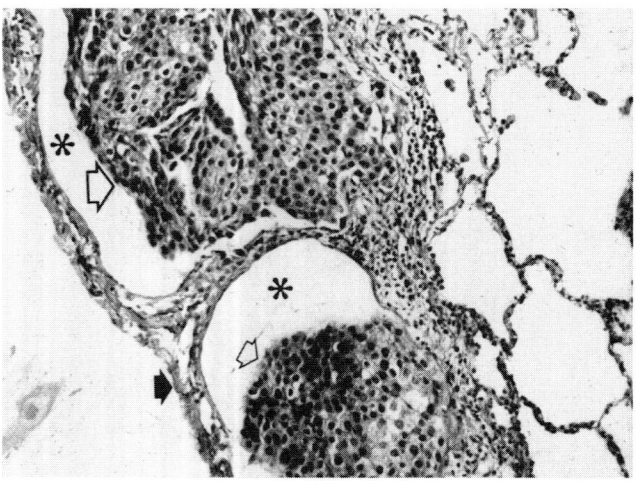

Figure 8–26. Histologic section of the periphery of the lung.

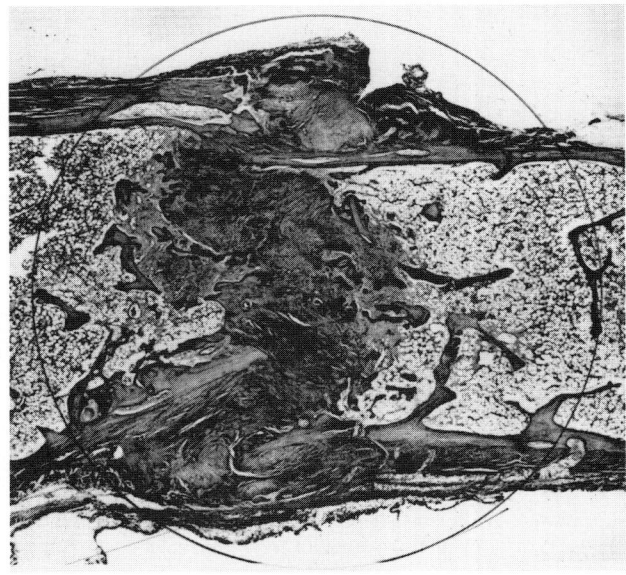

Figure 8–27. Photomicrograph showing section across a long bone.

 (C) healing of fracture
 (D) acute osteomyelitis
 (E) tuberculosis of the bone

789. The dense material extending through the shaft of the bone and continuing onto the periosteal surface is

 (A) osteoid seams in a sarcoma
 (B) hyalinized mature fibrous tissue
 (C) acute suppurative inflammatory exudate
 (D) provisional new bone (callus)
 (E) amyloid

790. Which of the following events is most likely to interfere with proper resolution of the illustrated process?

 (A) high doses of vitamin C
 (B) immobilization of the bone
 (C) foreign material and associated inflammation
 (D) high doses of vitamin D
 (E) high content of calcium in the diet

Questions 791 and 792. (Refer to Figures 8–28 and 8–29.)

791. Which of the following is the best description of the events illustrated?

(A) infarction
(B) lobar pneumonia
(C) lung abscess
(D) benign neoplasm
(E) malignant neoplasm

792. Which of the following is the most likely preceding event?

(A) cigarette smoking
(B) asbestos exposure
(C) deep venous thrombosis with embolus formation

(D) aspiration of infected materials
(E) septicemia

Questions 793 through 796. (Refer to Figure 8–30.)

793. The pale stroma areas are

(A) metastatic liposarcoma
(B) lipid accumulation in liver cells
(C) lipoid granulomas
(D) viral inclusions in liver cells
(E) alcoholic hyalin accumulation in liver cells

794. The condition is best described as

(A) fatty metamorphosis
(B) hepatocellular carcinoma
(C) passive venous congestion
(D) acute viral hepatitis
(E) miliary tuberculosis of the liver

795. Which one of the following is most likely to produce the depicted changes?

(A) metastatic carcinoma
(B) macronodular cirrhosis
(C) alcoholism
(D) bile stasis
(E) miliary tuberculosis

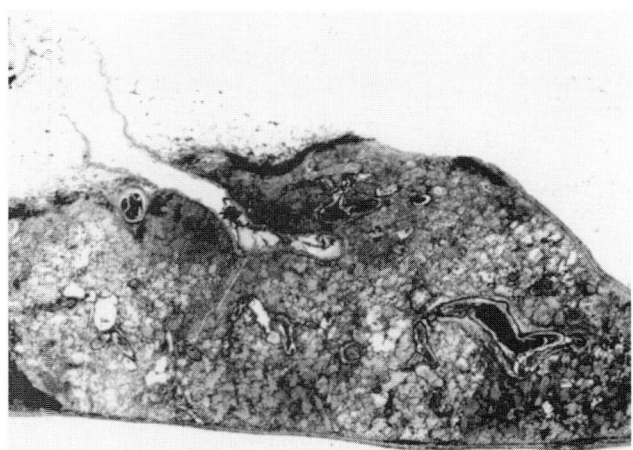

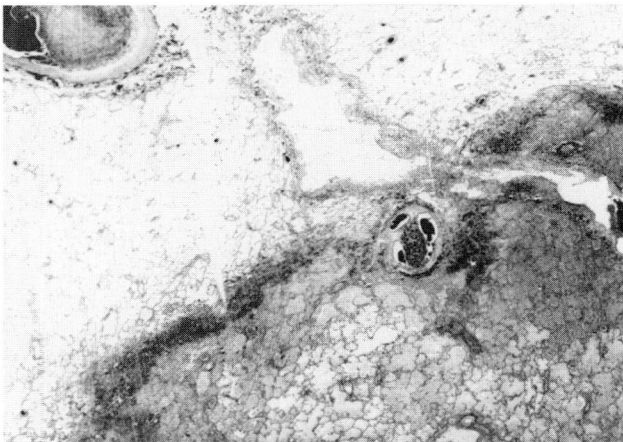

Figures 8–28 (*top*) and 8–29 (*bottom*). A lung shows a form of well-circumscribed consolidation.

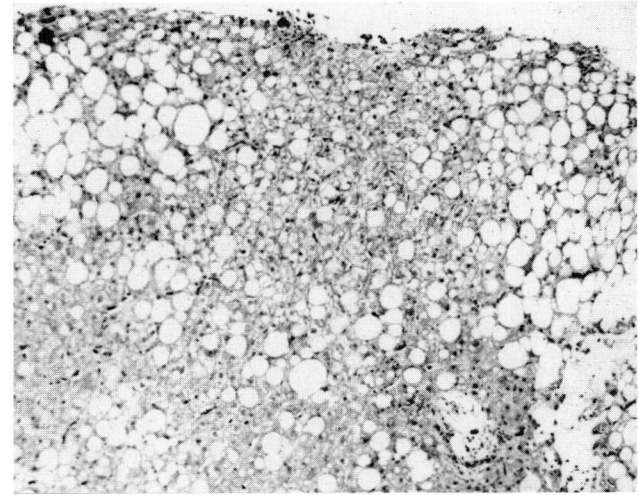

Figure 8–30. Photomicrograph from a liver biopsy.

796.   Which of the following is/are correct concerning the depicted process?

(A) The condition may be seen in choline deficiency.

(B) The condition may be seen in severe malnutrition.

(C) The condition may be seen in children.

(D) There are multiple possible causes.

(E) All of the above are correct.

Question 797. (Refer to Figure 8–31.)

797.   The lesion of the kidney in Figure 8–31 represents

(A) an infarct

(B) a benign tumor

(C) a cyst

(D) tuberculosis of kidney

(E) a malignant neoplasm

Question 798. (Refer to Figure 8–32.)

798.   What is the most common cell type of renal cell carcinoma?

(A) papillary carcinoma

(B) collecting duct carcinoma

(C) chromophobe renal cell carcinoma

(D) clear cell carcinoma

(E) transitional carcinoma

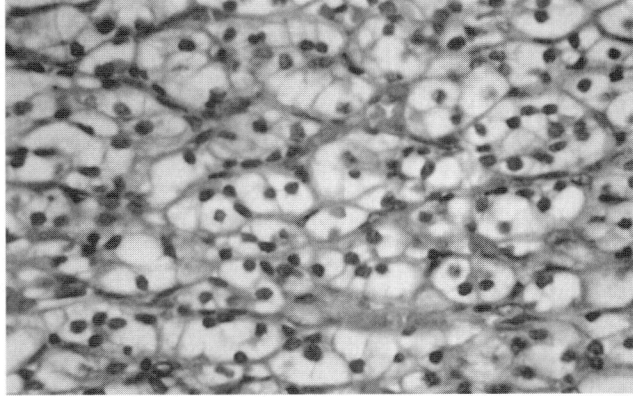

Figure 8–32. High power photomicrograph of the lesion of kidney (see color plate).

Questions 799 and 800. (Refer to Figure 8–33.)

799.   Most commonly this disease in Figure 8–33 becomes symptomatic

(A) in early childhood

(B) in the 2nd decade of life

(C) after the 7th decade

(D) after the 4th decade

(E) in the 3rd decade of life

800.   This disease is

(A) autosomal dominant

(B) autosomal recessive

(C) x-link dominant

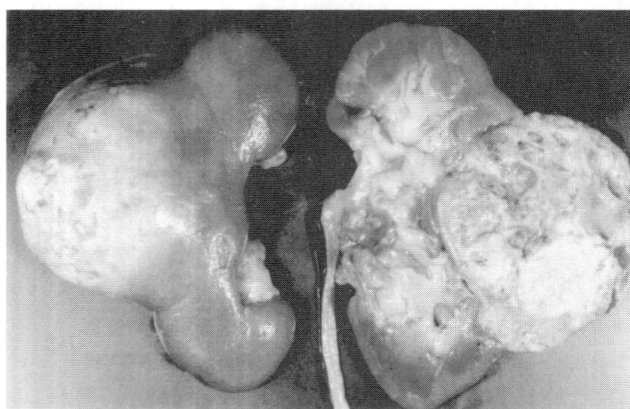

Figure 8–31. Bisected section of kidney (see color plate).

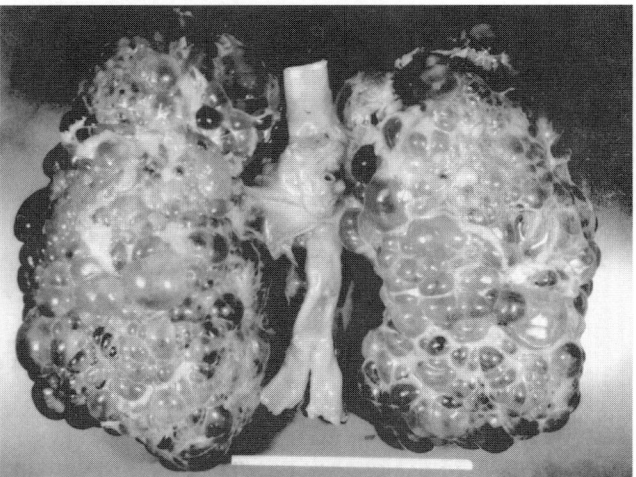

Figure 8–33. Gross appearance of kidneys of an adult person dying with renal failure (see color plate).

(D) x-link recessive

(E) not a hereditary disorder

Questions 801 and 802. (Refer to Figures 8–34 and 8–35.)

801.　The most likely diagnosis is

    (A) intestinal volvulus

    (B) intussusception

    (C) parasitic infestation

    (D) ulcerative colitis

    (E) malignant neoplasm

802.　The microscopic appearance of this lesion is appropriately described as

    (A) diffuse pattern

    (B) follicular pattern

    (C) marginal pattern

    (D) mixed follicular and diffuse pattern

    (E) starry sky appearance

Questions 803 and 804. (Refer to Figure 8–36.)

803.　The gross appearance of this brain demonstrates

    (A) an intracerebral (intraparenchymal) hemorrhage

    (B) congenital abnormality

    (C) infection

    (D) metabolic disease

    (E) parasitic infection

804.　The pathological changes depicted in this gross photograph are most likely related to

    (A) Alzheimer's disease

    (B) hypertension

    (C) metabolic encephalopathy

    (D) multiple metastases

    (E) "respirator brain"

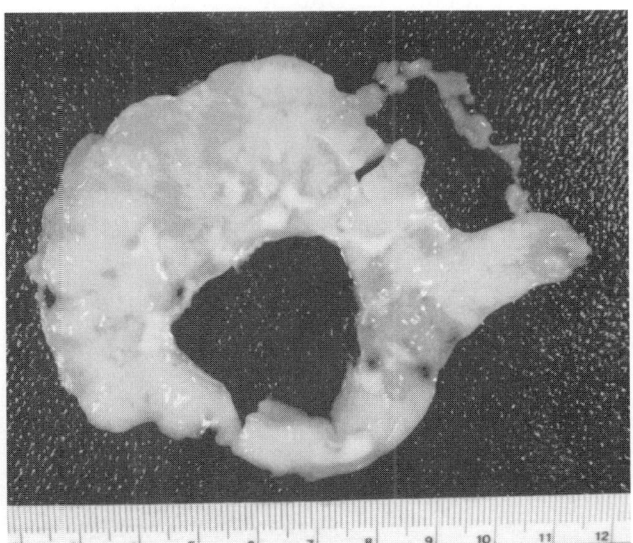

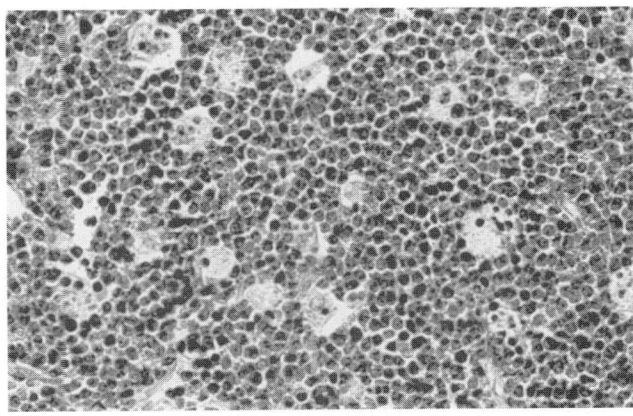

Figures 8–34 (*top*) and 8–35 (*bottom*). Cross section of small intestine (ileum) in a young child that developed an intestinal occlusion (see color plate).

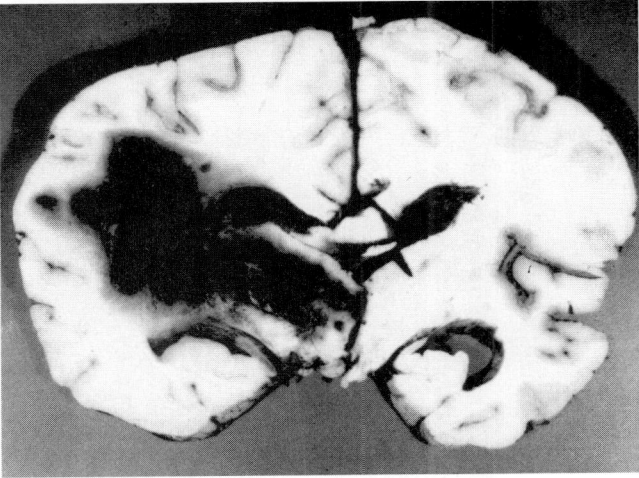

Figure 8–36. The gross specimen of a coronal section of the brain (see color plate).

Questions 805 and 806. (Refer to Figures 8–37 and 8–38.)

805. The lesion shown in this photomicrograph most likely represents

   (A) a malignant neoplasm
   (B) bone spur
   (C) osteochondroma
   (D) osteomyelitis
   (E) Paget's disease

806. Microscopic examination of this tumor demonstrates

   (A) cartilage
   (B) inflammatory cells
   (C) malignant osteoblasts producing woven bone
   (D) microcyst formation
   (E) normal marrow elements

Questions 807 and 808. (Refer to Figures 8–39 and 8–40.)

807. The most likely diagnosis of this lesion found in the prostate (marked by the arrow) is

   (A) neoplasm
   (B) abscess
   (C) hemorrhage
   (D) infarct
   (E) parasite

808. The neoplasm exhibited in this photomicrograph is

   (A) adenocarcinoma
   (B) adenoma
   (C) angiosarcoma
   (D) papillary carcinoma
   (E) squamous cell carcinoma

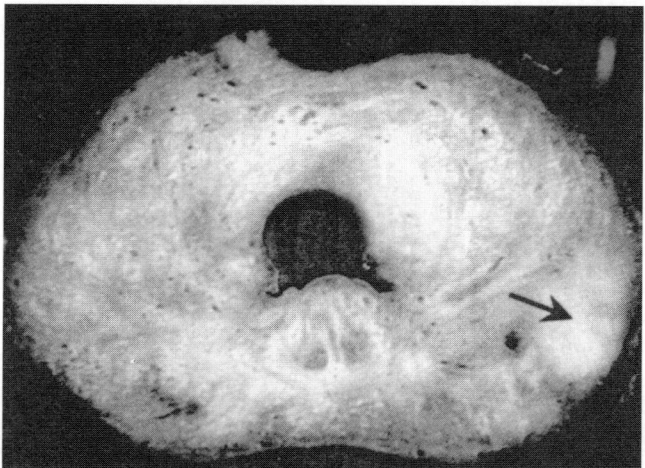

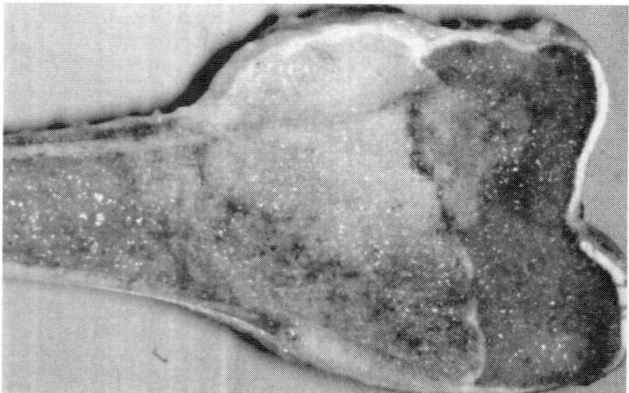

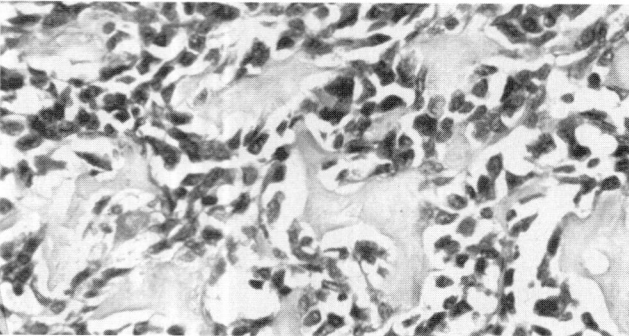

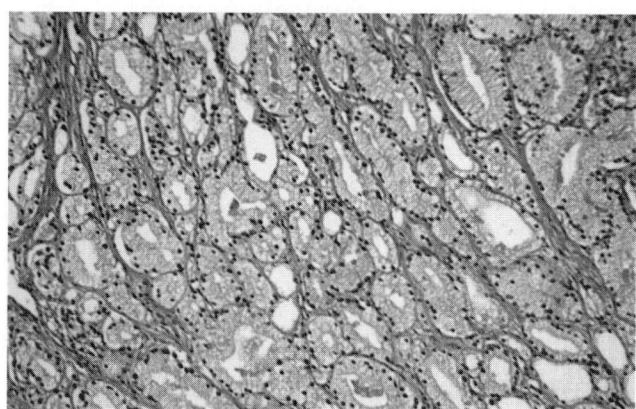

Figures 8–37 (*top*) and 8–38 (*bottom*). The gross specimen corresponds to a cross section of the distal part of the femur. The photomicrograph is a representative section of the lesion (see color plate).

Figures 8–39 (*top*) and 8–40 (*bottom*). The gross specimen in this photograph is a cross section of the prostate. The photomicrograph is a representative section of the lesion found in the prostate (see color plate).

Questions 809 and 810. (Refer to Figure 8–41.)

809. The lesion of this larynx located on the supra-glottic area is

(A) a benign ulcer
(B) a foreign object
(C) a malignant neoplasm
(D) a papilloma
(E) fungal infection

810. The lesion depicted in the larynx is related to

(A) laryngeal nodule degeneration
(B) parasite infestation
(C) cigarette smoking
(D) repeated infections
(E) viral laryngitis

Questions 811 and 812. (Refer to Figure 8–42, A and B.)

811. Looking at the external appearance of this ovarian mass, is it possible discern that

(A) it is benign
(B) it is multilocular
(C) it is malignant
(D) it is solid
(E) none of the above

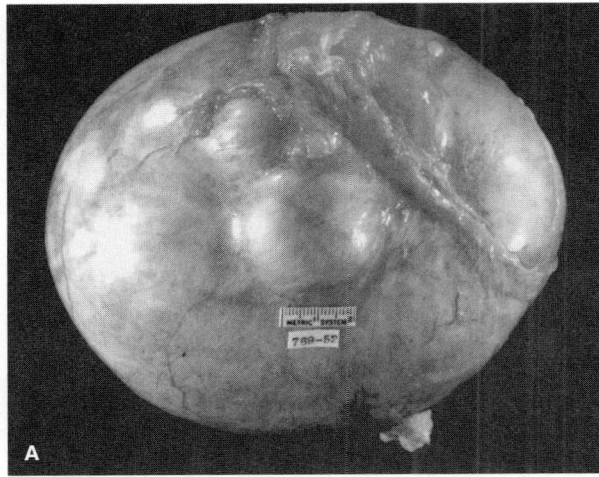
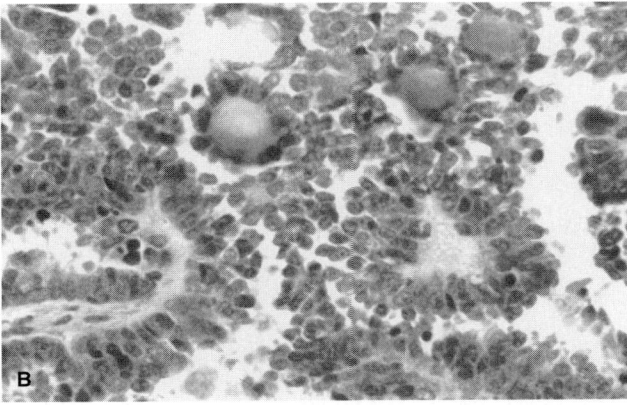

Figure 8–42. A and B, The gross specimen represents an ovarian cyst which has not been opened. The photomicrograph is a representative section of the lesion (see color plate).

812. Looking at this photomicrograph, is it possible to discern if this tumor is

(A) benign cystic teratoma
(B) serous
(C) mucinous
(D) dysgerminoma
(E) Sertoli–Leydig cell tumor

Questions 813 and 814. (Refer to Figures 8–43 and 8–44.)

813. This large tumor located on and adherent to the soft tissues of the thigh represents

(A) angiosarcoma
(B) leiomyosarcoma
(C) liposarcoma, low grade
(D) rhabdomyosarcoma
(E) squamous cell carcinoma

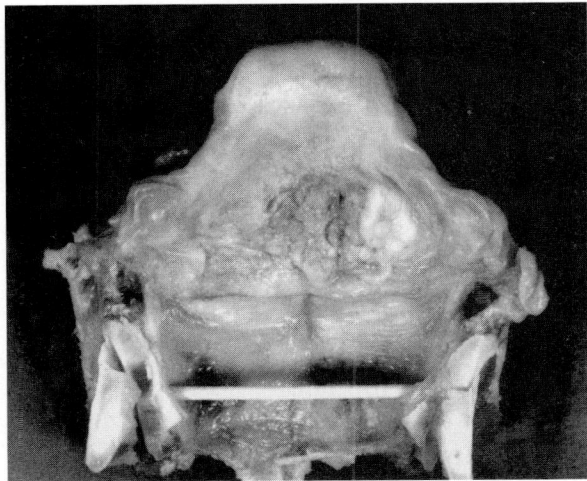

Figure 8–41. The gross specimen is a larynx, which has been opened from the posterior aspect (see color plate).

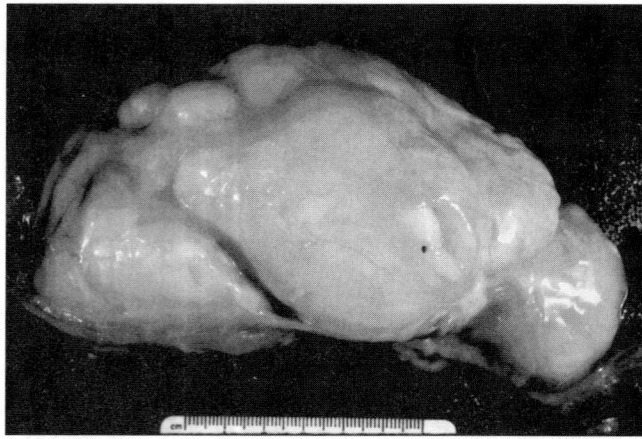

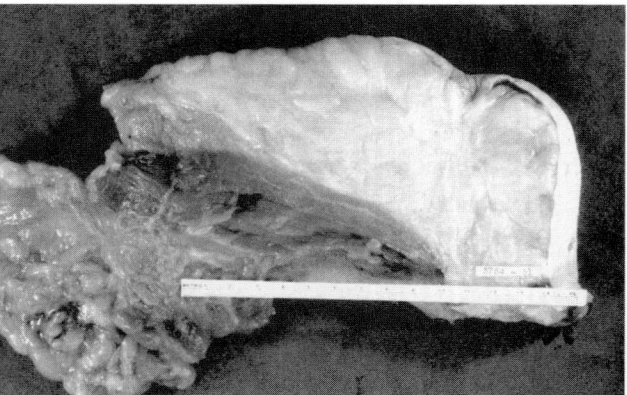

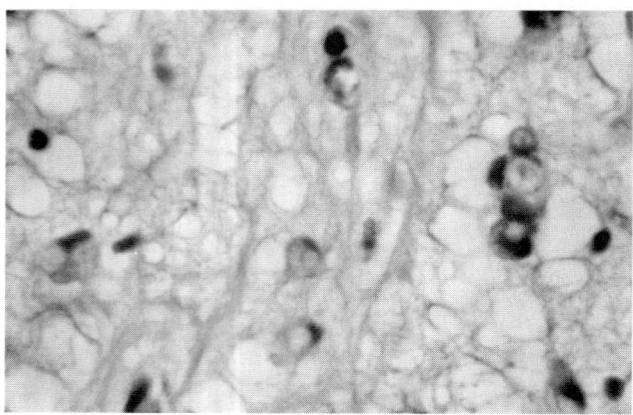

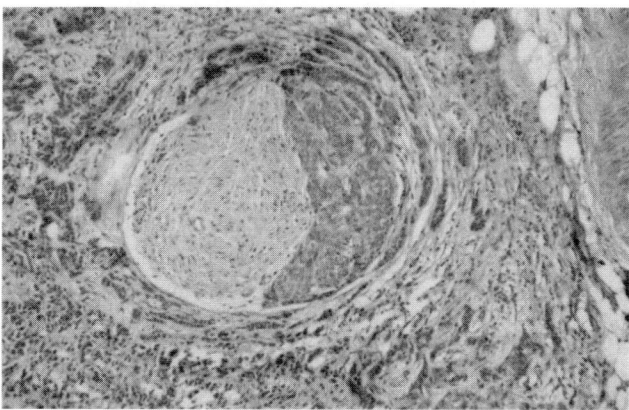

Figures 8–43 (*top*) and 8–44 (*bottom*). The gross specimen represents a tumor removed from the thigh of the 55-year-old male. The photomicrograph is a representative section of the lesion (see color plate).

Figures 8–45 (*top*) and 8–46 (*bottom*). This gross specimen exhibits a cross section of the breast. The photomicrographs represent different features of breast tumors (see color plate).

814. According to the histology display in this photomicrograph, this tumor could be classified as

    (A) well-differentiated liposarcoma
    (B) poorly differentiated liposarcoma
    (C) myxoid liposarcoma
    (D) angioliposarcoma
    (E) fibrous liposarcoma

Questions 815 through 818. (Refer to Figures 8–45 to 8–48.)

815. The lesion depicted in this cross section of the breast represents

    (A) phyllodes tumor
    (B) carcinoma NOS
    (C) fibrocystic disease

    (D) intraductal papilloma
    (E) fibroadenoma

816. This photomicrograph in Figure 8–46 represents

    (A) fibroadenoma
    (B) infiltrating ductal carcinoma, NOS
    (C) infiltrating ductal carcinoma, NOS with perineural invasion
    (D) phyllodes tumor
    (E) sclerosing adenosis

817. The pathological changes depicted in Figure 8–47 can be clinically described as

    (A) abscess formation
    (B) fibrocystic disease
    (C) inflammatory carcinoma of the breast
    (D) intraductal papilloma
    (E) perineural invasion

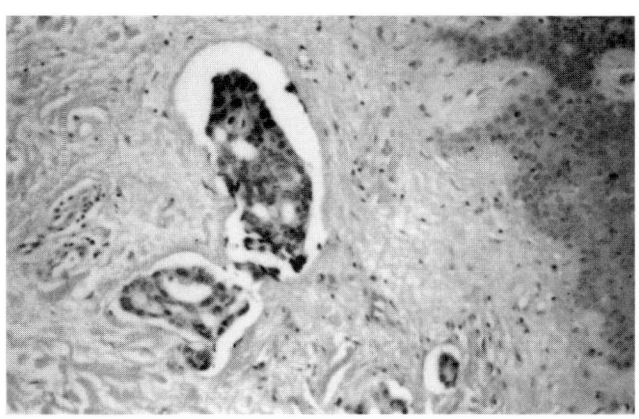

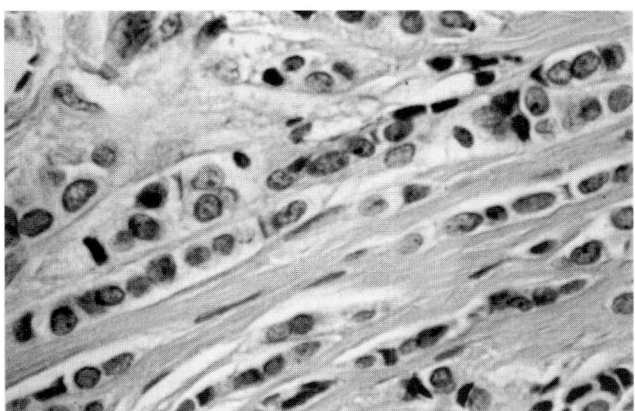

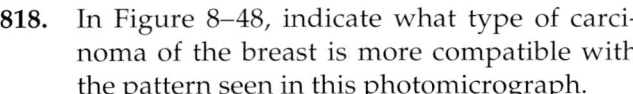

Figures 8–47 (*top*) and 8–48 (*bottom*). See caption to Figures 8–45 and 8–46.

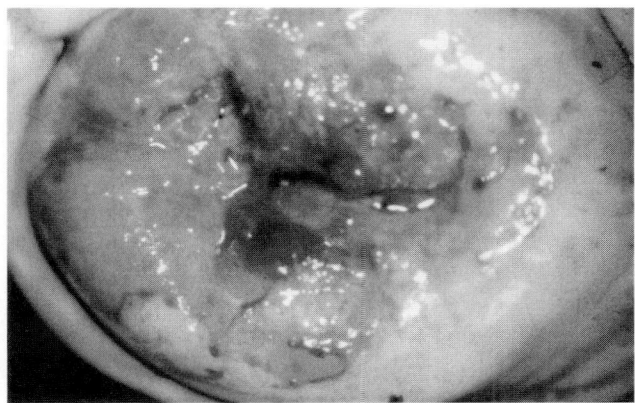

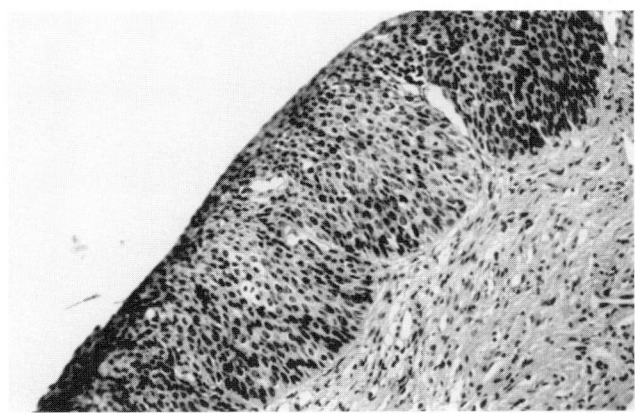

Figures 8–49 (*top*) and 8–50 (*bottom*). Colposcopic appearance of cervix. Microphotograph of a biopsy taken from the transitional zone (see color plate).

818. In Figure 8–48, indicate what type of carcinoma of the breast is more compatible with the pattern seen in this photomicrograph.

(A) colloid (mucinous) carcinoma

(B) infiltrating lobular carcinoma

(C) lobular carcinoma in-situ

(D) medullary carcinoma

(E) papillary carcinoma

Questions 819 and 820. (Refer to Figures 8–49 and 8–50.)

819. The lesion shown in Figure 8–49 will have to be further evaluated with

(A) cone biopsy

(B) multiple cervical biopsies

(C) cervical amputation

(D) laser surgery

(E) total hysterectomy

820. On the evaluation of this photomicrograph, your diagnosis will be

(A) CIN I

(B) normal

(C) squamous cell carcinoma in-situ

(D) adenocarcinoma

(E) invasive squamous cell carcinoma

Questions 821 and 822. (Refer to Figures 8–51 and 8–52.)

821. The lesion of the uterine cavity could be best characterized as

(A) infiltrating malignant neoplasm of the uterine cavity

(B) adenomyosis

(C) endometrial polyp

(D) leiomyoma

(E) tuberculosis of endometrial cavity

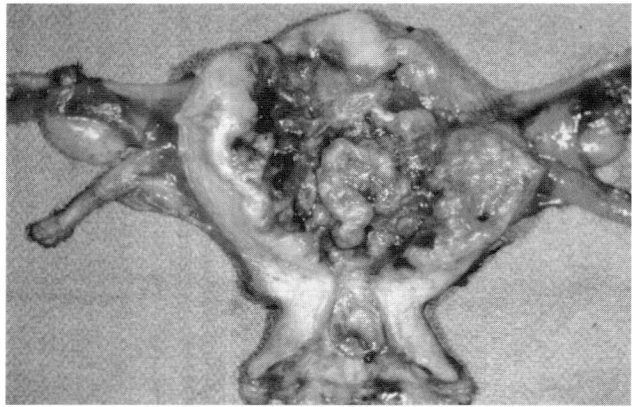

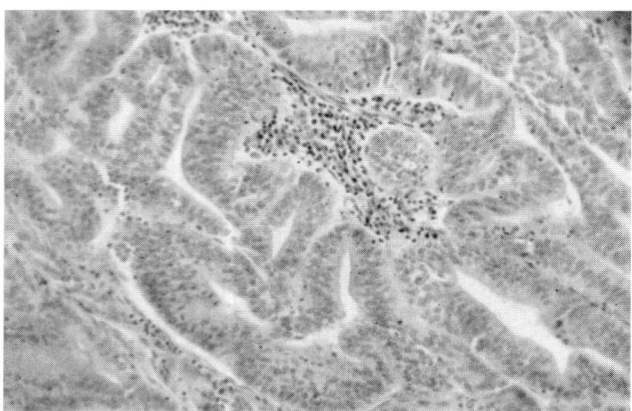

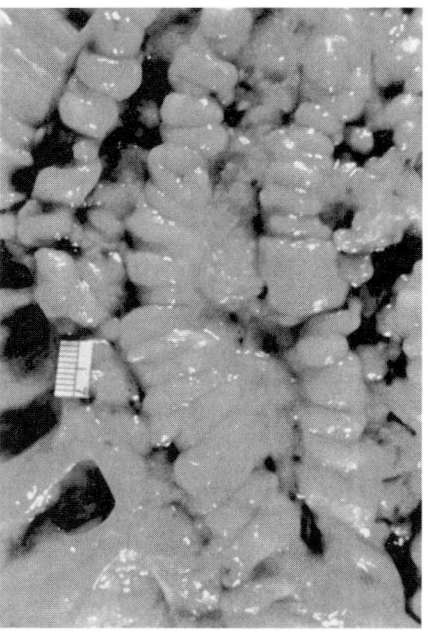

Figures 8–51 (*top*) and 8–52 (*bottom*). This is a gross photograph of the uterus from a total hysterectomy with bilateral salpingooopherectomy. The photomicrograph is a representative area of the lesion (see color plate).

822. The histological type of this endometrial carcinoma would be

    (A) adenosquamous carcinoma

    (B) clear cell type

    (C) endometrioid adenocarcinoma

    (D) papillary carcinoma

    (E) serous adenocarcinoma

Questions 823 and 824. (Refer to Figures 8–53 and 8–54.)

823. The pathological process involving this colon is most likely

    (A) diverticulosis

    (B) gangrene

    (C) a malignant neoplasm

    (D) a solitary ulcer

    (E) ulcerative colitis

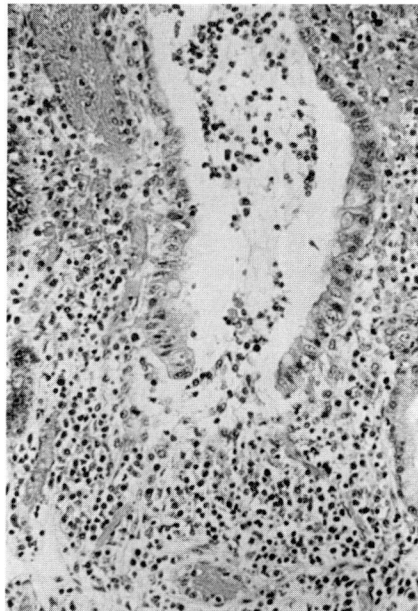

Figures 8–53 (*top*) and 8–54 (*bottom*). A segment of large bowel opened longitudinally (see color plate).

824. In this microphotograph (Figure 8–54), the lesion shown is

    (A) a crypt abscess

    (B) a malignant transformation

    (C) a pseudopolyp

    (D) an ulcer

    (E) metaplasia

Questions 825 and 826. (Refer to Figures 8–55 and 8–56.)

825. The lesion seen in the ileum in Figure 8–55 represents

(A) a benign tumor
(B) Crohn's disease
(C) diverticulosis
(D) ischemic disease
(E) a malignant tumor

826. The lesion that accompanies Crohn's disease seen in Figure 8–56 is better defined as

(A) abscess
(B) fistulous formation
(C) metaplasia
(D) microgranuloma
(E) ulceration

Questions 827 through 836. (Refer to Figures 8–57 to 8–70.)

827. In Figures 8–57 and 8–58, the presence of the ER + PR proteins in the nucleus of the cells is seen as

(A) a prognostic indicator
(B) a predicator of response to hormonal therapy
(C) frequently 50–85% of the tumors
(D) a common finding in postmenopausal women
(E) all of the above

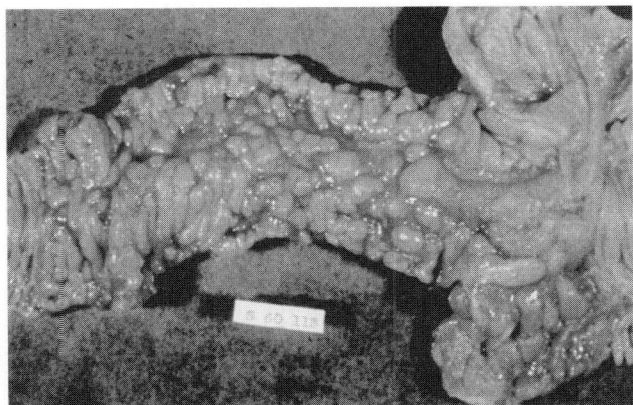

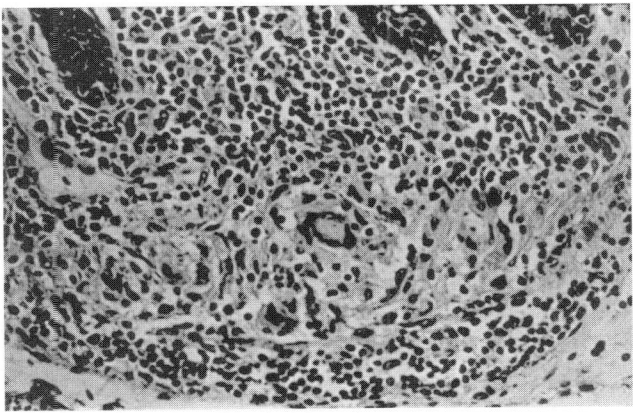

Figures 8–55 (*top*) and 8–56 (*bottom*). The gross specimen is a longitudinally opened terminal ileum with ileocecal valve. The photomicrograph is a representative area of the lesion (see color plate).

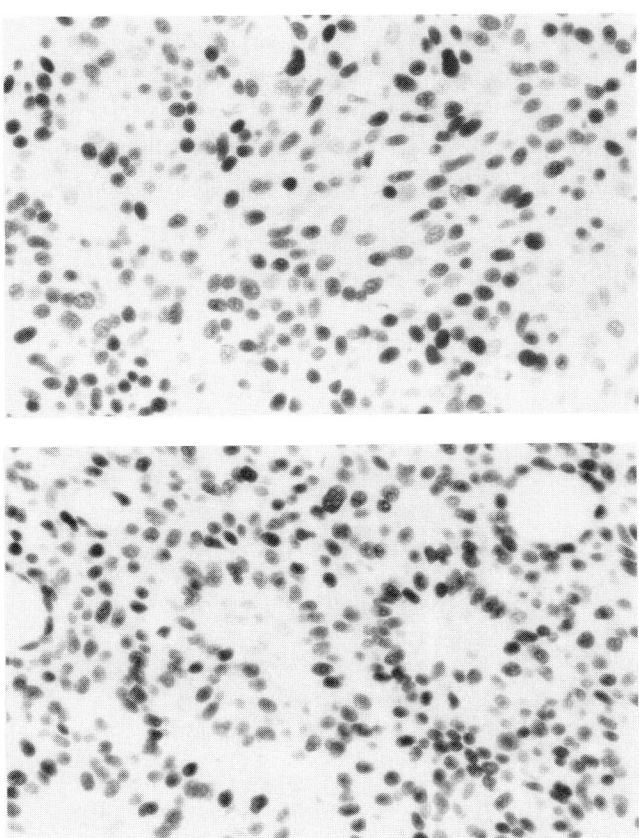

Figures 8–57 (*top*) and 8–58 (*bottom*). High-power photomicrographs representing a strong nuclear positivity for estrogen receptor protein (8–57) and progesterone (8–58) (see color plate).

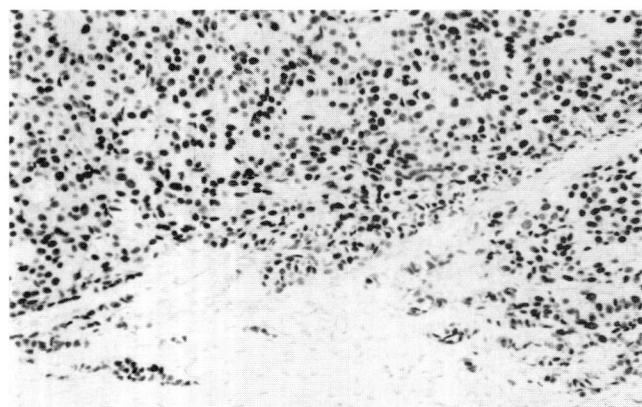

Figure 8–59. Photomicrograph with immunoperoxidase technique of expression of growth factor receptors related oncogenes (Her-2-Neu) (see color plate).

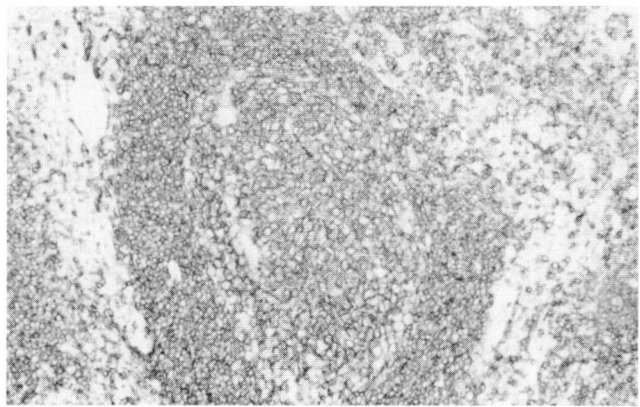

Figure 8–61. Intermedium-power photomicrograph of BCL-2 protein with immunoperoxidase technique with a strong cytoplasmic positivity (see color plate).

828. In Figure 8–59, the demonstration of positive Her-2-Neu overexpression will be most helpful in

(A) determining the type of breast cancer
(B) establishing an anti-Her-2-Neu therapy
(C) staging of the disease
(D) status of the lymphatic involvement
(E) not having any prognostic significance

829. In Figure 8–60, in the classic Hodgkin's disease the Reed–Sternberg cells are

(A) aneuploid cells
(B) positive for surface antigens for B lymphocytes
(C) occasional specific T lymphocyte receptors

(D) markers derived from the monocyte/macrophage series
(E) all of the above

830. In Figure 8–61, BCL-2 overexpression is most commonly seen in

(A) lymphoblastic lymphoma
(B) follicular lymphoma
(C) immunoblastic lymphoma
(D) Mantle cell lymphoma
(E) marginal lymphoma

831. In Figure 8–62, multiple myeloma is characterized by

(A) T cell proliferation
(B) plasma cell proliferation
(C) frequently originate in the soft tissue

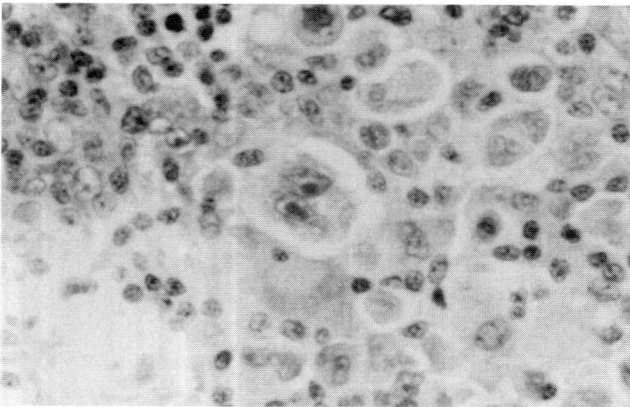

Figure 8–60. High-power photomicrograph depicts a classic binucleated Reed–Sternberg cell (see color plate).

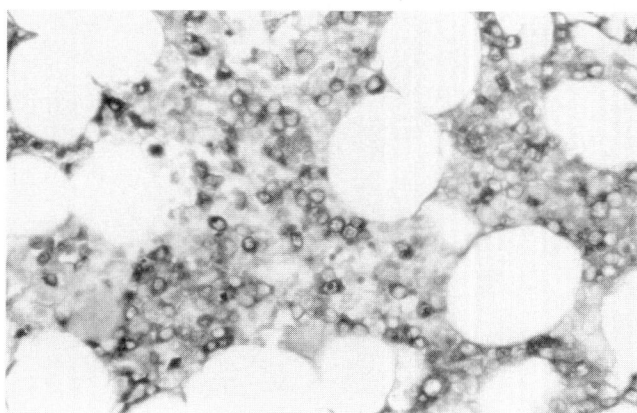

Figure 8–62. High-power photomicrograph of a bone marrow biopsy that has been treated with immunoperoxidase technique for lambda light chains (see color plate).

(D) natural killer lymphocytes origin

(E) prominent gastrointestinal symptomatology

832. In Figures 8–63 and 8–64, which subtype of Hodgkin's disease shows the lowest number of Reed–Sternberg cells?

(A) lymphocytic predominant Hodgkin's disease

(B) mixed cellularity

(C) nodular sclerosis

(D) nodular variant of cellular phase of NS Hodgkin's disease

(E) lymphocytic depleted Hodgkin's disease

833. In Figure 8–65, which of the following subtypes of Hodgkin's disease have the most favorable prognosis?

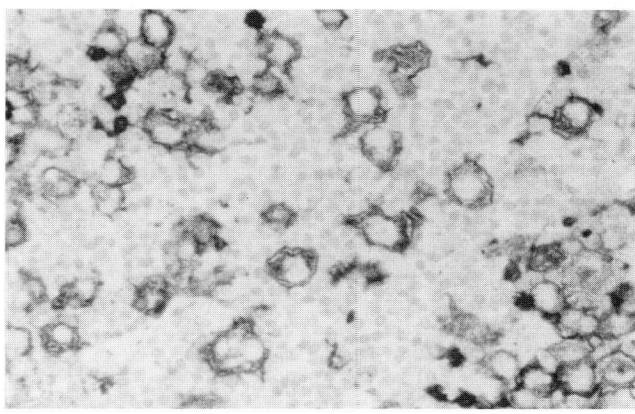

Figure 8–65. Photomicrograph of immunoperoxidase technique stained for CD20. The picture depicts the L-H cells characteristic of lymphocytic predominant Hodgkin's disease (see color plate).

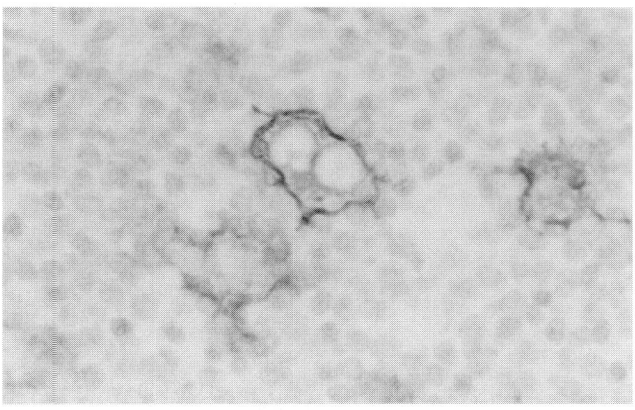

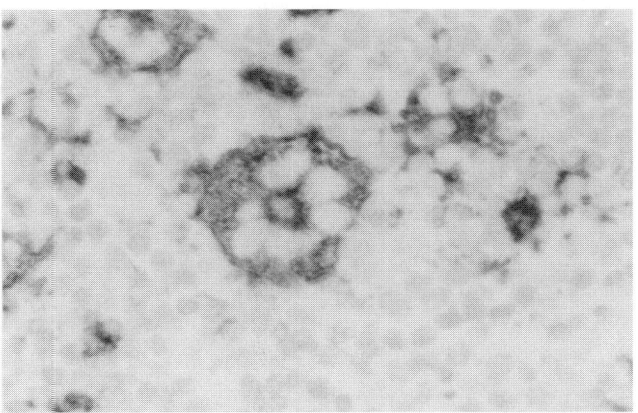

Figures 8–63 (top) and 8–64 (bottom). Photomicrographs of immunoperoxidase techniques for Reed–Sternberg cells and RS variant (polyploid). Figure 8–63 is stained for CD15 (Leu-M-1) and 8–64 is stained with CD30 (Ti-1) (see color plate).

(A) nodular sclerosing type

(B) lymphocytic depletion type

(C) mixed cellularity

(D) cellular phase of nodular sclerosing Hodgkin's disease

(E) lymphocytic predominant Hodgkin's disease

834. In Figure 8–66, which type of non-Hodgkin's lymphoma displays a characteristic 11,14 translocation?

(A) small cell lymphocytic

(B) follicular small cell lymphoma

(C) Mantle cell lymphoma

(D) marginal lymphoma

(E) diffuse large cell B cell lymphoma

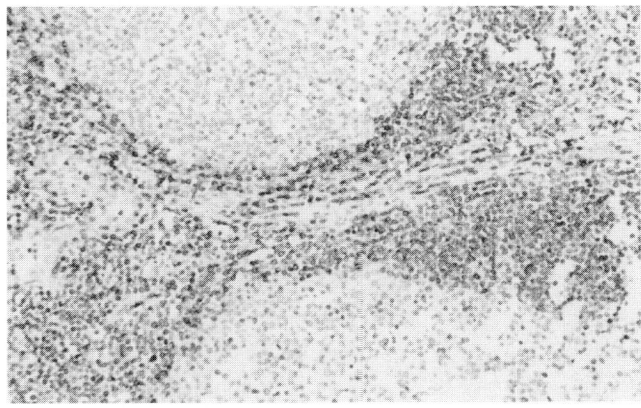

Figure 8–66. Photomicrograph of a lymph node which is stained with immunoperoxidase for cyclin-D1 (see color plate).

835. In Figures 8–67 and 8–68, which is the non-Hodgkin's lymphoma with a minority of neoplastic B cells in a background of normal T cells, with BCL-2 rearrangement?

(A) T cell-rich B cell lymphoma (TCRBCL)
(B) small cell lymphoma
(C) Burkitt's lymphoma
(D) lymphoblastic lymphoma
(E) diffuse large cell lymphoma

836. In Figures 8–69 and 8–70, the expression of kappa or lambda light chains is

(A) useful to determine the type of lymphoma
(B) useful to prove clonality
(C) useful to evaluate the mitotic index
(D) related to the staging of the tumor
(E) not helpful at all

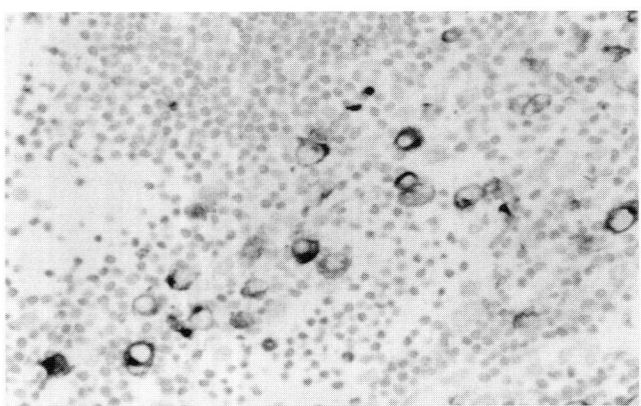

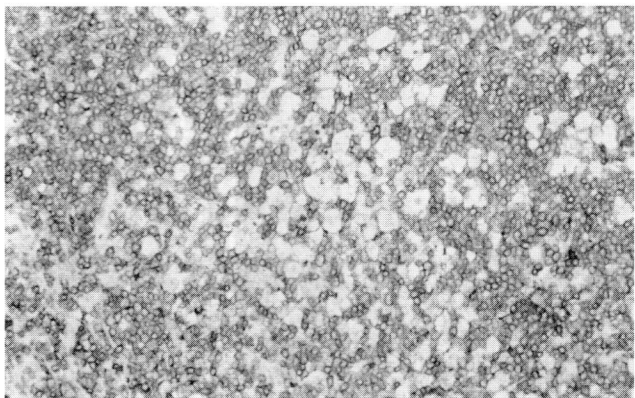

Figures 8–67 (*top*) and 8–68 (*bottom*). Photomicrograph (8–67) immunoperoxidase technique stained with CD20. Figure 8–68 low-power photomicrograph of same lymphoma stained with pan T antibodies (see color plate).

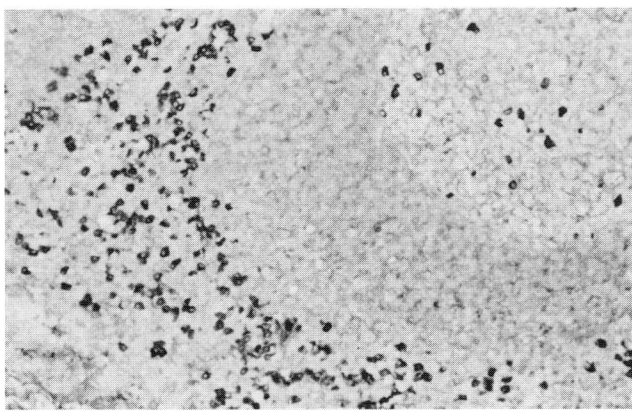

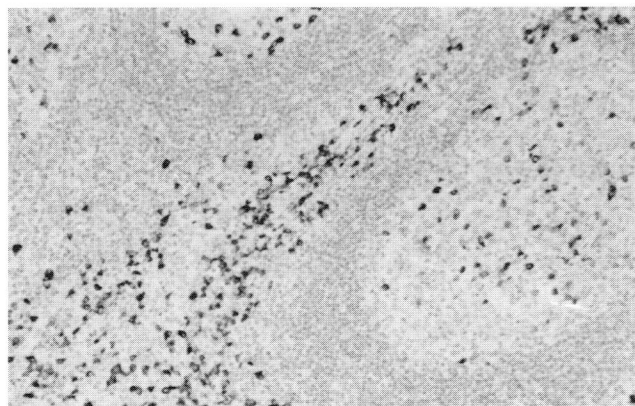

Figures 8–69 (*top*) and 8–70 (*bottom*). Figure 8–69 is a photomicrograph with the Kappa light chain stain, immunoperoxidase technique. Figure 8–70 photomicrograph of lambda light chain with immunoperoxidase (see color plate).

Answers and Explanations

Figure 8–1 shows a section of stomach with a peptic ulcer.

723. **(B)** Loss of continuity of an epithelial surface is the definition of ulceration. Figure 8–1 illustrates very clearly such a loss of continuity of the epithelium of the gastric mucosa. Therefore, the other listed alternatives are inappropriate. Although atrophic changes may precede or even occur after healing of such an ulcer, in the active stage, there is complete loss of epithelium. *(Chandrasoma and Taylor, pp. 577–580)*

724. **(B)** The diagnosis that most clearly matches the illustration is peptic ulcer. Hypertrophic gastritis and gastric carcinoma would result in an increase in the amount of cellular material in the epithelium. Intestinal metaplasia of gastric mucosa is not apparent in this case. Although gastric atrophy may occur in the healing phase of a peptic ulcer, congenital gastric atrophy clearly is not applicable in this instance. *(Chandrasoma and Taylor, pp. 577–580)*

725. **(C)** Peptic ulcers are thought to result from an overproduction of acid and pepsin, with autodigestion and destruction of the mucosa and persistence of the ulcer by the continued effect of such acid and pepsin. Chronic peptic ulcers cause continuous bleeding, often at a relatively low level, that is not apparent clinically but can result in iron deficiency anemia from chronic blood loss. *(Chandrasoma and Taylor, pp. 577–580)*

726. **(C)** The photograph depicts a peptic ulcer, a classic example of the ulcerative inflammation reaction. Chronic peptic ulcers grossly appear as solitary large punched out areas in the gastric mucosa with a smooth surfaced, firm base. The gastric rugae often radiate out from the ulcer bed. Microscopically, the ulcer demonstrates necrotic debris, inflammation, fibrin precipitates, and peripheral fibrosis. *(Chandrasoma and Taylor, pp. 577–580)*

727. **(E)** The potential long-term complications of gastric ulcers include hemorrhage, penetration, perforation, obstruction, and rarely, malignant transformation. Hypertension, pernicious anemia, atrophic gastritis, and gastric leiomyomatosis do not result from gastric peptic ulcers. *(Chandrasoma and Taylor, pp. 577–580)*

Figures 8–2 and 8–3 show gross and microscopic views of an appendix with acute inflammation, or acute appendicitis.

728. **(C)** With acute appendicitis, the inflammation extends through the wall of the appendix where there are many polymorphonuclear leukocytes that break down tissue, often with apparent exudate on the surface and within the lumen. This is, therefore, a good example of acute suppurative inflammation. There is no evidence of peptic ulceration or hyperplasia and chronic inflammation, granulomatous or nongranulomatous, does not produce this kind of picture. *(Rubin and Farber, pp. 748–749)*

729. **(C)** In most instances, untreated acute appendicitis, particularly if suppuration has taken place, does not heal spontaneously, and resolution certainly does not occur. Atrophy has been seen in the appendix but rarely as the result of an acute inflammation. Malignant transformation is an extremely unlikely event; whereas, ischemic necrosis with perforation is a frequently encountered complication, because the appendix has an end-artery system. The buildup of pressure resulting from the flow of venous blood increases the engorgement, and obstruction to the arterial supply and gangrene and perforation ensue. *(Rubin and Farber, pp. 748–749)*

730.   **(E)** Acute suppurative appendicitis, as depicted in Figures 8–2 and 8–3, demonstrates luminal suppurative debris, mural neutrophilic infiltration, focal necrosis, edema, vascular congestion, fecalith formation, and serosal exudates. *(Rubin and Farber, pp. 748–749)*

731.   **(C)** There is often an obstruction of the lumen of the appendix by a fecalith. This is a hard, inspissated, stonelike area of feces that initially causes irritation or ulceration of the mucosa. This is the portal of entry of intestinal bacteria and, in addition, creates an obstruction, which adds to the problem. Fecaliths occur relatively frequently. Acute appendicitis is much more frequently seen in the developed countries of the world than in the underdeveloped countries and is thought to be associated with dietary differences. Acute appendicitis rarely if ever resolves without treatment because of the vulnerability of the vasculature described in this answer and in the answer to Question 8. In addition to elderly patients, it is seen frequently in children and young teenagers. *(Rubin and Farber, pp. 748, 749)*

Figures 8–4 and 8–5 are photomicrographs of the lungs. The inflammatory process described extends evenly through all the alveoli with a distribution that is panlobular in type.

732.   **(B)** Lobar pneumonia is acute inflammation extending from one alveolus to the other through the pores of Kohn and extending to the interlobar septum and to the pleural surfaces. It differs from the other conditions in that diffuse interstitial pneumonia occurs in the alveolar walls and is usually a monocytic, lymphocytic response. Chronic granulomatous disease produces patchy areas of giant cell granulomas. Pulmonary fibrosis may be diffuse but results from the formation of collagen, not acute inflammatory cells and exudate. Lobular or bronchial pneumonia may be exudate. Lobular or bronchial pneumonia may be confluent, but there usually are some areas of normal alveoli between the consolidated areas that seem to concentrate around the terminal bronchioles and are, therefore, not panlobular as in lobar pneumonia. *(Cotran et al., pp. 717–721)*

733.   **(B)** *S. pneumoniae* is by far the most common organism to cause lobar pneumonia. Part of the disease process and the rapidity of spread throughout the entire lobe of the lung are thought to be associated with the immune response to the polysaccharide capsule of these organisms. Adenoviruses are more likely to produce interstitial pneumonia. Coliform organisms and other similar organisms more frequently produce bronchopneumonia. *M. tuberculosis* is characteristically the cause of granulomatous disease of the lungs, or tuberculosis. Asbestos particles may be associated with fibrosis. *(Cotran et al., pp. 717–721)*

734.   **(B)** Fibrin and large numbers of PMN in the alveoli are the hallmarks of acute lobular pneumonia; whereas, giant cells and lymphocytes are more frequently seen in granulomatous disease. Fibrous tissue would be the end result of these inflammatory conditions, not the acute phase. *(Cotran et al., pp. 717–721)*

735.   **(D)** It is of considerable interest that such extensive involvement of the lungs is not a frequently fatal disorder. In fact, it resolves completely, leaving no residual disease providing the alveolar walls have not been destroyed and architectural resolution can take place without fibrosis. Fibrosis does occur but rarely produces the dense fibrosis described here. Gangrene is extremely uncommon in the lungs, and calcification usually occurs as a result of granulomatous disease with fibrosis. *(Cotran et al., pp. 717–721)*

Figures 8–6 and 8–7 are photomicrographs of a lung with a patchy or lobular consolidation characteristic of bronchopneumonia, or lobular pneumonia. There are normal, recognizable alveoli between the areas of consolidation in contrast to Figures 8–4 and 8–5, where there was a diffuse inflammatory process.

736. **(C)** This lobular distribution is different from that of interstitial pneumonia and lobar pneumonia. Under low power, it might be confused with chronic granulomatous disease or patchy pulmonary fibrosis, but high power shows the presence of an acute inflammatory response rather than giant cell granulomas or fibrous tissue. *(Cotran et al., pp. 717–721)*

737. **(C)** *E. coli* is normally an inhabitant of the gastrointestinal tract and may cause aspiration into the lungs, such as a lobular distribution resulting from inflammation commencing around the terminal bronchioles. *S. pneumoniae* usually produces lobar pneumonia. Adenoviruses cause interstitial pneumonia, and *M. tuberculosis* cause granulomatous disease. Asbestos particles are the most likely to produce diffuse pulmonary fibrosis. *(Cotran et al., pp. 717–721)*

738. **(C)** PMNs are the hallmark of acute inflammation, whatever its distribution. The PMNs and their peribronchial and bronchial distribution indicate that the disease is bronchopneumonia. *(Cotran et al., pp. 717–721)*

739. **(D)** Partial resolution with some permanent damage to the bronchi and bronchioles is the most appropriate answer. Gangrene and calcification rarely occur, and complete resolution with no residual disease is very unlikely in bronchopneumonia, because there is usually damage to the terminal bronchioles and the alveolar walls communicating with them. *(Cotran et al., pp. 717–721)*

Figures 8–8 and 8–9 show discrete solid areas that are focal collections of liquefaction necrosis surrounded by polymorphonuclear leukocytes, with some localization characteristic of abscesses.

740. **(D)** These characteristics are those of abscesses. The picture is not diffuse, and, therefore, interstitial pneumonia and lobar pneumonia can be ruled out. The distinction between an abscess and lobular or bronchopneumonia can sometimes be difficult, because breakdown of tissue can complicate bronchopneumonia and produce abscesses. However, the distribution is independent of the terminal bronchioles and scattered through the lungs. Chronic granulomatous disease would produce giant cells and lymphocytes. *(Cotran et al., p. 722)*

741. **(C)** Abscesses can be caused by a number of organisms, both aerobic and anaerobic, that are pyogenic; i.e., they produce pus, which is the hallmark of an abscess. Adenoviruses cause interstitial pneumonitis. *M. tuberculosis* produces granulomas, asbestos particles produce diffuse fibrosis, and *M. pneumoniae* produces mostly interstitial but sometimes a bronchopneumonic type picture, and not characteristically a pyogenic response. *(Cotran et al., p. 722)*

742. **(B)** Abscesses can be caused by aspiration of infected material into the lungs, in which case they usually are associated with the bronchial tree. They can be the result of septicemic spread, a condition known as "pyemia," which is probably the most applicable in this instance. Asbestos and *M. pneumoniae* produce a different pattern in both distribution and the type of inflammatory cells involved. *(Cotran et al., p. 722)*

743. **(E)** Complete resolution is extremely unlikely, because there is liquefaction necrosis and, therefore, loss of tissue that would have to be replaced by fibrous tissue, which could result in pulmonary fibrosis. Abscesses may rupture into the pleural cavity, producing empyema, and may spread further via the bloodstream to produce brain abscess, which is one of the complications of lung abscess. *(Cotran et al., p. 722)*

Figures 8–10 and 8–11 illustrate the process of intravascular coagulation, or thrombosis.

744. **(B)** This is a thrombotic occlusion of a blood vessel and distinctly different from the haphazard arrangement of the elements of the blood seen in a postmortem blood clot. Although acute inflammation may complicate or even

precede thrombotic occlusion, there is no evidence in this case, nor is there chronic inflammation or tumor materials in an embolic form present. There is a distinct difference between a blood clot and a thrombus. A thrombus can occur only in a living blood vessel and in blood that is flowing. This creates the structure composed of layers of platelets, fibrin, and red cells in an orderly fashion. Blood may clot haphazardly after death and has no such structure. *(Cotran et al., pp. 124–129)*

745.   **(D)** The most probable outcome of thrombotic occlusion of a blood vessel, particularly an artery, is ischemic damage or infarction of the tissue supplied by that artery. Acute suppurative inflammation occasionally may complicate such a procedure but is not the most probable immediate outcome. Dissolution and dissipation of the blood clot may sometimes occur but are not the most probable occurrence. Chronic granulomatous inflammation and metastatic spread of tumor cells are not probable outcomes in this set of circumstances. *(Cotran et al., pp. 124–129)*

746.   **(E)** The final outcome of a thrombotic event depends on a complex interplay of a number of factors: the degree of collateral circulation, the type of artery occluded, the state of collateral circulation, the state of tissue oxygenation before the occlusion, the degree and rate of recanalization of the thrombus, and the activity of the fibrinolytic system. *(Cotran et al., pp. 124–129)*

747.   **(E)** Alteration of the blood flow, increased coagulability of the blood, and damage to the intima of the vessel wall are the classic Virchow's triad, which is the basis on which thrombosis may occur. *(Cotran et al., pp. 124–129)*

Figures 8–12 and 8–13 show gross and microscopic characteristics of a neoplasm of the colon, which is a well differentiated adenocarcinoma.

748.   **(C)** This is a malignant neoplasm demonstrating invasion of the bowel wall, with a variable degree of involvement of the adjacent mucosa. Hyperplasia would not produce such

an invasive process, nor would a benign neoplasm, which in the colon would probably be a polyp. There is no evidence of acute suppurative inflammation. *(Chandrasoma and Taylor, pp. 622–624)*

749.   **(C)** This is a malignant neoplasm, because there is lack of encapsulation. It is invasive, and the cells are recapitulating the glandular structure of the colonic mucosa. Therefore, by definition, this is a carcinoma and an adenocarcinoma in type. Ulcerative colitis would produce, as the name implies, multiple areas of ulceration and mucosal inflammation. Crohn's disease of the colon is a granulomatous disease that involves the full thickness of the colonic walls, and adenomatous polyp is a well-defined and not invasive process. Amebic dysentery would produce an inflamed, ulcerated lesion. *(Chandrasoma and Taylor, pp. 622–624)*

750.   **(E)** Such tumors will, in fact, grow and produce obstruction to the lumen, ulceration of the mucosa, and subsequent hemorrhage owing to invasion of the blood vessels in the submucosa. *(Chandrasoma and Taylor, pp. 622–624)*

751.   **(E)** Well-differentiated colonic adenocarcinoma is a malignant neoplasm. It occurs most frequently in the highly industrialized Western nations, in individuals over 45 years old, in individuals with low-fiber, high-fat diets, in association with chronic ulcerative colitis, and in association with familial polyposis. The malignancy arises from gland-forming epithelium and usually retains at least focal glandular architecture or secretion of mucin by individual tumor cells. *(Chandrasoma and Taylor, pp. 622–624)*

Figures 8–14 and 8–15 show the gross and microscopic appearances of a malignant tumor of the lung, or bronchogenic carcinoma.

752.   **(C)** The obvious invasive properties of this tumor and its poorly differentiated state indicate that it is malignant. There is no evidence of infarction, lung abscess, or granuloma, and the tumor does not have the characteristics of a benign lesion. *(Rubin and Farber, pp. 655–660)*

753. **(C)** The tumor cells appear to be differentiated in the direction of the squamous type of epithelium and, therefore, would be called a "squamous cell" or "epidermoid" carcinoma. An adenoma of the bronchus would be a well differentiated glandular tumor. Tuberculosis would produce the characteristic appearance of giant cell granulomas with caseous necrosis; these are not present. *(Rubin and Farber, pp. 655–660)*

754. **(E)** This type of tumor can produce obstruction to the bronchial tree, can ulcerate, and can produce hemorrhage. The obstruction will cause collapse and accumulation of materials, with infection and pneumonia distal to the obstruction. It is often these complications that first bring the tumor to the attention of the physician, particularly pneumonia that does not resolve or that recurs after treatment. The hemorrhage often produces the symptoms of hemoptysis or blood in the septum. *(Rubin and Farber, pp. 655–660)*

755. **(D)** Squamous cell carcinoma of the lung is strongly associated with cigarette smoking. Prior to most frank carcinomas there is squamous metaplasia of the bronchial epithelium with subsequent progressive dysplasia. Other factors that increase the risk for developing lung cancer include inhalation of asbestos, uranium, nickel, chromate, and gold. Low-fiber diets, hypercoagulable states, sickle cell anemia, and bacterial infections are not directly associated with pulmonary squamous cell carcinoma. *(Rubin and Farber, pp. 655–660)*

Figures 8–16 and 8–17 show aspects of the microscopic findings in a lump removed from the breast of a 45-year-old woman. It has the features of a poorly differentiated malignant tumor, a carcinoma of the breast.

756. **(A)** This is a malignant tumor of the breast. All of the other choices can mimic the gross appearance and the clinical features. Microscopy, therefore, is vital to the correct diagnosis. *(Chandrasoma and Taylor, pp. 822–829)*

757. **(A)** The microscopy shows this to be a tumor, and the similarity to ductal tissue of the breast would classify it as an adenocarcinoma. A fibroadenoma is a distinctly different well-circumscribed combination of duct and fibrous tissue. Fat necrosis produces areas of necrosis of fat, with responding inflammatory changes. Fibrosis and duct obstruction with abscess produce the classic liquefaction necrosis and many polymorphonuclear leukocytes. Tuberculous mastitis is a rare condition in developed countries of the world and produces the typical granulomatous lesion of tuberculosis. *(Chandrasoma and Taylor, pp. 822–829)*

758. **(D)** The stage of the disease is the single most important variable of the listed choices that affects the eventual outcome of breast carcinoma. This is supported by the observation that the 5-year survival rate for stage I, II, III, and IV is 85, 66, 41, and 10%, respectively. In a node-negative patient (all stage I and some stage II), the status of the steroid receptors, DNA ploidy, percent S phase, and oncogene status are additional independent factors affecting prognosis. *(Chandrasoma and Taylor, pp. 822–829)*

759. **(C)** Breast carcinoma is most likely to occur in first- and second-degree female relatives of known breast carcinoma patients. There is a fivefold increased likelihood of breast carcinoma developing in a female whose mother or sister has had breast carcinoma. In addition, there is an independent increased likelihood of breast carcinoma developing in individuals who are nulliparous, those with early menarche, those with late menopause, those who have never breastfed their children, and those whose first pregnancy was at a late age. Breast carcinoma is also more likely to occur in whites than Orientals, and in individuals with high fat diets. *(Chandrasoma and Taylor, pp. 822–829)*

Figures 8–18 and 8–19 show a uterus with a number of well-defined tumors, which are benign leiomyomas, or tumors arising from the uterine musculature.

760. **(B)** These are well-circumscribed, encapsulated, benign tumors of the uterus. The combination of the gross appearance and the microscopy allows these distinctions to be made. *(Rubin and Farber, pp. 998–999)*

761. (A) The correct diagnostic term is a benign leiomyoma. Leiomyosarcomas are much rarer and produce a more pleomorphic picture, with higher mitotic rate. Adenocarcinoma of the endometrium would have a glandular structure. Squamous cell carcinoma of the cervix or a teratoma of the uterus would be composed of a number of different cell types. *(Rubin and Farber, pp. 998–999)*

762. (E) These tumors are frequently multiple, and there is not a high incidence of malignant transformation. They are the most common neoplasm in the adult female genital tract and are benign lesions arising from the uterine myometrium. *(Rubin and Farber, pp. 998–999)*

Figure 8–20 is an electron micrograph that demonstrates swollen mitochondria with floccular densities that are seen as dense deposits. These are evidence of cell injury and disruption of oxidative phosphorylation.

763. (C) The condition is swollen damaged mitochondria. Apoptosis is a nuclear phenomenon, as are karyolysis and karyorrhexis. Viral inclusions have a distinct pattern that is not seen as floccular density as demonstrated. *(Rubin and Farber, pp. 5–8)*

764. (C) The best description of the condition is decreased respiration of the mitochondria with flocculation. Lipid peroxidation with cell membrane damage is not indicated in this instance. Clumping of chromatin is not present, and although there may be damage to the endoplasmic reticulum, it is not as appropriate an answer. Lysosomal changes with cell swelling are not present at this stage. *(Rubin and Farber, pp. 5–8)*

765. (B) Cell injury resulting from mercuric chloride poisoning or early ischemic changes in infarction can produce this kind of mitochondrial damage. Cytomegalovirus produces a characteristic inclusion, and saponification indicates complete disruption of the cell, with soap formation and calcium deposition. *(Rubin and Farber, pp. 5–8)*

766. (D) Disruption of oxidative phosphorylation in the mitochondria is the mechanism involved. Abnormalities of lipid storage would produce a different picture. Viral transformation of the cellular DNA is an unrelated phenomenon, and although toxic poisoning of the lysosomal system may produce similar effects, they occur at different stages in cell damage. *(Rubin and Farber, pp. 5–8)*

Figure 8–21 depicts an egg with a lateral spine, which is characteristic of Schistosoma mansoni.

767. (C) These parasites all produce different shape and size eggs that are clearly distinguishable. *(Rubin and Farber, pp. 440–443)*

768. (C) Humans are the most frequent host for the adult forms, which are the worms that produce eggs. The snail and the fish play a different role in the life cycle of the schistosomes. The mosquito and the dog are not involved at all. *(Rubin and Farber, pp. 440–443)*

769. (D) The intermediate host in the parasitic life cycle of schistosomiasis is the snail. Fertilized eggs exit infected humans via either urine or feces. These eggs develop into miracidium larva in water and infect snails, the intermediate host. Cercaria larva then exit out of the snail into the water and then infect humans by penetrating through the skin. The adult worms come to lodge in either the intestinal or bladder venous plexus, where they copulate and secrete fertilized eggs, repeating the cycle. *(Rubin and Farber, pp. 440–441)*

770. (E) This is, in fact, a very common cause of blood loss in underdeveloped countries or areas where schistosomiasis is frequent. The adult male and female worms copulate either in the veins of the gastrointestinal tract or in the urinary bladder plexus of veins. The eggs are then shed either through the bladder or through the large intestine. Schistosomiasis is a worldwide problem and an extremely common disease for which millions of people carry the parasite. *(Rubin and Farber, pp. 471–472)*

Figure 8–22 depicts the branching hyphae of a fungus characteristic of Aspergillus.

771. **(C)** The branching hyphae are so characteristic that this is quite distinguishable from bacteria or rickettsia, which are much smaller. Viruses are intracellular, and protozoa have different structures and are separate entities. *(Rubin and Farber, pp. 434–435)*

772. **(C)** This is characteristic of *Aspergillus,* although other fungi may look similar. *(Rubin and Farber, pp. 434–435)*

773. **(D)** Aspergillosis rarely is a primary infection but often complicates other infections and is regarded as an opportunistic infection in people with lowered resistance or immune deficiency. It is not of high virulence in normal circumstances, and the port of entry is usually the respiratory tract. *(Rubin and Farber, pp. 434–435)*

Figure 8–23 shows a renal tubule with many enlarged tubular epithelial cells and a large nucleus containing intranuclear inclusions with a surrounding halo (the owl eye appearance). This is characteristic of the intranuclear viral inclusions seen in cytomegalovirus infections.

774. **(B)** This is a characteristic representation of viral inclusion bodies and should not be confused with storage material, which would be in the cytoplasm of the cell. *(Cotran et al., pp. 236–251)*

775. **(D)** These viruses are normally of low virulence, and although they may occur in a congenital setting, they are not hereditary diseases. Although malnutrition also can contribute to immune deficiency, the immune deficiency itself seems to be the main problem. *(Cotran et al., pp. 236–251)*

776. **(C)** This condition is characteristic of cytomegalovirus infection. The clinical manifestations of the disease, with hepatosplenomegaly and microcephaly, are characteristic of a congenital infection from transplacental passage of the virus but may be seen in patients with severe immune deficiency. *(Cotran et al., pp. 236–251)*

777. **(D)** The disease is seen most commonly in immunologically compromised hosts, although it may occur because of transplacental passage of the virus. It is not seen in an epidemic form, nor is it confined to the tropics. It is not transmitted readily from patient to patient, as are the viruses of measles or smallpox. *(Cotran et al., pp. 236–251)*

Figure 8–24 shows the typical scolex of a tapeworm, with many hooklets discernible.

778. **(C)** The photomicrograph demonstrates the mouthparts (scolex) of a tapeworm. These diagnostic structures may be seen in hepatic hydatic cysts caused by *Echinococcus granulosus. (Rubin and Farber, pp. 476–478)*

779. **(A)** Hydatid disease is caused by the dog tapeworm, *E. granulosus.* Accidental ingestion of infected canine feces by humans liberates the larval stage of the organism which may lodge in the liver, bone, brain, or lung. In these sites, these larva may evoke a chronic cystic (hydatid cyst) foreign body response. *(Rubin and Farber, pp. 476–478)*

780. **(B)** The transmission is usually via infected feces that contain the ova of the tapeworm. *(Rubin and Farber, pp. 476–478)*

781. **(D)** Although humans may be the primary host, this is not the most frequent occurrence. The dog is usually the most frequent primary host of this type of tapeworm, and the sheep is often a secondary host. Humans become a secondary host by ingesting sheep that are infected with the parasite. *(Rubin and Farber, pp. 476–478)*

Figure 8–25 shows the characteristic corkscrew appearance of multiple spirochetes, which require special staining techniques for their demonstration.

782. **(D)** Gram-positive cocci and gram-negative bacilli usually do not show this particular morphology, and although *Actinomyces* may produce a number of different morphologic forms, it is basically different. Donovan bodies occur intracellularly and in a different condition entirely. *(Rubin and Farber, pp. 410–413)*

783. **(E)** The spirochete of syphilis taken from a penile ulcer is by far the most likely diagnosis in this case. Chancroid, granuloma inguinale, lymphogranuloma venereum, and gonorrhea all are caused by different types of organisms that have different morphology and characteristics. (*Rubin and Farber, pp. 410–413*)

784. **(B)** Syphilis is largely transmitted venereally, and the organism does not survive long outside the body. It is not transmitted by food contamination and does not survive in dust and debris, as do such organisms as the acid-fast bacillus. (*Rubin and Farber, pp. 410–413*)

Figure 8–26 shows the periphery of the lung with clusters of malignant cells in what appear to be dilated subpleural lymphatics. This is a metastatic carcinoma from a primary carcinoma in the breast.

785. **(B)** This is a characteristic appearance of metastatic carcinoma, in this instance in the subpleural lymphatics of the lung, but it could be seen in lymph nodes or other sites. There is not the granulomatous appearance of tuberculosis, nor is there evidence of intravascular coagulation or the liquefaction necrosis of an abscess or infarction. (*Cotran et al., pp. 749–750*)

786. **(C)** This tumor pattern is very characteristic of a primary source in the breast, with spread to the subpleural lymphatics and to other parts of the lung. Embolization could result in tumor cells in a different, more diffuse metastatic pattern within the lung. (*Cotran et al., pp. 749–750*)

Figure 8–27 shows a section of long bone. The dense material in the center and at the periosteal surface is new bone formation, or callus, characteristic of the healing phase of a fracture.

787. **(C)** This is a form of healing that, in many respects, is very similar to that seen in other tissues, with the exception that the collagen or fibrous tissue is converted into bone. (*Rubin and Farber, pp. 1354–1356*)

788. **(C)** The healing of a fracture is distinctly different from the appearances of an osteogenic sarcoma or an osteoid osteoma, which are neo-plastic transformations of bone. Acute osteo-myelitis or tuberculosis of the bone shows the characteristic features of inflammation, which are not present in this illustration. (*Rubin and Farber, pp. 1354–1356*)

789. **(D)** The appearance of the dense material that extends to the periosteal surface is the new bone, or provisional callus, which is the precursor of the final bone before remodeling occurs in a fracture. Although fibrous tissue may occur as a complication of fractures with non-union, this is not seen in this illustration, and the appearance of osteoid in a sarcoma can sometimes mimic this appearance, although not in its entirety. There is no evidence of inflammation. (*Rubin and Farber, pp. 1354–1356*)

790. **(C)** A number of factors will retard the normal healing of bony fractures: foreign material in the wound, active inflammation, widely apposed fractured ends, deficiency of vitamin C, deficiency of vitamin D, deficiency of calcium, scar formation, and movement of the fracture ends during healing. High doses of vitamin C or D, a diet high in calcium, and immobilization of the bone would all tend to assist in rapid healing of a fracture. (*Rubin and Farber, pp. 1354–1356*)

Figures 8–28 and 8–29 show a lung with an area of infarction in which the alveolar walls appear indistinct and the lung is filled with red cells, but there is no evidence of inflammatory cells, as seen in pneumonia. The real clue to the condition is the blood vessel leading into the lung, which has a thrombotic occlusion. This is characteristic of infarction.

791. **(A)** Lobar pneumonia would produce many polymorphonuclear leukocytes, as would lung abscesses, with liquefaction necrosis also present. There is no evidence of neoplasm in the photograph. (*Cotran et al., pp. 703–704*)

792. **(C)** Deep venous thrombosis with embolization to the pulmonary vessels is the most likely antecedent. The individual may have had multiple emboli or venous congestion because of right-sided heart failure in addition. Although cigarette smoking and asbestos may contribute to lung disease, they do not in this setting, and there is no evidence of septicemia, although this can in itself produce emboli. Aspiration of infected materials produces a bronchopneumonic type of inflammatory condition. (*Cotran et al., pp. 703–704*)

Figure 8–30 is a photomicrograph of a liver, in which the liver cells appear to be replaced by empty spaces characteristic of fat. The fat is removed during the processing, leaving these circular globules replacing most of the liver cells.

793. **(B)** Lipid accumulation in the liver produces the picture shown. (*Rubin and Farber, pp. 788–791*)

794. **(A)** This often is described as fatty metamorphosis, although some other terms, such as "fatty infiltration" or "fatty liver," also are used. There is no evidence of hepatocellular carcinoma or of passive congestion, although these may occur in the same liver as fatty metamorphosis. Acute viral hepatitis and tuberculosis, which are inflammatory and destructive processes, also may occur in livers in which fatty metamorphosis is present. (*Rubin and Farber, pp. 788–791*)

795. **(C)** Hepatic fatty metamorphosis is seen most commonly in alcoholism. Other conditions in which liver cell fatty change may be seen include carbon tetrachloride poisoning, diabetes mellitus, malnutrition, after ingestion of hepatotoxins, after administration of various therapeutic drugs, during pregnancy, and choline deficiency. (*Rubin and Farber, pp. 788–791*)

796. **(E)** This condition frequently is reversible. In fact, severe protein malnutrition, if corrected, will produce a normal liver with no such accumulations of lipid. There are multiple causes of as similar picture. The condition may well affect children, particularly those with malnutrition, as well as adults with other disorders. Choline deficiency is one of the known causes. (*Rubin and Farber, pp. 788–791*)

Figure 8–31 depicts a large tumor mass occupying the cortex and medullary area with capsular invasion. The tumor impinges into the caliceal system and is composed of solid, *yellowish-white areas, with focal areas of cystic degeneration and hemorrhage.*

797. **(A)** The renal cell carcinomas can appear in any portion of the kidney, although it is more common to see them in the upper pole. The tumor that infiltrates the renal parenchyma also infiltrates and invades into the pelvicaliceal system. Tumor invasion of the renal vein is commonly seen. The other answers do not apply to this gross characteristic findings of renal cell carcinoma. (*Cotran et al., pp. 991–1094*)

Figure 8–32 depicts the classic histologic features of a clear cell carcinoma. The cells are arranged in small nests and cords, separated by delicate capillaries with almost no stroma.

798. **(D)** Clear cell carcinomas are the most common cell type neoplasms of renal cell carcinomas. The cells are arranged in a solid pattern, or tubular structures, containing a small centrally located nucleus, surrounded by a clear empty cytoplasm. Most of the clear cell carcinomas are well differentiated; however, higher grades have been described. Other types of carcinomas, such as papillary carcinoma, chromophobe renal cell carcinoma, and collecting duct carcinoma, are less common variants. (*Cotran et al., pp. 991–1094*)

Figure 8–33 depicts a kidney showing the typical characteristics of the adult polycystic kidney that is markedly enlarged and with numerous dilated cysts. This is an autosomal dominant lesion.

799 and 800. (799-D, 800-A) The adult polycystic kidney is an autosomal dominant disease. On the external surface, the kidney is markedly enlarged and multiple dilated cysts are found. On microscopic evaluation, however, some functioning glomeruli can be found in between the cystic walls. The constant enlargement of these cysts encroach upon the functioning glomerular units, and leads to final renal failure. The patients remain asymptomatic until late adulthood with the appearance of renal failure. Another symptomatology could be hematuria or the larger kidney masses produce abdominal flank pain. This disease may be associated with other cysts affecting other organs particularly in the liver up to 40%. They may remain asymptomatic. (Cotran et al., pp. 937–940)

Figure 8–34 shows the lumen of the intestine, which is narrow and covered by necrotic debris. The entire wall of the intestine is infiltrated from the mucosa to the serosa by a fleshy neoplastic process showing whitish areas of necrosis and reddish areas of hemorrhage. Figure 8–35 shows a tumor characterized by neoplastic intermedium-sized lymphocytes with slightly irregular nuclear membrane, inconspicuous nucleoli, and indiscernible cytoplasm. The neoplastic cells are separated by benign macrophages containing nuclear dust in the cytoplasm. This appearance is known as starry-sky appearance characteristic of Burkitt's lymphoma.

801.   **(E)** This extensive irregular thickening of the intestinal wall, which also involves the mesenteric fat represents a malignant neoplasm, most precisely Burkitt's lymphoma. The lumen of the bowel at this level is also severely compromised and is probably responsible for the intestinal occlusion. The mucosa is completely ulcerated, and the muscular layer of the intestine is completely replaced by the fleshy neoplasm with focal areas of hemorrhage and necrosis. The other selections for this question do not match the gross appearance of this picture. (Cotran et al., pp. 662–663)

802.   **(E)** In this microphotograph, there is a characteristic "starry sky" appearance of Burkitt's lymphoma. This starry sky pattern is produced by benign macrophages scattered among the tumor cells and create clear spaces on this dark blue background. The tumor cells in Burkitt's lymphoma are B cells with a high mitotic index. The tumor cells may have multiple small nucleoli and an amphophilic or basophilic cytoplasm. The other patterns described for this question are related with another type of lymphoma. (Cotran et al., pp. 662–663)

Figure 8–36 depicts an extensive area of hemorrhage, which has produced a destruction of the internal capsule, basal ganglia, part of the temporal lobe, and is invading into the third ventricle.

803.   **(A)** Spontaneous intraparenchymal hemorrhage of the brain occurs in the late adult life. The peak age for this condition is about 60 years. These massive hemorrhages are most commonly related to hypertension and are secondary to the rupture of the small intraparenchymal vessels. In this gross picture, we can see that the hemorrhage into the brain substance has extended also to the ventricles and the midbrain. The abnormalities of the small vessels are related to aging (hyaline atherosclerosis) and sometimes to microaneurysms. Most frequently, the intraparenchymal hemorrhages are originated in the putamen in 60% of the cases. The abscesses of the brain do not show this dark discoloration, parasitic infestation are more discrete and in different foci. (Cotran et al., pp. 1310–1311)

804.   **(B)** Hypertension is the most common underlying cause of primary brain parenchymal hemorrhage. (Cotran et al., pp. 1310–1311)

Figure 8–37 shows a malignant tumor originating in the intramedullary area that is invading the cortex as well as the pifisis by breaking into the remnants of the cartilaginous growth plate. The tumor, which is of yellow–tan color, has almost completely destroyed the cortex of the bone and is circumferentially involving the entire distal part of the femur with the formation of Codman's triangle (periosteal reaction). Figure 8–38 shows a representative area of the tumor composed of neoplastic cells that are ovoid in shape showing all the characteristics of highly malignant neoplasm separated by small irregular islands of osteoid.

805.   **(A)** The resection of this distal portion of the femur contains a malignant tumor that extends from the medullary canal, breaks through the cortex, and bulges into the soft tissues. A small Codman's triangle in the inferior portion of the lesion is seen that constitutes a periosteal reaction. The tumor also breaks through the growth plate (cartilage) and extends to the epiphysis. The gross appearance of this lesion does not represent an osteomyelitis or any kind of the benign lesions listed. (Rubin and Farber, pp. 1384–1385)

806. **(C)** The osteosarcomas on histological examination, as the one shown in the microphotograph, exhibit a malignant proliferation of osteoblasts, which contain an enlarged, hyperchromatic, and pleomorphic nucleus with a scant cytoplasm. These cells are surrounding woven bone "new bone" with poorly formed bony spicules. The osteosarcomas will spread through the bloodstream and into the lungs. Sometimes areas of malignant cartilage formation are present, as well as calcifications. (*Rubin and Farber, pp. 1384–1385*)

Figure 8–39 shows a cross section of the entire prostate with a urethra in the center and in the base a small protrusion that represents the verumontanum. On the peripheral zone of the prostate (indicated by the arrow), there is a rather diffuse, infiltrating lesion that is yellowish in color, compact, and represents an adenocarcinoma. Figure 8–40 shows the lesion, which is composed of well-defined glands, lined by a single uniform layer of low columnar cells. The size of these glands varies from small (microglandular structures) to large and dilated. There is a minimal variation in the size and shape of the nucleus and no evidence of mitotic activity. This tumor is considered a well-differentiated adenocarcinoma and on the Gleason classification would be a score 4.

807. **(A)** The cross section of this prostate shows multiple modularity, as well as small cysts consistent with benign prostatic hypertrophy. However, at the area marked by the arrow and in the peripheral portion of the prostate, there is a dense area that is an adenocarcinoma. Usually on gross examination, the prostatic carcinoma appears as a hard nodular structure with ill-defined margins, and in 75% of the cases, occupying the outer part of the gland (the peripheral zone). (*Chandrasoma and Taylor, pp. 558–559*)

808. **(A)** The malignant cells originating in this prostatic gland are forming small glandular structures, which are packed together, and exhibiting small lumens. This is, by definition, an adenocarcinoma. The adenocarcinoma, however not in all cases, is well differentiated, and different grades can be assigned to the degree of differentiation. Several histological grades of the prostate have been used; however, the

most popular is the Gleason classification in which two different areas of the prostate cancer are evaluated, those that have the best differentiation and the worst differentiated patterns. Adding the two numbers will give a Gleason score that is the guidance for further treatment and prognosis. (*Chandrasoma and Taylor, pp. 558–559*)

Figure 8–41 shows an irregular, ulcerated, and partially vegetating lesion composed of granular yellowish–brown tissue. This lesion represents a squamous cell carcinoma of the larynx.

809. **(C)** This irregular area, located on the left supraglottic area represents an infiltrating squamous cell carcinoma of the larynx. In general, fungal infections are mostly Candidiasis and are diffusely extending over the mucosal surface. A papilloma will have clean margins, and it will be a polypoid mass, not an infiltrating tumor, as in this case. In general, these tumors have irregular borders, they are exophitic partially and partially infiltrating, and the surface could be white, granular, or tan. It commonly involves the vocal cords, the ventricles, and the false vocal cords. The supraglottic carcinomas originate in the ventricle and false cords, as in this case. Up to one-third of the laryngeal carcinomas arise in this location. Metastases are more common in those originating in the glottic area of the larynx. The treatment could be surgical or radiation therapy. (*Rubin and Farber, pp. 594–595*)

810. **(C)** It has been found that most squamous cell carcinomas of the larynx are related to cigarette smoking. There are dysplastic changes in the progression of the epithelial lining of the larynx that may last for years before they become malignant. The normal mucosa is altered to histological changes with squamous dysplasia, which follows by squamous cell carcinoma in-situ. This lesion, in turn, progresses to invasive squamous cell carcinoma. (*Rubin and Farber, pp. 594–595*)

Figures 8–42A and 8–42B represent a cystic ovary with distended, shiny capsule and no evidence of gross invasion. Partially, the fallopian tube is crossing over the spec-

imen. Solid areas of the tumor show a serous papillary adenocarcinoma. In the picture, three psammoma bodies are
present (lamellar calcifications) and multiple complex
papillary projections covered by multiple layers of epithelial low cuboidal cells with evidence of pleomorphism and
mitotic activity. Obvious invasion of the ovarian stroma
was present.

811.   **(E)** Looking at the external examination of this
ovarian tumor without palpation or gross examination it is not possible to tell what type of
tumor it represents. On cross section, this ovarian neoplasm was filled with amber serous
fluid. Multiple loculations were present and
some solid areas that constituted only 10% of
the tumor mass. The external appearance was
smooth, glistening, and there were not any
excrescences or papillary projections outside of
the capsule. (Cotran et al., pp. 1069–1071)

812.   **(B)** The epithelium seen covering the finger-
like projections of this photomicrograph are
compatible with the serous origin. There
are three varieties of serous ovarian tumors.
The first type is benign tumors, which are
composed of small papillary projections,
with a single row of cells, no overlapping, no
evidence of mitotic activity, pleomorphism
or stromal invasion. The second category is
represented by the tumors of low malignant
potential, which contain an increased amount
of papillary projections overlapping of the
cells, with increase in mitotic activity. However, this type of tumor fails to demonstrate
invasion of the stroma, which distinguishes
them from the malignant variety. The third
type is histologically characterized by stromal
invasion. (Cotran et al., pp. 1069–1071)

Figure 8–43 shows a deep seeded tumor mass that was
attached grossly to the surrounding tissue. The mass is
lobulated and partially encapsulated. On cross section,
it showed the yellowish appearance of a fatty tumor. Figure 8–44 exhibits the histological characteristic of well-
differentiated liposarcoma. The tumor is not highly cellular,
but some of the cells exhibit hyperchromatia, and they are
recognized as a lipoblast.

813.   **(C)** Liposarcoma is the second most common
sarcoma of adulthood. They usually arise in

the deep soft tissues of the proximal extremities and retroperitoneum. They exhibit a translocation between chromosomes 12 and 16. On
gross examination, the typical liposarcoma
measures from a few centimeters, to as large as
40 cm and may weigh a few pounds. On cross
section the tumor had a greasy yellow appearance. In cases of high grade, such tumors can
become fleshy with areas of hemorrhage and
necrosis. (Rubin and Farber, p. 1410)

814.   **(C)** The most common pattern of the liposarcoma is the one of variable differentiated cells
"signet ring" lipoblasts embedded in a vascularized myxomatous stroma. The vacuolated
cells are lipoblasts, and occasional mitotic figures can be found. (Rubin and Farber, p. 1410)

Figure 8–45 shows a gross specimen in which the whole
breast has been removed with the axillary contents and
portions of the pectoralis major. The cross section exhibits
a tumor mass located under the areola and nipple with
marked retraction. The tumor is irregular in shape, contain stellate borders infiltrating the surrounding fibroadipose tissue. Figure 8–46 exhibits small groups of cells that
are diffusely infiltrating the breast stroma with a large
nerve trunk in the center showing perineural invasion.
Figure 8–47 shows on the right-hand side a portion of
the skin with the basal layer and pseudoepitheliomatous
hyperplasia (the keratin layer is not seen). Multiple lymphatic vascular channels are dilated and contain tumor
embolus that are malignant cells arranged in a similar
fashion as seen in the primary tumor. This represents a
dermolymphatic invasion (inflammatory carcinoma of the
breast). Figure 8–48 shows the classic "Indian filing" that
is most commonly seen in lobular carcinoma in the breast.

815.   **(B)** Most of the breast cancers are composed of
dense fibrous stroma, with irregular borders
infiltrating the surrounding adipose tissue.
The size may vary, but in this particular case,
it shows an attachment of the overlying skin
and nipple, with a retraction, and depending
upon the location, also a retraction of the skin
could be seen. On cross section, it is almost cartilaginous in consistency, areas of hemorrhage,
calcification and necrosis can be demonstrated. Fibrocystic changes of the breast are dis-
perse areas of fibrosis throughout the breast,
without showing a solitary mass, as in the photograph. Intraductal papillomas, when large,

can be visible. They are sharply circumscribed, and they do not exceed more than 1 cm in diameter. Phyllodes tumors are stromal tumors showing a characteristic growth pattern that mostly resembles fibroadenomas. Many times, multiple sections must be examined to distinguish between the low-grade and benign lesions. *(Cotran et al., pp. 1107–1113)*

816.   **(C)** On histological evaluation infiltrating ductal carcinoma shows a variegated pattern most commonly seen in small nests, cords, or anastomosing branches. These epithelial islands are infiltrating the fibroadipose tissue of the breast. The differentiation into glandular structures and the nuclear appearance will be given the final grade of these tumors. Clearly, we see perineural invasion in the center of the slide in which tumor growth is occupying the perineural space and compressing the nerve. This phenomenon, however, is not related with lymphatic invasion. *(Cotran et al., pp. 1107–1113)*

817.   **(C)** In the picture, a segment of the epidermis is seen in one of the corners, and the lymphatics appear to be filled with tumor emboli, which is compatible with ductal carcinoma of the breast. The lymphatics are dilated, and clinically, it is manifested as an edematous, reddish appearance of the skin overlying tumor. These changes have been clinically called "inflammatory carcinoma of the breast." The pathological substrate for this clinical lesion is dermolymphatic carcinomatosis. *(Cotran et al., pp. 1107–1113)*

818.   **(B)** This is a classic appearance of invasive lobular carcinoma in which a parallel single row of tumor cells are seen in between the bundles of collagen. This phenomenon has been described as "Indian filing." The other possibilities are histologically quite different than the one depicted in this photomicrograph. *(Cotran et al., pp. 1107–1113)*

Figure 8–49 shows a colposcopic picture of the cervix exhibiting erosions and changes on the mucosal surface that granted a biopsy. Figure 8–50 shows the squamous metaplastic epithelium replacing the columnar epithelial cells normally seen in the endocervix. A full-thickness dysplasia of the epithelial cells is present, characterized by

the immaturity of the cells, which is carried to the surface, the loss of polarity, the hyperchromatism, and the mitotic activity, which is also present in the upper third. By definition, this represents a squamous cell carcinoma in situ.

819.   **(B)** The lesion is grossly highly suspicious for squamous cell carcinoma in situ (CIN III), and, therefore, biopsies of the transitional zone and the lesion are indicated. Further therapy will be initiated upon the anatomical pathological diagnosis of these biopsies. *(Cotran et al., pp. 1051–1055)*

820.   **(C)** The histological features of the epithelial lining shows no evidence of maturation. The cytological abnormalities show nuclear pleomorphism, with abnormal chromatin distribution, and increasing nuclear cytoplasmic ratio. These immature cells are also present in the surface. A high number of mitotic figures are found. The basement membrane, however, is intact, and there is no evidence of invasive squamous cell carcinoma. *(Cotran et al., pp. 1051–1055)*

Figure 8–51 depicts a vegetating, focally ulcerating, and infiltrating lesion that involves almost the entire uterus. On the cross section of the entire thickness of the wall of the uterus, it is possible to see more than 50% invasion of the myometrium, and the tumor is present close to the serosal surface. Areas of necrosis and hemorrhage are seen on the gross specimen. Figure 8–52 shows a complex growth of neoplastic glandular structures covered by multiple layers of low cuboidal cells exhibiting mitotic activity and pleomorphism. In many other areas, this tumor was solid and much anaplasia was present.

821.   **(A)** The endometrial adenocarcinoma is seen in older age group than cervical carcinoma. It is most commonly seen in females with obesity, diabetes, hypertension, and infertility. The gross morphologic appearance of the endometrial adenocarcinoma is polypoid tumor mass that diffusely involves the endometrial surface and spreads by direct myometrial invasion. On more rare occasions, it will be localized to the surface or in the form of small polyps in which the base is most commonly involved by the adenocarcinoma. *(Cotran et al., pp. 1061–1063)*

822. **(C)** Out of the multiple morphological types that can be seen in endometrial adenocarcinoma the most common is the endometrioid type. These are tumors that are forming more or less well-defined glandular structures, lined by multiple layers of columnar epithelial cells. Classically, they can be divided into well, moderate, and poorly differentiated. Sometimes the tumor may contain small elements of squamous differentiation. Papillary and serous adenocarcinomas, as well as clear cell carcinomas, are tumors that are considered poorly differentiated in reference to their behavior, regardless of the degree of cellular differentiation. The staging is related to the extension into the myometrium, or outside of the pelvic organs. *(Cotran et al., pp. 1061–1063)*

Figure 8–53 shows a close-up gross photo of the specimen in which a rather fully developed severe case of ulcerative colitis is seen. The mucosa shows areas of ulceration, with hemorrhage and small islands of regenerating mucosa, which bulge toward the lumen, creating pseudopolyps. This lesion is not transmural. Figure 8–54 depicts a single gland of the colonic mucosa showing infiltration by neutrophils in the epithelial areas and focal necrosis. The neutrophils that are ulcerating the base of the gland are collecting in the lumen, forming the characteristic, crypt abscesses. These crypt abscesses are nonspecific for ulcerative colitis and may be observed in Crohn's disease, as well as other inflammatory bowel disease.

823. **(E)** In acute ulcerative colitis, a rather diffuse process is present in the mucosa, which is characterized by edema, and extensive ulcerations, which are hidden by pseudopolyps. These pseudopolyps are formed by inflamed non-ulcerated mucosa, with regenerative changes. The wall of the intestine in ulcerative colitis does not appear to be markedly thickened, and the serosal surface, which is not seen in the picture, is normal. *(Cotran et al., pp. 818–820)*

824. **(A)** Ulcerative colitis is an inflammatory disease of the colon that affects the superficial layers of the organ. In contrast with Crohn's disease, it does not contain granulomas and is continuous in appearance without skipped areas. Microscopically, ulcerative colitis shows a diffuse and inflammatory infiltrate of the lam-

ina propria and sometimes the submucosa. The neutrophils, which are contained in the superficial layers, sometimes produce small collections in the colonic glands, which are called crypt abscesses. Although many of them are present in ulcerative colitis, they are not specific or pathognomonic. Epithelial changes can happen in ulcerative colitis that lead from significant dysplasia in progress to frank carcinoma. It is important, therefore, to characterize in the biopsies if we are in the presence of a low-grade or high-grade dysplasia. *(Cotran et al., pp. 818–820)*

Figure 8–55 shows the ileocecal valve and terminal ileum. The mucosa show areas of ulceration, which form the so-called serpentine linear ulcers. The intervening mucosa appear to be spared. These features are referred on gross description as a cobblestone appearance. In between these areas are fistulous tracts, and fissures can develop. The colonic mucosa was not affected, and skipped areas were present. Figure 8–56 depicts histological sections showing transmural inflammation with fissures, thickening of the muscularis mucosa, and fibrosis of the submucosa and subserosal areas. Small microgranulomas were formed in the submucosa, as the one shown in the picture, and in the center, there is a multinucleated giant cell surrounded by epithelioid cells and outside by a rather intense lymphocytic infiltrate.

825. **(B)** The gross morphological changes of this ileum are compatible with Crohn's disease, which is an idiopathic disorder, also known as regional enteritis or granulomatous colitis. The typical histological features of this disease are characterized by transmural inflammation of the small bowel, or occasionally the colon or other areas of the GI tract. Also, not always, the presence of noncaseating granulomas, as well as fistulous tracts may be seen. The lesion is characterized by alternating with normal areas of intestinal mucosa, so called "skipped lesions." *(Cotran et al., pp. 816–817)*

826. **(D)** Noncaseating granulomas are present in about 50% of the cases of Crohn's disease. Special stains for acid fast and fungi (GMS) have been consistently negative. Granulomas may occur in other parts of the alimentary canal,

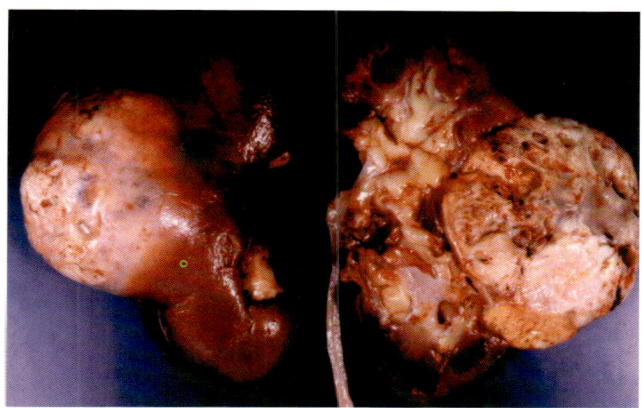

Plate 8–31.

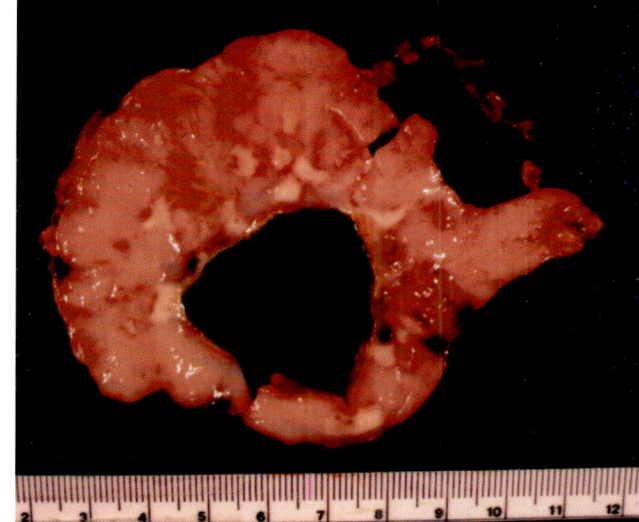

Plate 8–34.

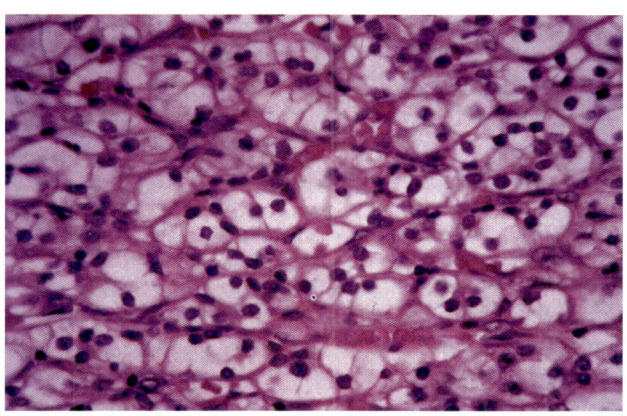

Plate 8–32.

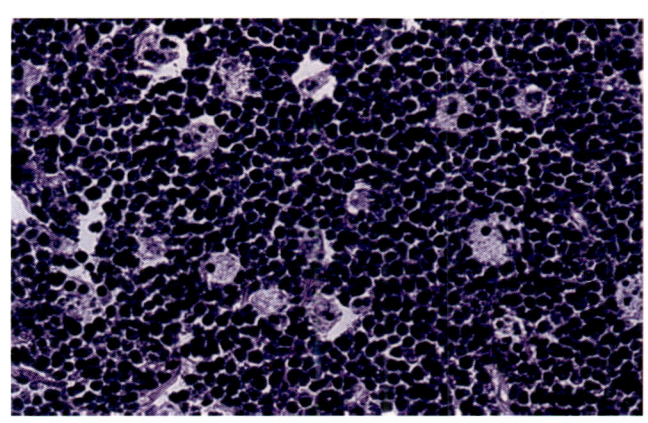

Plate 8–35.

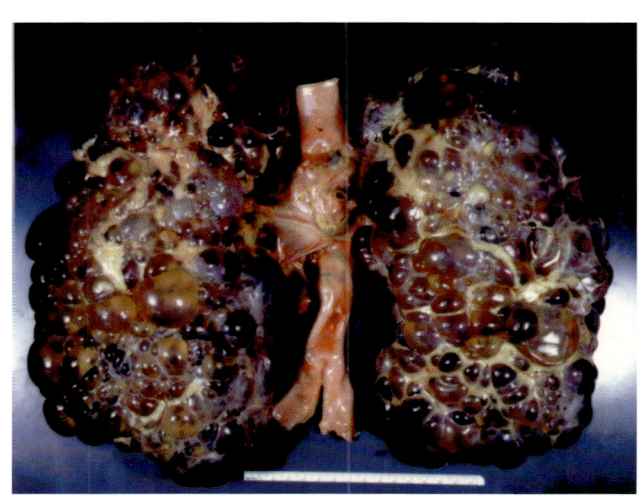

Plate 8–33.

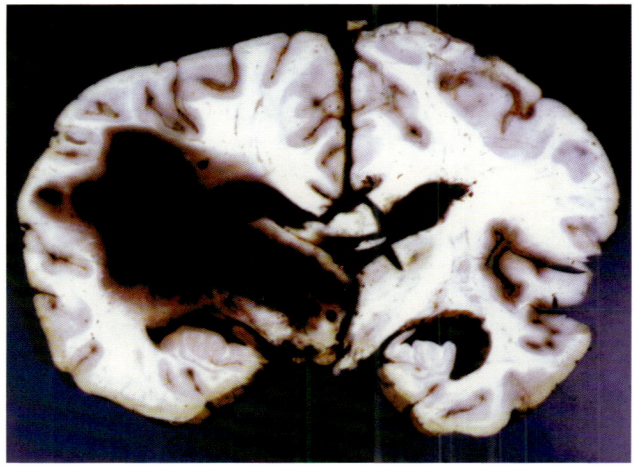

Plate 8–36.

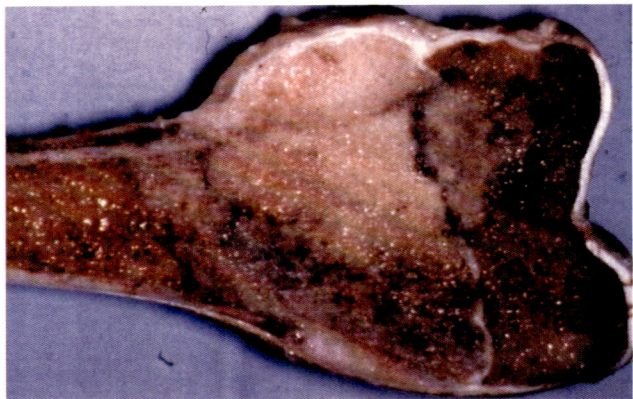

Plate 8–37.

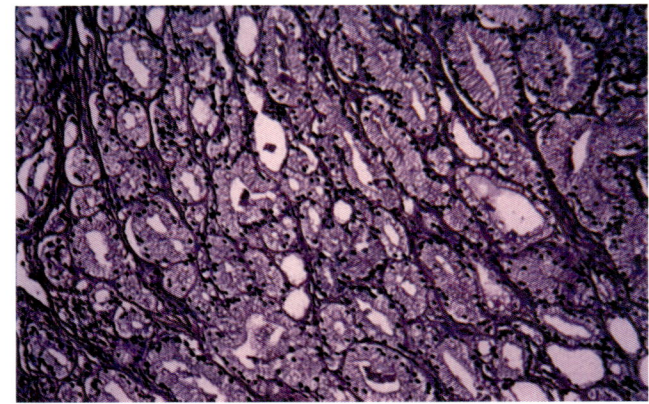

Plate 8–40.

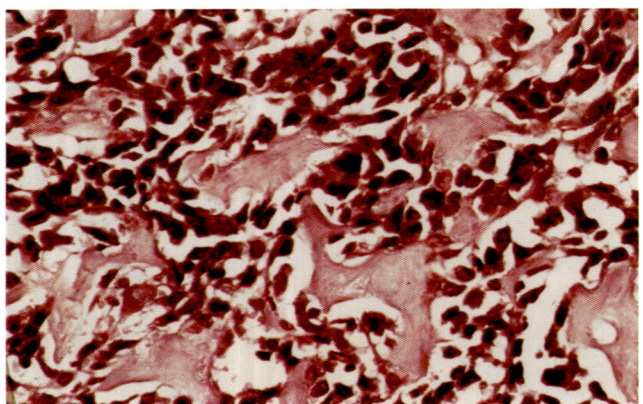

Plate 8–38.

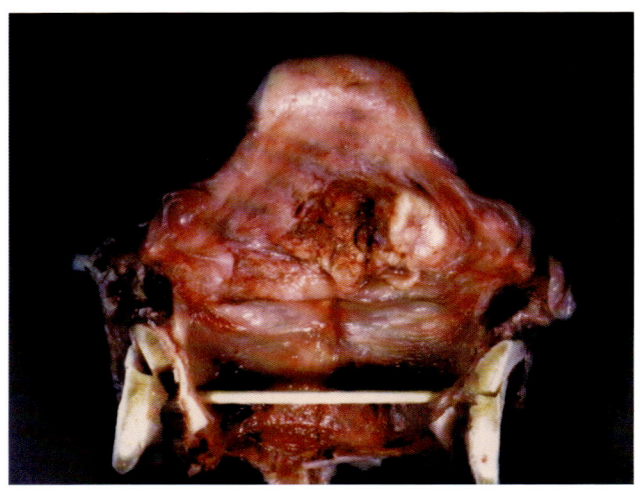

Plate 8–41.

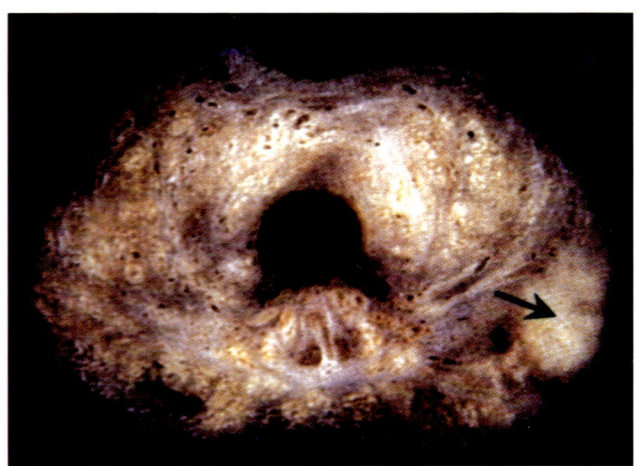

Plate 8–39.

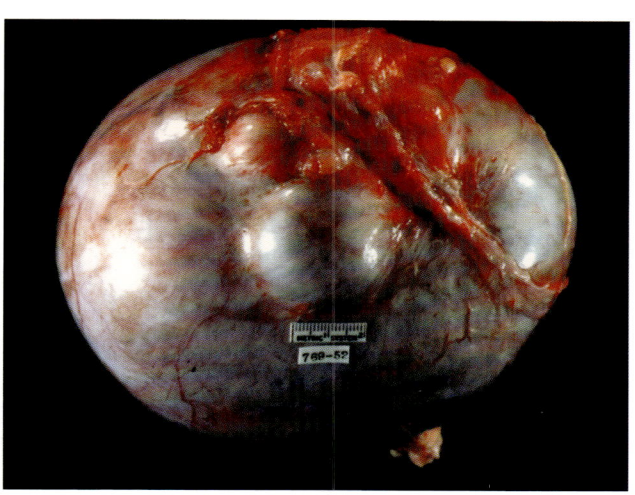

Plate 8–42A.

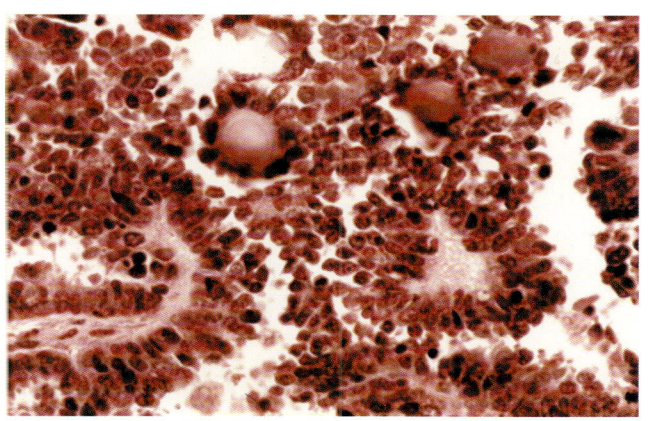

Plate 8–42B.

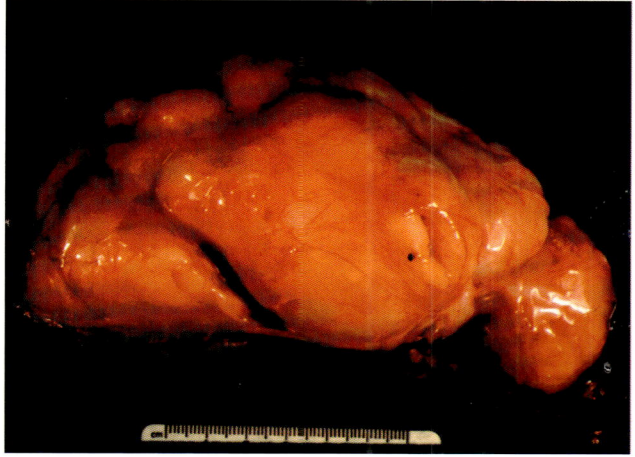

Plate 8–43.

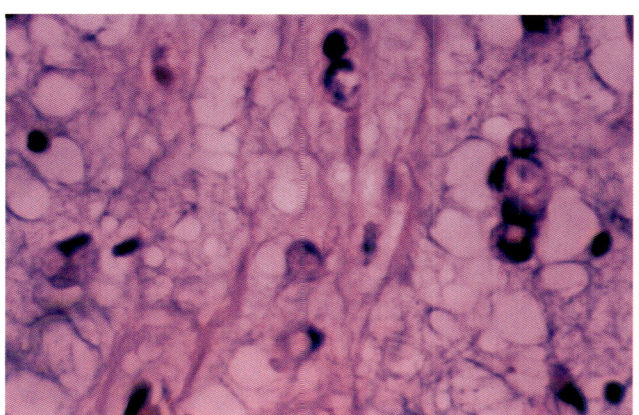

Plate 8–44.

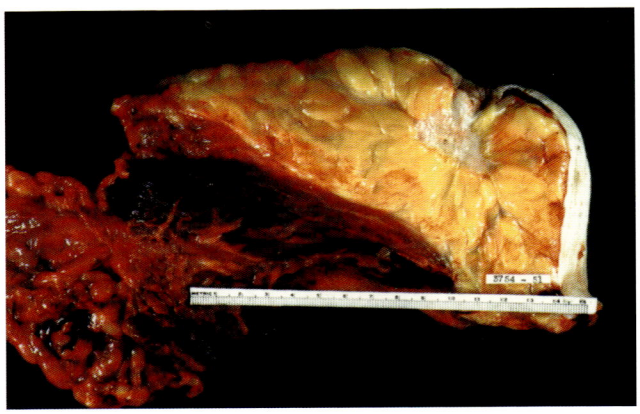

Plate 8–45.

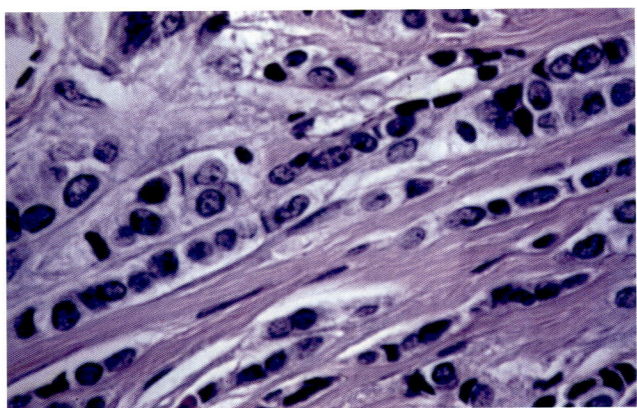

Plate 8–48.

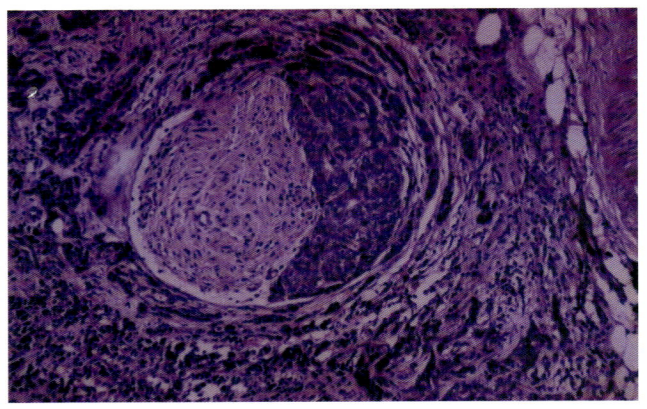

Plate 8–46.

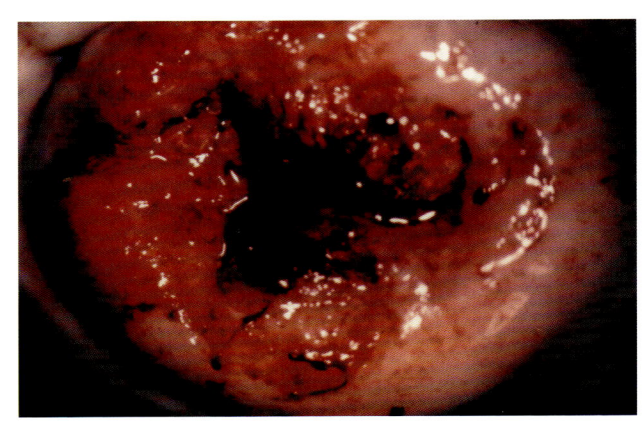

Plate 8–49.

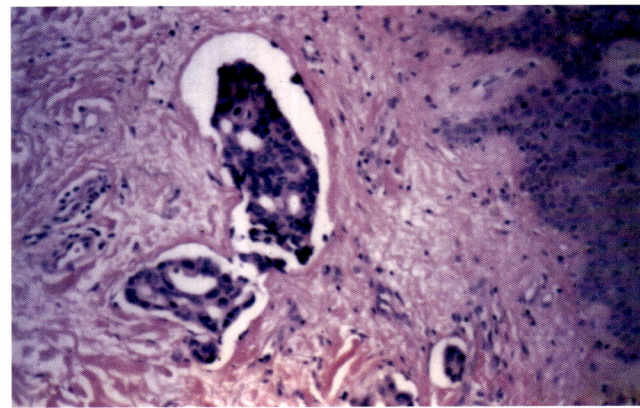

Plate 8–47.

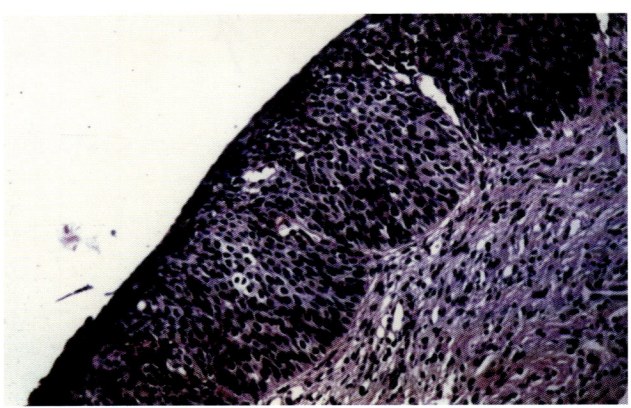

Plate 8–50.

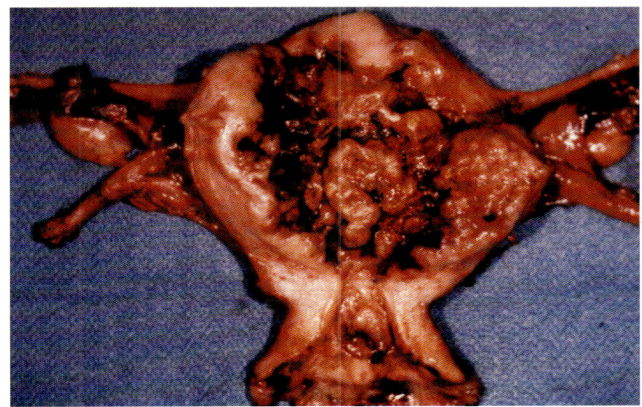

Plate 8–51.

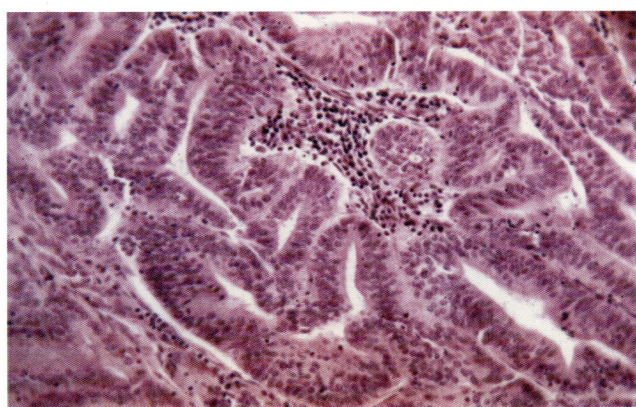

Plate 8–52.

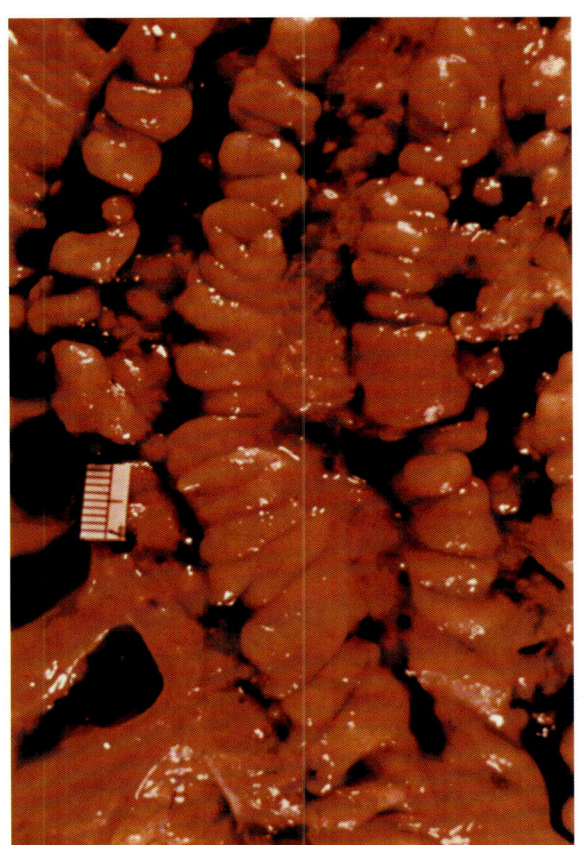

Plate 8–53.

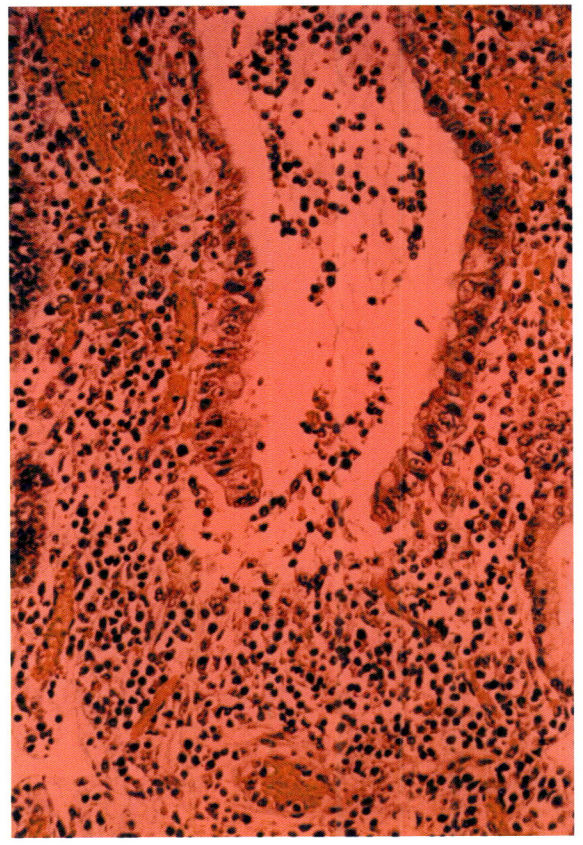

Plate 8–54.

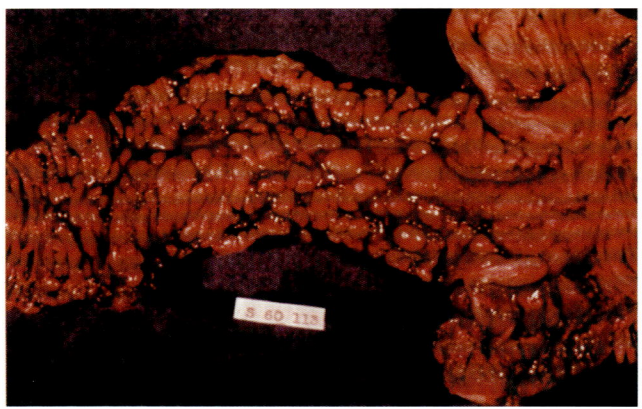

Plate 8–55.

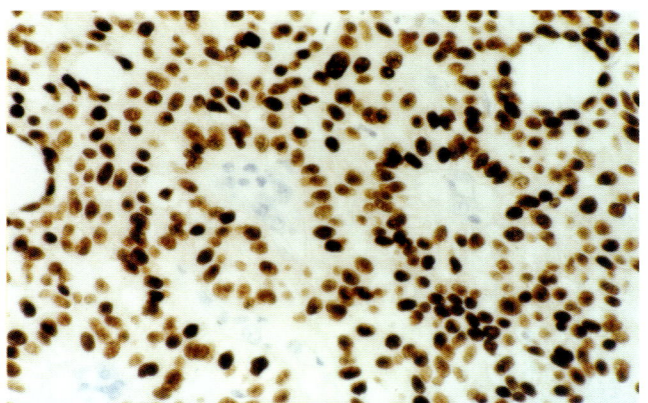

Plate 8–58.

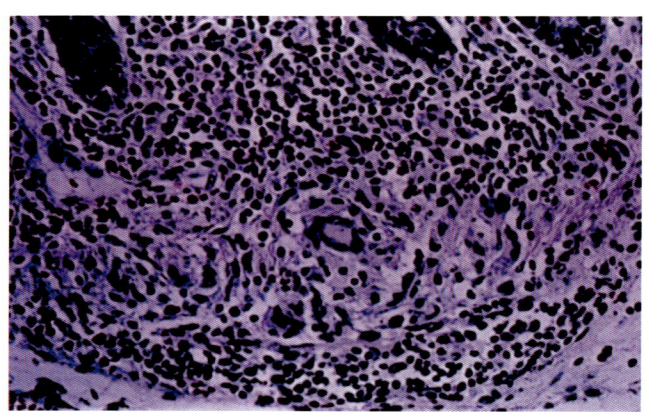

Plate 8–56.

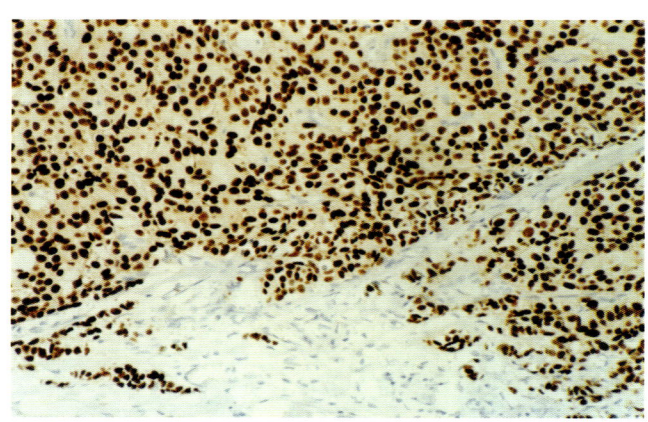

Plate 8–59.

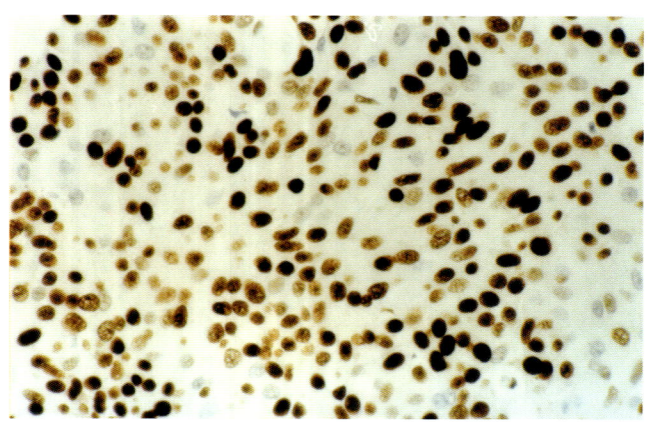

Plate 8–57.

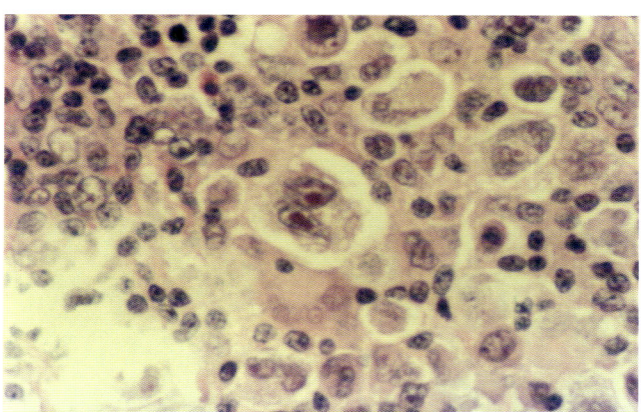

Plate 8–60.

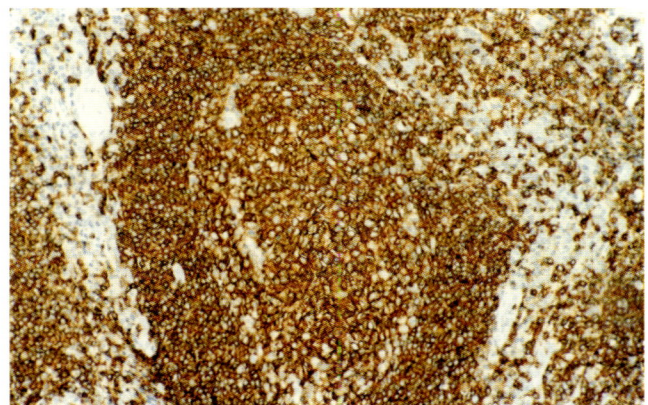

Plate 8–61.

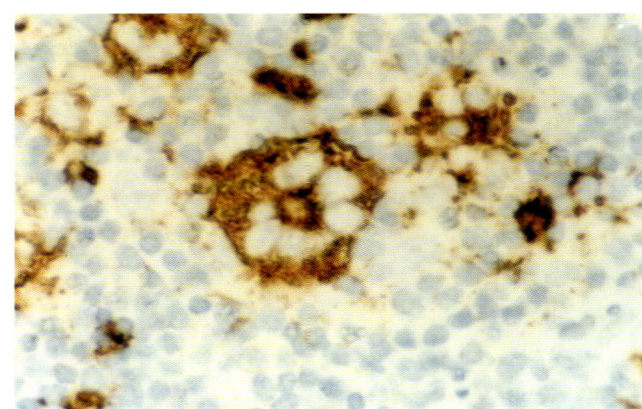

Plate 8–64.

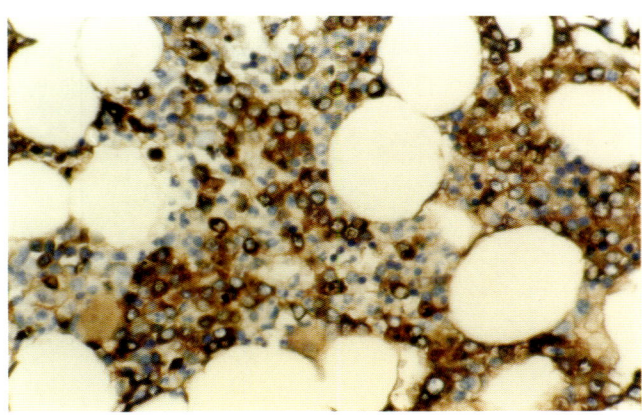

Plate 8–62.

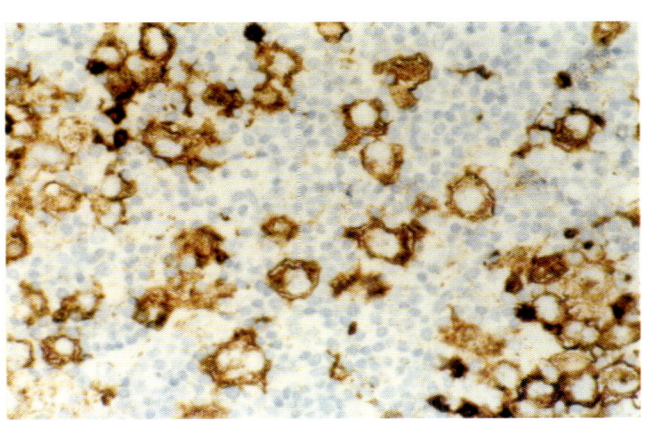

Plate 8–65.

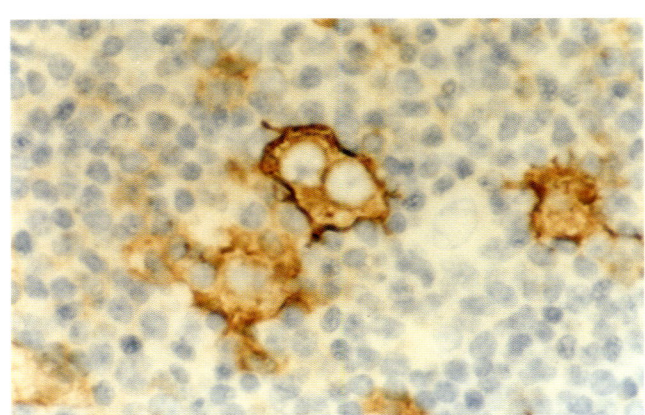

Plate 8–63.

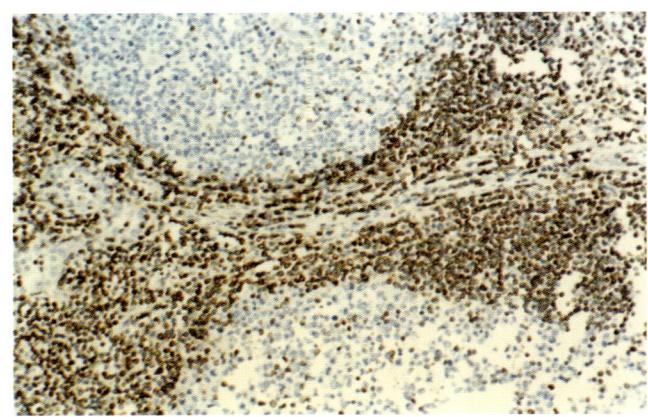

Plate 8–66.

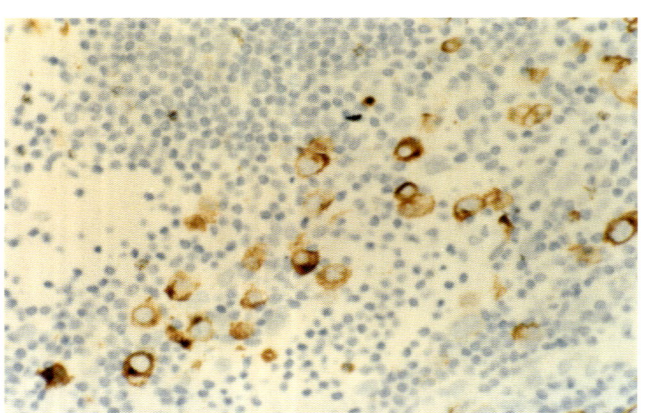

Plate 8–67.

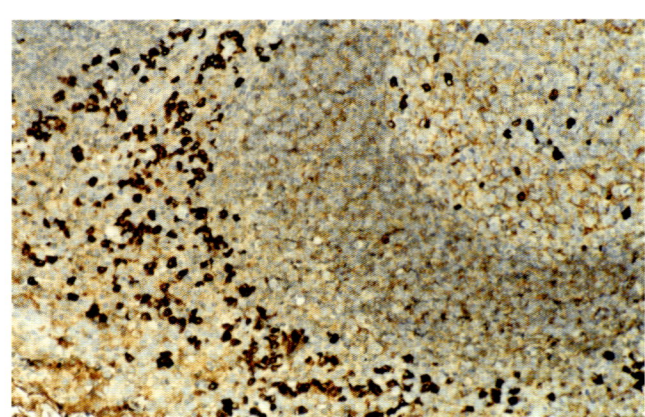

Plate 8–69.

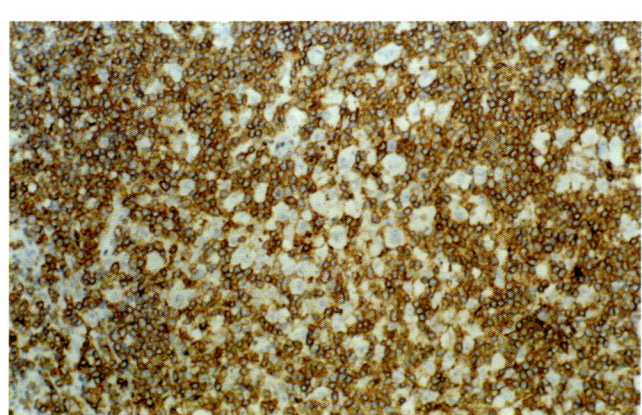

Plate 8–68.

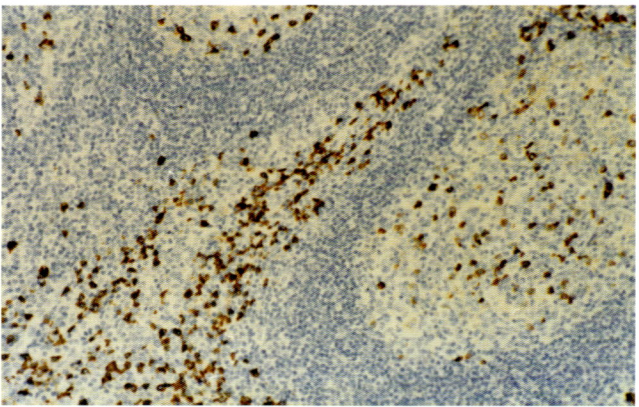

Plate 8–70.

from the mouth to the anus. The microgranulomas that are located in the lamina propria are characterized by a few giant cells, epithelial cells surrounded by lymphocytes. There is no evidence of central necrosis. These granulomas help to make the diagnosis of Crohn's disease, however they are not pathognomonic, of this disease. *(Cotran et al., pp. 816–817)*

827. **(E)** Approximately between 50–85% of the breast carcinomas exhibit estrogen and progesterone receptors. The presence of these proteins in the nucleus of the cells has been used as a prognostic indicator, because the positive tumors show a better prognosis, and they respond promptly to hormonal therapy. The cancer that possesses these positive receptors have been statistically proved to have long disease-free survival intervals, when compared to those negative for these receptors. The cancer with high levels of hormone receptors have a better prognosis than those that are negative. *(Cotran et al., p. 1045)*

828. **(B)** There has been a generation of new antibodies that inhibits the growth cells that possess activated Her-2/neu receptors. Her-2/neu overexpression is found in about 25% of human breast cancers and occurs by amplification and transcription of the C-erB-2/neu oncogene. This oncogene has been linked to early disease relapse and decrease on overall survival when these patients are positive. Cells that overexpress Her-2/neu are intrinsically resistant to the cytotoxic effects of tumor necrosis factor alpha. The patients who benefit the most from the therapy with anti-Her-2/neu antibodies are the ones with metastatic advanced breast cancer and positive Her-2/neu status. *(Cotran et al., p. 1115)*

829. **(E)** Recent studies have shown that Reed–Sternberg cells are aneuploid cells that contain clonal cytogenetic aberration. In multiple testing, the Reed–Sternberg cells are showing marked for B or T lymphocytes, as well as monocytes/macrophages cells. The molecular analysis on the immunoglobulin gene, rearrangement tends to support the B cell origin of the RS cells. *(Cotran et al., pp. 670–675)*

830. **(B)** The follicular lymphomas are characterized by a translocation (14,18). This translocation is mostly seen in some, but not all, follicular lymphomas and leads to expression of the BCL-2 protein. BCL-2 is known to be an antagonist of the apoptosis and the B cells in such matter remain immortal, promoting the survival of the cells in the follicular lymphoma. The reactive follicles contain numerous B cells undergoing apoptosis, but only the neoplastic follicles characteristically lacking of apoptotic cells show a marked overexpression of BCL-2. *(Cotran et al., p. 660)*

831. **(B)** Multiple myeloma is characterized by a proliferation of plasma cells, most commonly producing punch-out lesions in the bones of the entire skeleton. Microscopic examination of the bone marrow sections, as well as smears reveal an increased number of plasma cells that histologically vary from well differentiated, to cells with anaplastic nucleus and prominent nucleoli (plasmablasts). One of the major criteria for marrow involvement with multiple myeloma, is the counting of 30% of the total cellularity has to represent plasma cells or plasmablasts. Major, as well as minor criteria for making the definite diagnosis for multiple myeloma are required. *(Cotran et al., pp. 663–664)*

832. **(A)** The histologic appearance of lymphocytic predominant Hodgkin's disease is that of a prominence of mature lymphocytes with a few scattered histiocytes in the background. There is a paucity of typical Reed–Sternberg cells. Sometimes many sections must be obtained to make the diagnosis. Variants of RS cells, typical of this subtype (so-called L-H cells) were first described by Lukes and associates, and they are characteristic. The immunophenotype of these cells is different than the classic Hodgkin's disease in which the CD15 and CD30 are negative, and CD45 and B cell markers are positive. *(Rubin and Farber, pp. 1140–1147)*

833. **(E)** LP Hodgkin's is predominantly is a disease of the young adults and the majority of the patients are asymptomatic for a long time. The prognosis is very favorable, and in general, they present with stage I disease. The most

common area of involvement of the nodes is the cervical area to be followed by the inguinal area. The nodular variant of LP Hodgkin's disease has a positive pan B markers, CD20 and CD45. The cells are usually negative for CD15 and CD30. *(Rubin and Farber, pp. 1140–1147)*

834. **(C)** Mantle cell lymphoma is a neoplastic transformation of the cells in the mantle area of the lymph nodes, show a characteristic translocation for 11,14. This joins the BCL-2 oncogene on chromosome 11 to the immunoglobulin heavy-chain gene locus of chromosome 14. The gene product of BCL-1 is cyclin-D1 with immunoperoxidase technique can become evident with a bright positive cytoplasmic nuclear staining. This type of lymphoma is most commonly seen in elderly adults and is a rather aggressive B cell neoplasm which can undergo blastic transformation. *(Rubin and Farber, p. 1140)*

835. **(A)** On the pictures displayed, a minority of these cells are strongly positive (Figure 8–67) for cytoplasmic staining of CD20. Also, Figure 8–68 shows the reverse picture in which the mature T cells are showing strong staining for pan T markers, and the B cells are remaining unstained and surrounded by the T lymphocytes. The histologic feature of TCR-BCL is characterized by a predominance of T cells, which are small and with scant cytoplasm. In between these cells, a minority of

neoplastic cells are large B cells that stain by B cell markers. The neoplastic cells show an enlarged hyperchromatic nucleus with prominent nucleoli. The differential diagnosis of this non-Hodgkin's lymphoma will be with the lymphocytic predominant Hodgkin's disease, which can sometimes be very difficult. *(Rubin and Farber, pp. 1130–1149)*

836. **(B)** The histologic photomicrographs show germinal centers in which kappa and lambda cells appear to show scattered positivity in the follicles, as well as in the mantle zone. This appears to be a good balance of both cell types and, therefore, no neoplastic process is under consideration. Most of the time, the non-Hodgkin's lymphoma express evidence of light chain restriction, either kappa or lambda, which help to make the diagnosis in difficult cases. *(Rubin and Farber, pp. 1130–1149)*

REFERENCES

Chandrasoma P, Taylor CR. *Concise Pathology,* 3rd ed. Norwalk, CT: Appleton & Lange, 1998.

Cotran RS, Kumar V, Robbins SL. *Robbins Pathologic Basis of Disease,* 6th ed. Philadelphia: Saunders, 1999.

Rubin E, Farber JL. *Pathology.* Philadelphia: Lippincott, 1999.

CHAPTER 9

Heart and Blood Vessels

Study of the pathology of the heart has become more prevalent in the last decades with the evolution of medicine, because cardiac transplantation has become an important method of treatment of many cardiac diseases, which encompass the congenital heart diseases of childhood, storage diseases, sequels from infectious diseases, and atherosclerosis. Moreover, the importance of cardiovascular pathology should always be overemphasized, because the major causes of death in the United States are cardiovascular diseases. The weight of the adult human heart averages 300 g in males to 275 g in females ± 75 g. The adult heart weight is always related to body size and weight, and physiologic changes, as in the case of young athletes who will have a heart weight that approaches the upper limits and sometimes could exceed them. There are also changes related to age. For more specific details, pediatric pathology books contain charts for the weight of the heart of the fetus, infants, and adolescents.

Anatomically, the heart lies in the anterior mediastinum. Anteriorly, it is overlapped on the right and left side by the pleura and is also related in the anterior portion to the sternum. Laterally, it is related to the hilar structures of the right and left lung and on the posterior aspect, the posterior wall of the heart is in contact with the lower esophagus and descending aorta. The inferior wall rests to the diaphragm.

In addition, the heart is surrounded by the pericardium composed of a fibrous sac, microscopically covered by an endothelial lining. It contains between 20–40 cm of clear serous fluid. The leaflet of the pericardium that covers the heart is also called the epicardium. Both layers of the pericardium are covered by mesothelial cells forming a continuous layer, grossly a delicate membrane that is very smooth and moisturized by the epicardial fluid.

The myocardium constitutes the contractile section of the heart that is the live pump that makes possible the movement of the blood throughout the body. Basically, it is composed of striated muscle fibers that contain myofibrils composed of serially repeating contractile components called sarcomeres. The cardiac ventricular output is the product of the heart rate and the stroke volume, which is a function of the extent or shortening of the fibers of the ventricular myocardium.

CARDIAC VALVES

The atrial ventricular valves consist of the mitral and the tricuspid valve. The mitral valve is made up of the annulus, leaflets, chordae tendinae, and papillary muscles. The atrial ventricular valves are composed of three layers. The collagen bundles of the annulus are spread into the cusps of the mitral valve, and they continue into the chordae tendinae. The ventricular aspect is covered by the ventricularis on the ventricular surface. The atrial aspect is covered by the spongiosa, and this layer extends through the entire length of the leaflets.

CONDUCTION SYSTEM

These are specialized myocardial fibers in the conduction of the electric impulse to produce the contraction. The sinoatrial (SA) node is the primary pacemaker for the human heart. It is located at the junction of the superior vena cava and the lateral border of the right atrium.

The atrial ventricular (AV) node is located on the right side of the interatrial septum, by the opening of the coronary sinus. The atrial ventricular node is prolonged by a main bundle that is arranged parallel and terminates in the left and right bundle branches. Extensive and complex ramification of these bundles is present in the subendocardium of the right and left ventricles.

The blood supply is provided by the three coronary arteries, with the different branching and many different anatomical variations. The nerve supply is done by the sympathetic, as well as the parasympathetic system, and there are two networks of lymphatics in the heart, in the endocardium and epicardium.

BLOOD VESSELS

The blood vessels are structures that convey the fluids throughout the body, and according to their function, as well as size, the structure of the wall varies considerably. The vessels change in different ages of individuals. Because vascular abnormalities are the major cause of clinical disease, the pathology is based on different mechanisms: (a) for mechanical reasons, for obstruction of narrowing of the lumen; (b) for inflammatory and proliferative changes of the vessel wall; and (c) for weakening of the vessel wall and rupture.

The arteries are divided into three types: the large elastic arteries, the medium-sized muscular arteries, and the arterioles. Therefore, the walls of these arteries vary from mostly elastic tissue in the larger arteries, to predominantly smooth muscle cells in the muscular arteries, and the arterioles also contain a muscular wall that can be attenuated just proximal to capillary beds. All of the arteries, as well as the veins, are lined internally by a single layer of spindle-shaped endothelial cells. On light microscopy, these endothelial cells appear for the most part, flattened, and the cytoplasm is indiscernible. An external layer of tissue is present in the arteries as well as veins, which is called *adventitia*. The walls of the veins and venules as well as the lymphatics also differ from those of the arteries,

because adaptation to different pressures of the blood require a less layer; although, the intima, as well as the adventitia, remain similar.

DISEASES THAT MOSTLY AFFECT THE VASCULAR CHANNELS

Atherosclerosis is most common disease that affects the blood vessels, given that its incidence is common and frequent. Hypertension and vasculitis are also prevalent, although less common. Atherosclerosis not only affects the large vessels, with thickening of the intima and accumulations of lipid material forming the atheromatous plaque, it can also affect the smaller arteries in which a proliferation of the intima with cholesterol deposits can be seen. Marked narrowing and obstructions of the lumina is common. Marked variations of this morbid condition are related to age, sex, genetics, hyperlipidemia, and such secondary causes as, hypertension, cigarette smoking, and diabetes mellitus.

VASCULITIS

The inflammatory process affecting the blood vessels, which can be of different types, is called vasculitis. This pathological process leads to different clinical manifestations, according to the organ most affected. One of the most common noninfectious vasculitis is related to immune-mediated inflammatory changes. Different types of vasculitis can be divided into: (a) large vessel vasculitis; (b) giant cell (temporary) arteritis; (c) Takayasu arteritis; (d) medium-size vessel vasculitis; (e) polyarteritis nodosa; (f) Kawasaki disease; and (g) small vessel vasculitis, which includes, Wegener's granulomatosis, Churg–Strauss syndrome, microscopic polyangitis, Henoch–Schönlein purpura, essential cryoglobulinemia vasculitis, and cutaneous leukocytoclastic angitis.

Questions

837. Which is the most frequent factor that may predispose children to bacterial endocarditis?

    (A) congenital heart disease
    (B) myocarditis
    (C) pericardial effusion
    (D) rheumatic fever
    (E) viral infections

838. Pulmonary effects of ventricular septal defect (VSD) are principally attributable to which of the following?

    (A) associated pulmonic valve dysfunction
    (B) associated tricuspid valve dysfunction
    (C) pressure overload of the right ventricle
    (D) right to left shunt in utero
    (E) volume overload of the pulmonary circulation

839. A 32-year-old male has a brachial artery blood pressure of 210/140 mm Hg, and weak pulses and low blood pressure in the lower extremities. Which is the most likely diagnosis?

    (A) postductal coarctation of the aorta
    (B) preductal coarctation of the aorta
    (C) tetralogy of Fallot
    (D) transposition of the great vessels
    (E) VSD

840. Irreversible pulmonary vascular sclerosis typically is a late result which of the following?

    (A) large left-to-right shunt
    (B) large right-to-left shunt
    (C) long-standing tricuspid valve insufficiency
    (D) prolonged cyanosis
    (E) severe right ventricular outflow obstruction

841. Hypertension most commonly in the early stages is manifested by which of the following?

    (A) cardiovascular disease
    (B) cerebral edema
    (C) few symptoms, if any
    (D) renal disease
    (E) stroke

842. In malignant hypertension, where can early changes can be detected?

    (A) in the aorta
    (B) in the cerebral arteries
    (C) in the coronary arteries
    (D) in the renal arteries
    (E) in the retinal arterioles

843. Which is the most common change in giant cell (temporal) arteritis?

    (A) granulomatous inflammation throughout the wall
    (B) granulomatous inflammation of the intima only
    (C) eosinophilia
    (D) lymphocytic infiltrate
    (E) plasma cell infiltrate

844. Which is a life-threatening complication of abdominal aortic aneurysm (AAA)?

(A) infection
(B) embolism
(C) occlusion of major blood vessels
(D) rupture
(E) impingement of vital structure

845. Which arteries are most prominently affected in polyarteritis nodosa?

(A) larger sized arteries
(B) capillaries
(C) aorta
(D) small- and medium-sized muscular arteries
(E) coronary arteries

846. Which characterizes the term "leukocytoclastic angitis?"

(A) granulomatous inflammation
(B) medium-sized arteritis
(C) large vessel arteritis
(D) fragments of neutrophils along the vessel walls
(E) microinfarcts

847. Which is most clearly associated with hypercholesterolemia?

(A) atherosclerosis
(B) hypertension
(C) vasculitis
(D) liver failure
(E) aortic cystic medial necrosis

848. Causes of hypercholesterolemia include which of the following?

(A) cigarette smoking
(B) genetic abnormalities of low-density lipoprotein (LDL) receptor
(C) hypertension
(D) genetic abnormalities of lipoprotein lipase
(E) genetic abnormalities of platelet-derived growth factor (PDGF)

849. Atherosclerosis most often affects which of the following?

(A) brachial and radial arteries
(B) femoral arteries
(C) intramural arteries of the left ventricle
(D) small pulmonary arteries
(E) infrarenal abdominal aorta.

850. What is believed to be the earliest event in atherogenesis?

(A) intimal thickening and lipid accumulation
(B) platelet activation
(C) triglycerides increase
(D) vasoconstriction
(E) increased vascular permeability

851. Of the following, which is the MOST important risk factor for atherosclerosis?

(A) alcohol use
(B) systemic hypertension
(C) multiple pregnancies
(D) diabetes insipidus
(E) autoimmune diseases

Answers and Explanations

837. **(A)** Children who develop bacterial endocarditis have an underlying cardiac anomaly that is a predisposing factor. Because rheumatic heart disease has been successfully treated, and the sequels of that disease are lower, the majority of the cases of bacterial endocarditis in children are seen in cases of congenital heart disease. The valves more commonly affected by this process are the mitral and aortic valves. The most frequent congenital heart disease in children that are affected by bacterial endocarditis are patent ductus arteriosus, Tetralogy of Fallot, and ventricular septal defect. The most common pathological change on the leaflets of the valves are vegetations, which, on microscopic examination, appear to be composed of fibrin, cellular debris, and platelets with bacterial colonies. *(Rubin and Farber, pp. 571–572)*

838. **(E)** Ventricular septal defects are the most common of all congenital heart diseases. In the development of the fetal heart, there is a muscular septum that grows in between the two ventricles. The growth is upward from the apex to the base of the heart. This is joined by a down-growth of a membranous septum that joins the muscular septum and separates the right and left ventricles. Failure to develop completely the membranous portion of the septum forms an abnormal communication between the right and left ventricles. Defects of the muscular portion of the septum can also be seen. This defect of the closure of the interventricular chamber will lead to left ventricular hypertrophy and congestive heart failure, which are the most common complications of this disease consistent in a left-to-right shunt.

This will create an increase in pulmonary flow. *(Rubin and Farber, pp. 543–544)*

839. **(A)** Coarctation of the aorta is a local constriction of this vessel that, for the most part, is seen immediately below the origin of the left subclavian artery at the site of the ductus arteriosus. This anomaly is two to five times more frequently found in males than in females and is also associated with another malformation, which is bicuspid aortic valve. The pathogenesis of the coarctation of the aorta is believed to be secondary to the pattern of flow in the ductus arteriosus during the fetal life. The discrepancy between the blood pressure in the upper and lower extremities is the hallmark of the coarctation of the aorta. *(Rubin and Farber, pp. 549)*

840. **(A)** The left-to-right shunts of the blood happen in different congenital heart diseases, such as ventricular septal defect, atrial septal defect, patent ductus arteriosus, and anomalous pulmonary vein drainage. All of these congenital abnormalities will lead to easy fatigue, dyspnea, and changes in the pulmonary vasculature, secondary to pulmonary hypertension and sclerosis. *(Rubin and Farber, pp. 543–549)*

841. **(C)** Most patients who are hypertensive in the early stages only show a few symptoms. Many times, the first manifestation of hypertension is myocardial infarction, stroke, and chronic renal disease. About 20% of the population of the industrialized countries are affected by hypertension with subsequent consequences. *(Rubin and Farber, pp. 509–513)*

842. (E) Malignant hypertension is manifested by rapidly progressive vascular compromise with the onset of symptomatic disease of the brain, heart, or kidney. It could not be defined by the degree of blood pressure elevation, and with the modern therapy of antihypertensive drugs malignant hypertension has become a rare disorder. The pathological changes are detected particularly at the microvascular level. On examination of the retina, the arterioles in cases of a malignant hypertension show changes that help in the diagnosis. These changes are microaneurysm, focal hemorrhage, necrosis, edema, and scarring. *(Rubin and Farber, pp. 512–513)*

843. (A) Giant cell arteritis tends to be a condition characterized by headaches and throbbing temporal pain. Sometimes such constitutional symptoms as malaise, fever and weight loss can be present. On histological examination, there is a granulomatous inflammation of the media and intima, but the adventitia can also be affected. These inflammatory changes are consistent with lymphocytes, plasma cells, and occasional giant cells. The internal elastic lamina appears fragmented. The lumen of the artery is considerably narrowed. `(Rubin and Farber, pp. 516–517)*

844. (D) The abdominal aortic aneurysms that most commonly develop secondary to atherosclerosis are positioned, for the most part, below the renal arteries and above the bifurcation of the aorta. They might be fusiform or saccular, and they may remain largely asymptomatic. Occasionally the aneurysm may affect such organs as the kidney, and atherosclerotic plaques can be dislodged and carried to the vessels of the kidney or lower extremities (embolism). Infections of the aortic aneurysms are rare unless they represent a mycotic abdominal aneurysm, which is an aneurysm that has been infected secondary, with further destruction of the media. Rupture of the aneurysm into the retroperitoneal or the peritoneal cavity usually leads to a massive hemorrhage, and without immediate surgical care can have a rapid fatal outcome. *(Cotran et al., pp. 524–527)*

845. (D) Polyarteritis nodosa affects most prominently the small and medium-sized vascular arteries and the distribution of the inflammatory process is focal. On occasion, however, this inflammatory patchy infiltrate can be extended to the larger-sized arteries, such as renal, splenic, and coronary arteries. The characteristic finding on the walls of the arteries is fibrinoid necrosis, with an inflammatory cell infiltrate that includes neutrophils, lymphocytes, plasma cells, and eosinophils. Polyarteritis nodosa affecting the small vessels is frequently associated with the presence of antineutrophil cytoplasmic antibodies (ANCA). In patients who survive the disease, with intensive treatment, areas of scarring are present affecting mostly the media as well as the intima. *(Rubin and Farber, pp. 515–516)*

846. (D) Hypersensitivity, or leukocytoclastic vasculitis affects generally the smaller arterioles, capillaries, and venules. These lesions are thought to represent hypersensitivity reaction and involve the skin, mucous membranes, lungs, brain, heart, gastrointestinal tract, kidneys, and muscles. The clinical picture when these organs are affected is hemoptysis, hematuria, proteinuria, abdominal pain, and muscle weakness. Histologically, we could see occasional fibrinoid necrosis of the wall of the small vessels, and there is a characteristic infiltrate of neutrophils that are fragmented, and they follow around the vessel wall. Immunoglobulin and complement components may be present in the vascular lesions and in the skin. *(Cotran et al., pp. 521–522)*

847. (A) There is a significant correlation between the severity of atherosclerosis and the levels of total plasma cholesterol or low-density lipoproteins (LDL). This has been demonstrated in an epidemiologic analysis, as judged by the mortality rate from myocardial infarctions. The higher level of cholesterol, the higher the risk for coronary artery disease. When levels of serum cholesterol are lowered by diet or drugs, the rate of progression of atherosclerosis disease is slowed. Moreover, it has been shown that some atherosclerotic plaques have also regressed, therefore, the risk of cardiovascular disease is also reduced. Many studies have proved that lowering cholesterol levels in the blood reduces the risk of atherosclerotic-related events. *(Cotran et al., pp. 505–506)*

848.   **(B)** Atherosclerosis is considered one of the most common complications of hyperlipidemia. Hypertriglyceridemia plays a less significant role in atherosclerosis. The fraction implicated in the atherosclerotic process is low density lipoprotein (LDL). Genetic defects in lipoprotein metabolism and hyperlipidemia are associated with accelerated atherosclerosis. Familial hypercholesterolemia is caused by defects in the LDL receptor leading to inadequate hepatic uptake of the LDL and markedly increased circulating LDL. *(Cotran et al., pp. 504–505)*

849.   **(E)** Atherosclerosis is characterized by the atheromatous plaques, which are lesions that consist of an accumulation of cholesterol and cholesterol esters covered by fibrous cap and in contact with the intima. They vary in size and sometimes may become ulcerated. The most affected artery is the abdominal aorta, below the renal arteries. Although all of the other arteries listed in the question can be affected by atherosclerotic process, they are not as prominent or as severe as those seen in the abdominal aorta. *(Cotran et al., pp. 499–500)*

850.   **(A)** The earliest lesion in atherosclerosis is endothelial injury with thickening of the intima as well as lipid accumulation that produces the characteristic atheromatous plaques. These plaques can progress, protruding through the lumen and weaken the medial of the arteries, which obviously leads to complications. Triglyceride increase is not a primary event in atherogenesis, nor is the platelet activation or increase in vascular permeability. *(Cotran et al., pp. 497–499)*

851.   **(B)** Hypertension has been considered for many years the major risk factor for atherosclerosis, and after age 45, hypertension is a stronger factor than hypercholesterolemia. When blood pressure exceeds a 170/95 mm Hg, the risk of ischemic heart disease increases fivefold. Cigarette smoking and diabetes mellitus also increase the risk of atherosclerosis. *(Cotran et al., pp. 498–509)*

REFERENCES

Cotran RS, Kumar V, Robbins SL. *Robbins Pathologic Basis of Disease*, 6th ed. Philadelphia: Saunders, 1999.

Rubin E, Farber JL. *Pathology*. Philadelphia: Lippincott, 1999.

CHAPTER 10

Respiratory System

The respiratory system can be divided into air passages that include the nasal cavity, the pharynx, larynx, trachea, and bronchi. The second portion would be the lungs which are built to carry out their most important function of the exchange of gases between the air and the blood. The beginning of the air passages on the mucosal area are histologically covered by nonkeratinizing squamous epithelium. The surface of the larynx, as well as the trachea and major bronchi, are lined by respiratory epithelium and in the submucosa contain small mucinous-secreting glands. Progressing into the division of the bronchi, they become the bronchioles, which lack cartilage on the wall. The bronchioles further divide in terminal bronchioles, connected to several alveolar sacs. The alveoli and the respiratory bronchioles form the acinous (terminal respiratory unit). The alveolar sacs are composed of a wall 5–10 microns thick and is covered by type II pneumocytes over 90% of the surface and type I pneumocytes on the remainder. The type I pneumocytes are particularly vulnerable to injury. The type II pneumocytes are in charge of dividing and differentiating into the new type I cells that reconstruct the alveolar surface. Also, the type II pneumocytes are the source of pulmonary surfactant.

In this chapter, the focus is mainly on the lung, and the questions are related to pulmonary infections, chronic obstructive pulmonary disease, interstitial diseases of the lung, including pneumoconiosis and tumors.

Questions

DIRECTIONS (Questions 852 through 861): Each of the numbered items or incomplete statements in this section is followed by answers or by completions of the statement. Select the ONE lettered answer or completion that is BEST in each case.

852. What condition(s) are related to cigarette smoking?

   (A) centriacinar emphysema
   (B) chronic bronchitis
   (C) increased risk of death from coronary artery disease
   (D) primary lung carcinoma
   (E) all of the above

853. Which neoplasm causes abdominal cramps, diarrhea, bronchospasm, and episodic flushing of the skin?

   (A) bronchial carcinoid
   (B) cardiac myxoma
   (C) colonic adenocarcinoma
   (D) gastric lymphoma
   (E) uterine leiomyoma

854. Occupational exposure to asbestos can result in which of the following?

   (A) calcified plaques of the pleura
   (B) increased risk of lung carcinoma
   (C) increased risk of malignant mesothelioma
   (D) symptomatic pulmonary interstitial fibrosis
   (E) all of the above

855. Which malignant neoplasm of the lung is most commonly associated with ectopic hormone production?

   (A) adenocarcinoma
   (B) bronchiolo–alveolar cell carcinoma
   (C) large cell carcinoma
   (D) small cell carcinoma
   (E) squamous cell carcinoma

856. An elderly patient, a heavy smoker with chronic productive cough shortness of breath, develops cyanosis and edema. The last two events are secondary to which of the following?

   (A) dilatation of bronchial walls due to chronic persistent infection
   (B) enlargement of air spaces with decreased diffusion capacity
   (C) heart failure secondary to pulmonary hypertension
   (D) hypertrophy of bronchial mucus glands
   (E) narrowing of airways due to bronchial smooth muscle contraction

857. What is the type of lung cancer with a high rate of mortality?

   (A) adenocarcinoma
   (B) bronchioloalveolar carcinoma
   (C) large cell carcinoma
   (D) small cell anaplastic carcinoma
   (E) squamous cell carcinoma

858. Which is the finding that occurs in the bronchial epithelium of cigarette smokers?

(A) basal cell hyperplasia

(B) carcinoma in situ

(C) dysplasia

(D) squamous metaplasia

(E) all of the above

859. Within the following pneumoconiosis, which is the one related to malignant mesothelioma?

(A) anthracosis

(B) asbestosis

(C) berylliosis

(D) coal workers' pneumoconiosis

(E) silicosis

860. An elderly patient presented with unproductive cough and dyspnea. His past medical history indicates that he was a sandblaster. The chest x-ray reveals patchy fibrotic nodules in the upper lobes of the lung with peripheral calcifications. What is your diagnosis?

(A) asbestosis

(B) berylliosis

(C) coal workers' pneumoconiosis

(D) sarcoidosis

(E) silicosis

861. What is the most likely finding in an individual who has alpha$_1$-antitrypsin deficiency?

(A) centriacinar emphysema and cirrhosis

(B) centriacinar emphysema only

(C) cirrhosis only

(D) panacinar emphysema and coronary artery disease

(E) panacinar emphysema only

DIRECTIONS (Questions 862 through 866): For each numbered word or phrase, select the ONE lettered option that is most closely associated with it. Each lettered option may be selected once, more than once, or not at all.

(A) acute eosinophilic pneumonia

(B) extrinsic asthma

(C) idiopathic pulmonary fibrosis

(D) panacinar emphysema

(E) pulmonary alveolar proteinosis

862. Inherited alpha$_1$-antitrypsin deficiency

863. IgE-mediated bronchospasm

864. Parasitic infection

865. Circulating and pulmonary immune complexes

866. Surfactant excess and cellular debris

DIRECTIONS (Questions 867 through 874): Each of the numbered items or incomplete statements in this section is followed by answers or by completions of the statement. Select the ONE lettered answer or completion that is BEST in each case.

867. In a paraneoplastic syndrome, the production of corticotropin (ACTH) is seen more commonly in what type of malignant neoplasm?

(A) adenocarcinoma of the lung

(B) bronchioloalveolar carcinoma of the lung

(C) malignant mesothelioma

(D) small cell carcinoma of the lung

(E) squamous cell carcinoma of the lung

868. Which malignant primary tumor of the lung do most of the patients survive for less than 2 years?

(A) adenocarcinoma

(B) bronchial carcinoid

(C) bronchioloalveolar carcinoma

(D) small cell anaplastic carcinoma

(E) squamous cell carcinoma

869. Which primary lung tumor is not treated surgically?

(A) adenocarcinoma

(B) bronchial carcinoid

(C) large cell carcinoma

(D) small cell anaplastic carcinoma

(E) squamous cell carcinoma

870. Which lung neoplasm is less likely to metastasize?

   (A) adenocarcinoma
   (B) atypical carcinoid (neuroendocrine carcinoma)
   (C) carcinoid tumor
   (D) large cell anaplastic carcinoma
   (E) small cell carcinoma

871. Which micro-organism is most commonly related to lobar pneumonia?

   (A) *Chlamydia trachomatis*
   (B) *Pseudomonas aeruginosa*
   (C) *Staphylococcus aureus*
   (D) *Streptococcus pneumoniae*
   (E) *Treponema pallidum*

872. Which congenital anomaly of the lung does not have a normal connection to the airway system, and the blood supply comes from the aorta or its branches?

   (A) a bronchogenic cyst
   (B) a bronchopulmonary sequestration
   (C) a pulmonary hamartoma
   (D) atelectasis
   (E) bronchopulmonary dysplasia

873. Of the conditions listed, which is the most likely to progress to an end-stage lung disease?

   (A) asthma
   (B) bronchiectasis
   (C) hypersensitivity pneumonitis
   (D) Löffler's syndrome
   (E) primary pulmonary hypertension

874. Chronic exposure to asbestos leads to the development of which malignant tumor?

   (A) acute myelogenous leukemia
   (B) angiosarcoma
   (C) malignant melanoma
   (D) malignant mesothelioma
   (E) papillary thyroid carcinoma

DIRECTIONS (Questions 875 through 879): For each numbered word or phrase, select the ONE lettered option that is most closely associated with it. Each lettered option may be selected once, more than once, or not at all.

   (A) asthma
   (B) bronchopulmonary dysplasia
   (C) Caplan's syndrome
   (D) emphysema
   (E) Löffler's syndrome

875. Permanent enlargement of airspaces distal to terminal bronchioles with destruction of alveolar walls

876. Mucous plugs within the bronchi; bronchial smooth muscle and mucous gland hypertrophy; bronchial inflammation with numerous eosinophils; Charcot–Leyden crystals within airways

877. Pneumoconiosis and rheumatoid arthritis

878. Pulmonary eosinophilia

879. Oxygen dependence in infants

DIRECTIONS (Questions 880 and 881): Each of the numbered items or incomplete statements in this section is followed by answers or by completions of the statement. Select the ONE lettered answer or completion that is BEST in each case.

880. Which is the most common micro-organism implicated in bronchopneumonia?

   (A) *Histoplasma capsulatum*
   (B) *Staphylococcus aureus*
   (C) *Streptococcus hemolyticus*
   (D) *Streptococcus pneumoniae*
   (E) *Toxoplasma gondii*

881. A patient developed left-sided chest pain, chills, fever, and cough with hemoptysis. On chest x-ray, a diffuse infiltrate of the entire lobe was seen. Which is the most logical diagnosis?

   (A) interstitial pneumonia
   (B) Legionella pneumonia
   (C) pneumococcal pneumonia
   (D) staphylococcal pneumonia
   (E) viral pneumonia

Answers and Explanations

852. **(E)** Tobacco smoking has been related to lung cancer for many years. Cigarette smoking increases the incidents of the risk of developing lung cancer tenfold, and in heavy smokers with more than 40 cigarettes per day, the increase is up to 20-fold. Quitting smoking for over 10 years reduces the risk to control levels. Also, cigarette smoking related to many cancers of the respiratory, as well as the GI tract, is also known to cause such non-neoplastic diseases as high risk for coronary artery disease, centracinar emphysema, and chronic bronchitis. *(Cotran et al., pp. 741–742)*

853. **(A)** Carcinoid tumors represent only a small portion of lung tumors (1–5%). The bronchial carcinoids are histologically composed of small nests with intermediate-type of cells containing a round nucleus and eosinophilic cytoplasm. Occasionally, they may form rosettes. On special stains, the bronchial carcinoids show neuroendocrine granules, which can be detected for immunoperoxidase technique, as well as with electron microscopy. These tumors may produce a carcinoid syndrome characterized by flushing, asthma-like attacks, cyanosis, and diarrhea. *(Cotran et al., pp. 747–748)*

854. **(E)** Classically, exposure to asbestos has been described as having a marked increase in incidence of malignant tumors of the pleura (mesothelioma). Also, a high risk of lung carcinoma is present in people working with asbestos, because they are also associated with significant cigarette smoking. The long-term exposure to asbestos also can lead to calcified plaques of the pleura, as well as symptomatic pulmonary interstitial fibrosis. *(Cotran et al., pp. 551–552)*

855. **(D)** The origin of the small cell carcinoma is the neuroendocrine cells (Kulchitsky cells). These cells, which are present along the bronchial epithelial lining, can also be seen in the alveolar spaces. The small cell carcinoma is pleomorphic highly malignant neoplasm, in which the classic pattern is the so-called oat cell carcinoma. Other varieties have been described, such as spindle cell, polygonal cells, and intermediate type cells. On special immunoperoxidase stains or electron microscopy, these cells contain dense-core neural secretory granules. These tumors are most commonly associated with paraneoplastic syndrome; they are the most aggressive of the lung tumors and most likely have metastasis at the time of diagnosis. *(Cotran et al., pp. 743–745)*

856. **(C)** Pulmonary hypertension could be primary or secondary; however, more frequently, it is secondary. Increasing the pulmonary blood flow or pulmonary vascular resistance will be secondary to chronic obstructive or interstitial lung disease, congenital heart disease, or recurrent thromboemboli. Once the portal hypertension is established as in the example given secondary to pulmonary disease, heart failure may ensue. *(Cotran et al., pp. 704–705)*

857. **(D)** Refer to the explanation in Answer 855. *(Cotran et al., pp. 743–745)*

858. **(E)** Cigarette smoking acting over the respiratory epithelium produces many morphological changes that can also be identified with the histology. Loss of the cilia, basal cell hyperplasia, and squamous metaplasia, which can be followed by dysplasia and carcinoma in situ. Given time, carcinoma in situ of the bronchial mucosa breaks into the basement membrane and invades into the parenchyma, the regional lymph nodes, and produces distant metastases. (*Rubin and Farber, p. 312*)

859. **(B)** Asbestos, with its widespread use for insulation, flooring, and roofing materials, as well as pipes among others, has become a significant risk for developing malignant neoplasms. Even low level exposure of asbestos shows a significant risk for asbestos-related neoplasms. Among the most common tumors associated with asbestosis are bronchogenic carcinoma and malignant mesothelioma. The other answer listed, pneumoconiosis, does not have the same risk for developing mesothelioma. (*Chandrasoma and Taylor, pp. 541–542*)

860. **(E)** Silicosis is caused by inhalation of crystalline silicone dioxide (silica). Workers in such risky occupations as sandblasting are exposed to silica and may develop diseases related to deposition of silica in the lung. While in the alveoli, the silica crystals are phagocytized by macrophages. The toxic effect of silica produces cell death and liberation of the free silica particles. Inflammation and fibrosis follows leading to the formation of nodules composed of hyalinized collagen around the crystals. Silica crystals can also be carried in the lymphatics to hilar lymph nodes. (*Chandrasoma and Taylor, p. 540*)

861. **(E)** Severe alpha$_1$-antitrypsin deficiency occurs in homozygotes that have no alleles at the locus (PiZZ). Usually, the onset of symptoms becomes apparent during childhood. Histologically in the liver biopsies, it appears as eosinophilic globules in the cytoplasm of the hepatocytes. These globules are of alpha$_1$-antitrypsin, which can be better visualized using immunoperoxidase techniques of PAS stain. The persons with alpha$_1$-antitrypsin deficiency develop panacinar emphysema by age 40. The development of cirrhosis is rare. (*Chandrasoma and Taylor, p. 533*)

862. **(D)** Refer to Answer 861. (*Chandrasoma and Taylor, p. 533*)

863. **(B)** Bronchial asthma is considered a response of the tracheal bronchial tree to the exposure of stimuli. Bronchospasm produces obstruction of the airflow usually of short duration, which is reversible. Serum IgE is increased and mediates the bronchospasm. (*Chandrasoma Taylor, p. 529*)

864. **(A)** Eosinophilic pneumonia is a group of diseases characterized by pulmonary interstitial infiltrates by eosinophils, as well as peripheral eosinophilia. This disorder encompasses different pathological process that include parasitic infections, allergic bronchopulmonary aspergillosis, and drug reactions. (*Chandrasoma and Taylor, p. 539*)

865. **(C)** Idiopathic pulmonary fibrosis encompasses a group of diseases that histologically show features of widening of the septae, alveoli walls, by fibrous tissue and scattered inflammatory infiltrates. This disease, of unknown cause, has a presence of circulating immune complexes with deposition in the interstitium, which has been proved by the immunofluorescence, in many cases. This suggests an immunologic basis of the disease. (*Chandrasoma and Taylor, p. 536*)

866. **(E)** Pulmonary alveolar proteinosis is histologically characterized by filling of the alveolar spaces with homogenous, amorphous, and eosinophilic material rich in lipids. This material is considered to be surfactant, because of either overproduction or decrease in clearance. The patients with alveolar proteinosis clinically present with dyspnea and dry cough, and x-ray shows a consolidation affecting, mostly in the beginning, the lung bases. (*Chandrasoma and Taylor, p. 544*)

867. **(D)** Paraneoplastic syndromes produced by bronchogenic carcinoma are often a complication of the neoplasm, and they may produce adrenocorticotropic hormone (ACTH) antidiuretic hormone (ADH), parathyroid hormone, calcitonin, gonadotropins, or serotonin. Of all tumors in the lung that produce hormones, the

most common is the small cell anaplastic carcinoma. *(Chandrasoma and Taylor, p. 746)*

868. (D) Untreated, the survival rate for small cell cancer is 6–17 weeks. This particular tumor is not effectively removed surgically; therefore, the treatment of choice is chemotherapy and radiation. Using this modality, up to 15–25% have reported cure rates; although, many patients at the time of diagnosis have distant metastases. *(Cotran et al., pp. 745–746)*

869. (D) Refer to Answer 868. *(Cotran et al., pp. 745–746)*

870. (C) Carcinoid tumors of the lung are not classically considered encapsulated, and there is infiltration of the surrounding tissues. The spread is either a local metastasis or distant metastasis. Most bronchial carcinoids, however, have no secretory activity, and they do not metastasize, following a relatively benign course for a long period of time. *(Cotran et al., pp. 747–748)*

871. (D) The etiology of lobar pneumonia, which is a bacterial infection, is most commonly caused by *Streptococcus pneumoniae*. Pathologically, lobar pneumonia is a fibrinosuppurative consolidation of large areas or the entire lobe of the lung. Different stages have been described, having the first stage of congestion, second of red hepatization, followed by gray hepatization and the last resolution. *(Chandrasoma and Taylor, pp. 515–516)*

872. (B) Bronchopulmonary sequestration is defined as a present of lobes or segments of lobes of the lung without a normal connection to the airway system. The blood supply originates in the aorta, or in its branches, not from the pulmonary arteries. Sequestration can be extralobal or intralobal, which are found within the lung, per se. *(Cotran et al., p. 699)*

873. (C) Hypersensitivity pneumonitis are diseases of the lung characterized by damaging the alveolar walls of the individuals reacting to either organic dusts or occupational antigens. Numerous syndromes have been described of this type, such as farmers' lung, pigeons' breathers lung, humidifier, or air conditioner lungs. This type of hypersensitivity must be promptly recognized because of the possibility of a progression to a serious damage of the lung with fibrosis. *(Cotran et al., p. 737)*

874. (D) Refer to Answer 859. *(Chandrasoma and Taylor, pp. 541–542)*

875. (D) Emphysema by definition is characterized by a permanent enlargement of the alveolar spaces, which is followed by destruction of the walls without creating major fibrous scarring. Many types of emphysema have been described, according to its anatomic distribution. Centriacinar, panacinar, paraseptal, and irregular are some of the different forms of emphysema. *(Cotran et al., p. 707)*

876. (A) Asthma is a chronic lung disease characterized by periodic episodes of airflow obstruction secondary to reversible bronchospasms. The histologic substruct of asthma is characterized by hypertrophy of the bronchial wall smooth muscle, increase in submucosal glands, edema and inflammation of the bronchial wall with a prominence of eosinophils, thickening of the basement membrane, and bronchial epithelium. Curschmann spirals and Charcot–Leyden crystals in the sputum can be found. *(Cotran et al., pp. 715–716)*

877. (C) Caplan's syndrome is characterized by the development of nodular pulmonary lesions that are similar to rheumatoid nodules. Histologically, the nodules in the Caplan's syndrome have a central necrosis around the fibroblasts, macrophages, and collagen. Caplan's syndrome occurs as in association with known pneumoconiosis, and patients develop rheumatoid arthritis. *(Cotran et al., p. 730)*

878. (E) The infiltration of eosinophils in the lung could be secondary to different diseases, which could be primary, as well as secondary. In primary eosinophilia, which is also called Löffler's syndrome, is characterized by a pulmonary lesion that shows a thickened alveolar septae and with an inflammatory infiltrate composed mostly of eosinophils. This is also accompanied by a peripheral eosinophilia. *(Cotran et al., p. 738)*

879. **(B)** Bronchopulmonary dysplasia is defined as an oxygen dependence at 20 days of age and characterized by a persistent respiratory distress for up to 3–6 months. Pathologically, it shows a epithelial hyperplasia and squamous metaplasia. Alveolar thickening of the walls, and peribronchial as well as interstitial fibrosis are present. Bronchopulmonary dysplasia is present in 50% of infants under 1,000 g body weight at birth. Because high concentrations of oxygen produces a high mortality on this disease, alternative methods have been employed. *(Cotran et al., pp. 472–473)*

880. **(B)** Bronchopneumonia is characterized by focal areas of consolidation of the lung with acute inflammation. The most common pathogen for bronchopneumonia is staphylococci. Other organisms can also be implicated, such as streptococci, Pneumococci, and *Haemophilus influenzae*, etc. *(Chandrasoma and Taylor, pp. 514–518)*

881. **(C)** Lobar pneumonia is an acute bacterial infection of a large part of the lung or the entire lobe. Classic lobar pneumonia is produced by *Streptococcus pneumoniae*, and different stages of this disease can be seen with different histological patterns. In the first stage of congestion, it is histologically characterized by vascular congestion and interalveolar fluid with neutrophils. The second stage or red hepatization is characterized by a massive confluent exudation with red cells and neutrophils into the alveolar spaces. The third stage or gray hepatization is progressive disintegration of the red cells and persistent of the fibrin suppurative exudate. At the stage of resolution, the consolidated areas and the exudate of the alveolar spaces disappear by insigmatic digestion. *(Chandrasoma and Taylor, pp. 514–518)*

REFERENCES

Chandrasoma P, Taylor, CR. *Concise Pathology*, 3rd ed. Norwalk, CT: Appleton & Lange, 1998.

Cotran RS, Kumar V, Robbins SL. *Robbins Pathologic Basis of Disease*, 6th ed. Philadelphia: Saunders, 1999.

Rubin E, Farber L. *Pathology*. Philadelphia: Lippincott, 1999.

CHAPTER 11

Gastrointestinal System, Liver, and Pancreas

The foregut is formed from the endoderm. By 5 to 6 weeks of gestation, the separation between the esophagus and the trachea is almost completed. The esophagus is lined by nonkeratinized squamous epithelium. The muscular wall of the esophagus consists of an outer longitudinal layer and inside a circular layer. Under the epithelial layer, a submucosa is present and a muscularis mucosa composed of longitudinal smooth muscle fibers. The intra-abdominal portion of the esophagus is lined by a serosa, although the majority of the esophagus is surrounded by fascia that condenses on the outer layer forming a sheath-like structure. The stomach is divided into five different anatomical regions: the cardia, the fundus, the body (corpus), the antrum, and the pyloric sphincter. The gastric wall consists of: mucosa, submucosa, muscularis propria, and serosa.

The folded gastric mucosa is punctuated by millions of gastric foveolae, leading to the mucosal glands. The entire surface is covered by foveolar cells (mucin-secreting cells). Mitoses are frequent since the mucosa is totally replaced every 2–6 days. The gastric glands vary according to anatomical regions. The cell types of the gastric glands are composed of a) mucous cells (antral and cardia regions); b) parietal cells (fundus), which contain in the cytoplasm the hydrogen ion pump and also secrete intrinsic factor; c) chief cell (base of gastric fundus), which secretes proteolytic proenzymes; and d) endocrine cells (body, fundus, and antrum), pouring their secretions directly to the blood.

The small intestine is divided grossly into three different segments; the duodenum, the jejunum, and the ileum. The histology of the small intestine has a variegated pattern that adapts to the different functions along the different segments. Because the principal function of the small intestine is absorption, several architectural adaptations are present to increase the amount of surface, grossly infoldings of the mucosa, and microscopically, is seen as delicate mucosal projections (villous epithelium). The lamina propria is well defined. The muscularis propria is formed by a longitudinal, as well as circular layer of smooth muscle, with a myenteric plexus of Auerbach located at the interface of the inner and outer smooth muscle layers of muscularis externa. The serosa and subserosa region cover and encircle the wall of the intestine.

The colon is an intraperitoneal segment of intestine measuring 1–1.5 meters, except for the most distal part, which is the rectum and is not covered by serosa. It begins in the ileocecal valve and is divided into different portions, such as cecum with appendix, ascending right colon, hepatic flexure, transverse colon, splenic flexure, descending colon, and the S-shaped sigmoid colon, which is connected to the rectum. The cross section of the entire wall of the colon reveals a mucosal surface composed of a single layer of tall columnar epithelium and a lamina propria with thin muscularis mucosa. There is also a muscularis propria that has two different layers. The serosa and subserosa area almost entirely covers the organ except for the rectum at the perineal reflection.

In all of the organs described, the reader will become familiarized with questions in reference to the most common neoplasms originating in the gastrointestinal mucosa, the benign tumors, inflammatory diseases of the colon, as well as some of the gastrointestinal infections so prevalent in developing countries. Acute appendicitis, which is the most common surgical emergency and reflux esophagitis, peptic ulcer disease, which are so prevalent in today's gastrointestinal clinic consultations are also referenced.

Diseases of the liver and the most common pathology of the pancreas are also be discussed in this chapter.

Questions

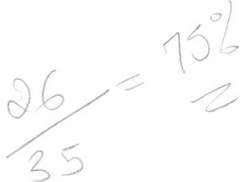

$$\frac{26}{35} = 75\%$$

DIRECTIONS (Questions 882 through 916): Each of the numbered items or incomplete statements in this section is followed by answers or by completions of the statement. Select the ONE lettered answer or completion that is BEST in each case.

882. In squamous cell carcinoma of the esophagus, which is the most important factor to consider in the prognosis?

   (A) degree of differentiation
   (B) duration of symptoms
   (C) method of treatment
   (D) stage at the time of diagnosis
   (E) type of symptoms

883. Which is the most frequent malignant neoplasm of the esophagus?

   (A) adenocarcinoma
   (B) leiomyoma
   (C) squamous cell carcinoma
   (D) squamous cell papilloma
   (E) mucoepidermoid carcinoma

884. Reflux of gastric juice into the esophagus may cause which of the following?

   (A) neoplasia in the lower esophagus
   (B) peptic ulceration in the lower esophagus
   (C) stenosis of the lower esophagus
   (D) replacement of squamous epithelium by columnar epithelium in the lower esophagus
   (E) all of the above

885. Which is the most common cause of death in Mallory–Weiss syndrome?

   (A) massive hemorrhage at the esophago-gastric junction
   (B) obstruction of the esophagus
   (C) perforation of a peptic ulcer in the upper stomach
   (D) rupture of a paraesophageal hernia
   (E) septicemia

886. Loss of ganglial cells in the myenteric plexus of the esophagus is known as which of the following?

   (A) achalasia
   (B) hiatal hernia
   (C) Mallory–Weiss syndrome
   (D) Plummer–Vinson syndrome
   (E) Zenker's diverticulum

887. Which is the most likely severe complication of Barrett's esophagus?

   (A) Mallory–Weiss syndrome
   (B) Plummer–Vinson syndrome
   (C) adenocarcinoma
   (D) leiomyosarcoma
   (E) squamous cell carcinoma

888. Duodenal and gastric ulcerations, intractable to usual modalities, are characteristic of which of the following?

   (A) alcohol abuse
   (B) aspirin effect
   (C) severe shock
   (D) Peutz–Jegher syndrome
   (E) Zollinger–Ellison syndrome

889. Infection with Helicobacter pylori is commonly associated with which of the following?

(A) chronic active gastritis
(B) congenital pyloric stenosis
(C) Crohn's disease
(D) Cushing's ulcer
(E) gastric stress ulcer of the stomach

890. Adenocarcinoma of the colon may be seen most frequently associated with which of the following?

(A) Crohn's disease
(B) diverticulosis
(C) hamartomatous polyps
(D) pseudomembranous colitis
(E) ulcerative colitis

891. Which of the following pathology conditions is most commonly associated with adenocarcinoma of the colon?

(A) tubular adenoma
(B) villous adenoma
(C) hyperplastic polyp
(D) juvenile retention polyp
(E) Peutz–Jegher polyp

892. A biopsy of a contracted and rigid wall stomach will show which of the following?

(A) multifocal carcinoids
(B) signet ring cell carcinoma (linitis plastica)
(C) chronic atrophic gastritis
(D) Menetrier's disease
(E) Zollinger–Ellison syndrome

893. Cytoplasmic granules that stain positive on immunoperoxidase technique for neuron specific enolase and chromogranin are characteristics of which of the following?

(A) glioblastoma
(B) lymphoma
(C) adenocarcinoma
(D) squamous cell carcinoma
(E) carcinoid tumor

894. What produces clinical symptoms of abdominal cramps, diarrhea, and bronchospasm in a carcinoid tumor?

(A) carcinoembryonic antigen
(B) chorionic gonadotropin
(C) serotonin
(D) alpha-fetoprotein
(E) alpha₁-antitrypsin

895. In comparing different prognostic features in a patient with gastric carcinoma, which is the most important?

(A) histologic subtype
(B) depth of invasion
(C) microscopic growth pattern
(D) anatomic site within the stomach
(E) extent of lymph node metastasis

896. Which is the most common malignant neoplasm that accounts for the highest number of deaths in the United States?

(A) gastric carcinoma
(B) pancreatic carcinoma
(C) colorectal carcinoma
(D) hepatocellular carcinoma
(E) small bowel carcinoma

897. Which of the following is a complication of diverticulosis of the colon?

(A) infection
(B) hemorrhage
(C) perforation
(D) obstruction
(E) all of the above

898. A patient previously treated with certain antibiotics develops an overgrowth of *Clostridium dificile*. Which is the most common pathological event that may follow?

(A) diverticulitis
(B) Crohn's disease
(C) ischemic colitis
(D) pseudomembranous colitis
(E) ulcerative colitis

899. Which inflammatory bowel disease is characterized by segmental involvement (skipped areas), transmural inflammation, fistulous tracts, and often granulomas?

   (A) diverticulitis
   (B) Crohn's disease
   (C) ischemic colitis
   (D) pseudomembranous colitis
   (E) ulcerative colitis

900. Which is the most frequent location of Crohn's disease?

   (A) ileum
   (B) rectum
   (C) ascending colon
   (D) colon and rectum
   (E) small bowel and colon

901. In celiac sprue, which is the most common etiologic factor?

   (A) vitamin D deficiency
   (B) hypersensitivity reaction to milk proteins
   (C) inability to digest milk sugars
   (D) hypersensitivity reaction to components of grains
   (E) overgrowth of normal intestinal bacterial flora

902. Which are the most common histological findings of Crohn's disease?

   (A) transmural hemorrhagic necrosis
   (B) macrophages in the mucosa
   (C) ulcers undermining the mucosa
   (D) transmural chronic inflammation often with granulomas
   (E) absence of ganglion cells in the muscularis propria

903. Histological examination of an acute appendix will display which of the following?

   (A) viral inclusion
   (B) infiltration by neoplasm
   (C) full-thickness (transmural) acute inflammation

   (D) granulomatous infiltration of the appendiceal tip
   (E) fibrous obliteration of the appendiceal mucosa

904. Why do cancers of the pancreas have a poor prognosis?

   (A) They destroy the islets of Langerhans.
   (B) They invade nerves in the early stage.
   (C) They are usually poorly differentiated.
   (D) They often cause migratory thrombophlebitis.
   (E) They remain clinically silent until unresectable.

905. Acute pancreatitis is histologically characterized by which of the following?

   (A) fibrosis
   (B) hemorrhage
   (C) acute inflammation
   (D) proteolytic destruction of parenchyma
   (E) mucus plugs in the pancreatic duct

906. The factor(s) that predispose to acute pancreatitis is/are which of the following?

   (A) hyperlipidemia
   (B) gallstones
   (C) alcohol abuse
   (D) viral infections
   (E) all of the above

907. What liver disease shows the greatest predominance in females?

   (A) hemochromatosis
   (B) alcoholic cirrhosis
   (C) Wilson's disease
   (D) primary biliary cirrhosis
   (E) primary sclerosing cholangitis

908. Cirrhosis predisposes to which of the following?

   (A) gynecomastia
   (B) hemorrhoids
   (C) splenomegaly
   (D) hepatocellular carcinoma
   (E) all of the above

909. What is the most common cause of micronodular cirrhosis in the United States?

    (A) hemochromatosis
    (B) alpha$_1$-antitrypsin deficiency
    (C) chronic alcohol consumption
    (D) hepatitis B virus infection
    (E) hepatitis C virus infection

910. Damage to the liver parenchyma in cases of viral hepatitis is secondary to which of the following?

    (A) direct cytopathic effect of the virus
    (B) cytotoxic effect of antibodies to viral antigens
    (C) cytotoxic T-cell reaction against infected hepatocytes
    (D) infection of vascular endothelium leading to vasculitis and ischemia
    (E) circulating immune complexes producing damage to both infected and noninfected hepatocytes

911. Which tumor is most commonly associated with high elevations of alpha-fetoprotein?

    (A) carcinoma of the head of the pancreas
    (B) choriocarcinoma
    (C) cirrhosis
    (D) hepatocellular carcinoma
    (E) massive hepatic necrosis

912. In a patient with hepatitis A, what are the chances of developing chronic hepatitis?

    (A) about 10%
    (B) about 30%
    (C) about 50%
    (D) almost 100%
    (E) 0%

913. Hepatic adenoma is most likely to happen in whom?

    (A) alcoholics
    (B) those with hepatitis D
    (C) those who use oral contraceptives
    (D) those with diets poor in fiber
    (E) diabetics

914. The most likely progression from chronic liver disease to cirrhosis is secondary to which of the following?

    (A) cytomegalovirus
    (B) hepatitis B
    (C) hepatitis C
    (D) hepatitis D
    (E) human immunodeficiency virus

915. Which is the most common pathological process to develop when a gallstone obstructs the cystic duct?

    (A) acute cholecystitis
    (B) ascending cholangitis
    (C) bile stasis in the liver
    (D) carcinoma of the gallbladder
    (E) cirrhosis of the liver

916. Colonic adenocarcinoma is one of the most frequent neoplasms that metastasize to the liver. Which results most commonly from these metastases?

    (A) complete occlusion of the large hepatic duct
    (B) cystic degeneration of the metastatic tumor
    (C) massive hemorrhage due to tumor necrosis
    (D) multiple nodules of similar sizes
    (E) rupture of the liver capsule

Answers and Explanations

882. **(D)** Carcinoma of the esophagus is a highly lethal tumor and is a disease of the elderly. Etiology factors include alcoholism, cigarette smoking, hot drinks, aflatoxins, and smoked fish. Seventy-five percent of the esophageal carcinomas are squamous cell carcinomas. Adenocarcinomas, in general, arise from Barrett's esophagitis. The overall prognosis is very poor, with 70% of the patients dying within 1 year after diagnosis of the disease. The most important parameter of the prognosis is the stage at the time of diagnosis, because over 80% 5-year survival is present in the tumors detected during the surveillance of Barrett's esophagus. *(Chandrasoma and Taylor, pp. 568–570)*

883. **(C)** Refer to Answer 882. *(Chandrasoma and Taylor, pp. 568–570)*

884. **(E)** Reflux of gastric juice into the lower esophagus occurs even in normal individuals without producing many symptoms. However, in some patients, they become symptomatic, and the prolonged exposure to the acidity of the gastric fluid to the mucosa in excess amounts can histologically produce all of the changes listed in the answers. *(Chandrasoma and Taylor, pp. 563–565)*

885. **(A)** Mallory–Weiss syndrome is pathologically characterized by a longitudinal tear of the mucosa of the esophagus in the lower third. In general, it is induced by prolonged vomiting, and is common in alcoholics. Severe hemorrhage with hematemesis can cause death. *(Chandrasoma and Taylor, p. 567)*

886. **(A)** Achalasia is a disease of the esophagus in which there is a loss of ganglial cells in the myenteric plexus throughout the esophageal wall. The lack of propulsive peristaltic waves without proper relaxation of the cardiac sphincter creates a dilated and tortuous esophagus. Hiatal hernia is a herniation of part of the stomach through the diaphragmatic hiatus. For Mallory–Weiss syndrome, please refer to Answer 885. Plummer–Vinson syndrome consists of dysphagia that occurs in patients with severe iron deficiency anemia. The dysphagia results from atrophy of the pharyngeal mucosa and web-like mucosal folds are present in the upper esophagus in some patients. Zenker's diverticulum is an out-pouching of the lumen of the esophagus in which the epithelial sac herniates through a weakened defective muscle wall of the esophagus. *(Chandrasoma and Taylor, pp. 565–567)*

887. **(C)** Barrett's esophagus is defined as intestinal metaplasia of the normal nonkeratinizing squamous epithelium of the esophagus, characterized by the presence of goblet cells. Malignant tumors that originate in the Barrett's esophagus are adenocarcinomas. Dysplastic changes on the mucosa of the Barrett's esophagus are considered precancerous lesions. None of the other answers listed is considered a complication of Barrett's esophagus. *(Chandrasoma and Taylor, p. 564)*

888. **(E)** The multiple endocrine neoplasia (MEN) with multiple endocrine adenoma syndromes are characterized by the familiar occurrence of multiple endocrine neoplasms. In type I, it consists of pituitary adenoma, parathyroid hyperplasia or adenoma, pancreatic islet cell neoplasm, including gastricnoma. Multiple peptic ulcerations occur in these patients probably related to gastrin production (Zollinger–Ellison syndrome). (*Cotran et al., p. 927*)

889. **(A)** H. pylori is a small, rather curved rod organism that is present in the surface mucus layer that covers the epithelium of the gastric glandular elements. It can be seen in routine H&E sections, without special stains. It is easily found in the areas where there is chronic active (neutrophils) inflammatory changes. Helicobacter gastritis is associated with chronic duodenal ulcer in almost 100% of the cases. An increase in gastric adenocarcinoma and malignant lymphomas, has been noted with H. pylori infection. (*Chandrasoma and Taylor, pp. 576–577*)

890. **(E)** Ulcerative colitis is an inflammatory disease of uncertain etiology and has a chronic relapsing course. As a complication of ulcerative colitis, the patients have a higher chance to develop colon carcinoma, in approximately 10% of the cases. Carcinomas, in general, are originated in epithelial dysplasia. The carcinomas originating in ulcerative colitis are known to be poorly differentiated, deeply infiltrating into the muscularis, they are aggressive and multiple, with poor prognosis. (*Chandrasoma and Taylor, pp. 614–616*)

891. **(B)** Villous adenomas are approximately 10% of the colonic adenomas. Most of the villous adenomas are soft and flat-surfaced. Histologically, they are composed of a proliferation of colonic epithelial cells organized into papillary projections. Thirty to seventy percent of the villous adenomas harbor a focal area of carcinoma. In tubular adenomas, although considered a premalignant lesion, only 3–5% are considered to be able to be transformed into an infiltrating carcinoma. Hyperplastic polyps are controversial, but most authorities do not believe that they are preneoplastic lesions. In Peutz–Jegher polyp, there is only a slight increased risk in carcinoma. (*Chandrasoma and Taylor, pp. 620–622*)

892. **(B)** Linitis plastica or leather-bottle stomach is the name given to a diffusely infiltrating adeno-

carcinoma that produces thickening and contracted gastric wall. The mucosa shows flattened folds and in general, is not ulcerated. Chronic atrophic gastritis may have an atrophic folds of the mucosa, but they do not show the rigidity of the wall. Menetrier's disease is characterized by thickening and increase in the amount of rugal folds. Multifocal carcinoids and Zollinger–Ellison syndrome do not show the characteristics described for the linitis plastica. (*Chandrasoma and Taylor, p. 582*)

893. **(E)** Carcinoid tumors originate in the neuroendocrine cells present throughout the gastrointestinal tract. The appendix is most frequently involved, to be followed by the ileum. On the histological examination, the carcinoids are composed of uniform, round cells that are formed in small nests and cords and growing without encapsulation. Special stains can be performed to demonstrate the neurosecretory granules in the cytoplasm such as, chromogranin, neuron specific enolase or, can also be detected by electron microscopy. Lymphomas, glioblastoma, and adenocarcinoma, as well as squamous cell carcinoma do not contain neurosecretory granules in the cytoplasm. (*Chandrasoma and Taylor, p. 627*)

894. **(C)** Carcinoid tumors can present with a carcinoid syndrome, which results from release of serotonin into the blood. However, in most of the carcinoid tumors of the GI tract, serotonin, although released to the blood, does not produce carcinoid syndrome, because it is inactivated in the liver. Only when the carcinoids have metastasized to the liver, will the serotonin be produced by the hepatic metastasis and reach the systemic circulation. Carcinoid syndrome is clinically manifested by abdominal cramps, diarrhea, bronchospasm, and dilatation of the vessels of the skin, causing episodic redness of the face and other parts of the body. (*Chandrasoma and Taylor, p. 628*)

895. **(B)** The diagnosis of gastric carcinoma is established by endoscopy with biopsy. This sample will allow us to diagnose the cell type and then radiologic changes, as well as computerized tomography, will allow us to provide informa-

tion about the extent of surgical resectability. The prognosis depends almost entirely on the depth of invasion of the neoplasm. (*Chandrasoma and Taylor, pp. 582–583*)

896. **(C)** Colorectal carcinoma is second only to lung cancer as a cause of death in the United States. The other answers listed for this question; although for some of them, the prognosis is worse than colorectal carcinoma, the incidence is much lower to account for the same number of deaths. (*Chandrasoma and Taylor, pp. 622–623*)

897. **(E)** Colonic diverticulosis is a very common disease, and it is estimated that 50% of the patients over the age of 60 years have diverticulosis. The sigmoid colon is the most common area involved. Many cases of sigmoid colon diverticulosis are asymptomatic, but complications such as, infection, hemorrhage, perforation, and obstruction can be frequently seen. (*Chandrasoma and Taylor, pp. 598–599*)

898. **(D)** Treatment of the infections with clindamycin, ampicillin, tetracyclin, or other antibiotics alter the bacterial flora of the colon and permits the overgrowth of *Clostridium dificile*. The powerful exotoxin of this bacteria produces effects on the mucosal epithelium of the colon that results in pseudomembranous enterocolitis. Patchy areas of the mucosa are necrotic, and the exudate remains attached to the surface. The other answers listed in this question are not related to *Clostridium dificile* toxin. (*Chandrasoma and Taylor, pp. 603–604*)

899. **(B)** Crohn's disease is a chronic inflammatory disorder of unknown etiology that has the potential to involve the different portions of the GI tract from the mouth to the anus. It is characterized by a transmural inflammation with skipped areas in which the intestinal wall is not affected. Frequently, the presence of non-caseating epithelioid granulomas is seen. Ischemic colitis histologically shows, in the acute phase, coagulation necrosis of the intestine. When chronic, the presence of granulation tissue with acute and chronic inflammation is seen, accompanied by fibrosis of the submucosa. Pseudomembranous colitis has

been described in the previous question, and ulcerative colitis shows no transmural inflammation or granulomas. Diverticulitis is an inflammation of the diverticulum and contains no histological resemblance with Crohn's disease. (*Chandrasoma and Taylor, pp. 610–611*)

900. **(A)** The most common site of involvement by Crohn's disease is the ileum. Although Crohn's disease can involve the entire GI tract, the most characteristic location is in this part of the small intestine. (*Chandrasoma and Taylor, pp. 610–612*)

901. **(D)** Celiac disease, which is caused by a high immunologic hypersensitivity, most often affects and is restricted to the small intestinal mucosa. Celiac disease is caused by the action of acidic peptides contained in the wheat protein gluten and affecting the intestinal mucosa. The exact mechanism of the damage is not certain. (*Chandrasoma and Taylor, p. 590*)

902. **(D)** Refer to Answer 899. (*Chandrasoma and Taylor, pp. 610–611*)

903. **(C)** Acute appendicitis, which is the most common surgical emergency, occurs at any age, with peak incidence in young adulthood. Inflammation of the appendix is preceded by obstruction of the appendiceal lumen by a fecalith, by submucosal lymphoid hyperplasia, or another cause. The pathogens include *E. coli* and *Streptococcus faecalis*. Histological examination on microscopy reveals transmural acute inflammatory changes of the entire appendix, which is infiltrated by polymorphonuclear cells. In early cases of acute appendicitis, only an erosion of the surface of the mucosa is present with abundant polymorphonuclear cells. (*Chandrasoma and Taylor, p. 599*)

904. **(E)** Carcinoma of the pancreas is referred to adenocarcinoma that originates in the ductal system of the pancreatic tissue. The etiology is unknown; however, some causes such as cigarette smoking, have a fivefold increase in incidences of pancreatic carcinoma. Microscopically, it is is characterized by a well-differentiated adenocarcinoma, which are associated with marked desmoplastic reaction. When the

carcinoma is located on the head of the pancreas, the clinical symptomatology appears early, and in general, the first symptom is obstructive jaundice. When located on other portions of the pancreas, it remains silent, and most of the time, the evidence of the carcinoma is manifested for the appearance of metastasis, often to the liver. (*Chandrasoma and Taylor, pp. 677–678*)

905. **(D)** Acute pancreatitis is a syndrome resulting from the permeation of activated pancreatic digestive enzymes from the ductal system of the pancreas into the parenchyma. It is associated with an extensive destruction of the peripancreatic tissue and acute inflammation. There is a widespread necrosis of the tissues subject to the effect of the extravasated pancreatic enzymes. (*Chandrasoma and Taylor pp. 672–673*)

906. **(E)** Many factors have been associated with acute pancreatitis, including biliary tract calculi, alcoholism, hypercalcemia, and hyperlipidemia, as well as viral infections. (*Chandrasoma and Taylor, pp. 672–673*)

907. **(D)** Primary biliary cirrhosis, which is a chronic progressive disease of the liver characterized by destruction (nonsuppurative) of the intrahepatic bile ducts with scarring and progression to cirrhosis and liver failure. Lymphocytes and plasma cells surround and destroy the walls of the bile ducts. Granulomas are present in up to 30% of the cases. The terminal phase shows disappearance of bile ducts and portal fibrosis. Middle-aged women are mostly affected, with a ratio of 6:1. (*Chandrasoma and Taylor, p. 653*)

908. **(E)** Cirrhosis of the liver can have variegated etiologic factors, but it is characterized by extensive fibrosis of the portal triads and involving also the central veins, with a greater or lesser degree of activity and the presence of regenerative nodules. Scarring of the liver is accompanied by a constellation of clinical features related to chronic liver failure, as well as portal hypertension. Hemorrhoids, splenomegaly, hepatocellular carcinoma, and gynecomastia are some of the common

effects of liver failure or portal hypertension. (*Chandrasoma and Taylor, pp. 653–656*)

909. **(C)** Alcohol is the most frequent cause of cirrhosis in the United States. Typically, it shows extensive scarring of the liver parenchyma with micronodular regeneration of the hepatocytes. Biopsy shows that there is an extensive replacing of the liver parenchyma with fibrous tissue, with micronodular formation. Also, Mallory bodies, as well as different degrees of fatty metamorphosis can be present in alcoholic cirrhosis. (*Chandrasoma and Taylor, p. 655*)

910. **(C)** All the hepatitis viruses replicate within the hepatocytes and cause damage. This damage is either caused as a direct effect of the virus or as an immunologic response against the cell bearing the viral antigens that will be the T-cells. (*Chandrasoma and Taylor, p. 644*)

911. **(D)** Hepatocellular carcinoma often secretes alphafetoprotein into the blood. Elevated serum levels of alphafetoprotein is present in 90% of the patients with hepatocellular carcinoma. The alphafetoprotein could be slightly elevated in cases of hepatitis and cirrhosis, as well as in germ cell neoplasms of the gonads. However, they do not reach the level of a hepatocellular carcinoma. Immunohistochemical stains can be done on the biopsy to show the presence of alphafetoprotein in the neoplastic cells. (*Chandrasoma and Taylor, p. 60*)

912. **(E)** Hepatitis A that is caused by an RNA enterovirus is usually transmitted via the fecal–oral route with a short incubation period of 2–6 weeks. Hepatitis A is usually a mild acute illness with recovery in a few weeks. This type of hepatitis A does not progress to chronic hepatitis or cirrhosis and there are no chronic carriers of this disease. (*Chandrasoma and Taylor, p. 641*)

913. **(C)** Hepatocellular adenoma is a rare benign tumor that occurs mainly in women taking oral contraceptives and sometimes in athletes on anabolic steroids. On light microscopy, the benign hepatocytes are arranged in thick cords. There is not evidence of portal tracks. Hemor-

rhage and infarctions are common complications. *(Rubin and Farber, pp. 658–659)*

914. **(C)** Hepatitis C, which is caused by a single-stranded RNA virus, is responsible for over 90% of the cases of hepatitis associated with transfusion of blood and blood products in the United States. The disease also occurs in drug abusers and transplant recipients, as well as renal dialysis patients. It is associated with a higher incidence of chronic hepatitis, which occurs in 50% of those affected and cirrhosis complicates 20%. *(Chandrasoma and Taylor, p. 643)*

915. **(A)** Acute cholecystitis, in 80% of the cases, is caused by an obstruction of the cystic duct by a gallstone. Once obstructed, the gallbladder becomes susceptible to infection by bacteria. *(Chandrasoma and Taylor, p. 666)*

916. **(D)** Metastatic lesions to the liver account for the majority of malignant neoplasms involving the organ. The most common tumors that metastasize to the liver are those from the gastrointestinal tract, breast, and lung, as well as malignant melanoma. Grossly, the nodules of metastatic carcinoma often show central necrosis, and, although the size may vary, for the most part, many nodules are about the same size. *(Chandrasoma and Taylor, p. 662)*

REFERENCES

Chandrasoma P, Taylor CR. *Concise Pathology,* 3rd ed. Norwalk, CT: Appleton & Lange, 1998.

Cotran RS, Kumar V, Robbins SL. *Robbins Pathologic Basis of Disease,* 6th ed, Philadelphia: Saunders, 1999.

Rubin E, Farber JL. *Pathology,* Philadelphia: Lippincott, 1999.

CHAPTER 12

Male Genital Tract and Kidney

The renal pelvis, ureters, bladder, and urethra are covered by a special form of epithelium that is transitional (three to five layers thick) and could even be thicker in part of the urinary bladder. These pseudostratified cells are covered by special cells on the surface called "umbrella cells." The ureter, as well as the urinary bladder, contain layers of smooth muscle, which in the urinary bladder is well-defined and thicker. The ureters, urinary bladder, and urethra can show congenital abnormalities, inflammation, and tumors.

The prostate, which is a retroperitoneal organ surrounding the neck of the urinary bladder and the urethra, is also the site of numerous pathological processes, the most common being, benign prostatic enlargement (prostatic hypertrophy or hyperplasia); inflammatory processes and last, malignant neoplasm (adenocarcinoma), which is the most common form of cancer in men. Several etiologic factors, have been identified, such as, age, race, family history, hormonal levels, and environmental influence. Most cases are adenocarcinomas graded following the Gleason score. It is calculated by evaluating two different areas of the prostate, the least differentiated and the most differentiated. The values are added, and a score is assigned from 2 to 10.

In the testicles, congenital abnormalities, inflammatory processes, and neoplasms must be considered. Such inflammatory processes as mumps, tuberculosis, syphilis, and nonspecific orchitis have been described.

Neoplasms that involve the testicles are related to the germ cells. The WHO classification is based on the fact that most testicular tumors originate in intratubular testicular germ cells. The germ cell tumors are divided in seminoma, with a spermacytic variant, embryonal carcinoma, yolk sac tumor, polyembryoma, choriocarcinoma, and teratomas were mature or immature.

Special consideration should be given to tumors showing more than one histologic pattern, such as embryonal cell carcinoma, plus teratoma, or choriocarcinoma. The second type of tumors originating in the testicles are the sex cord stromal tumors, such as Leydig cell, Sertoli cell, and the granulosa cell tumors.

DISEASES OF THE KIDNEY

The specific structural and functional unit of the kidney is the nephron. The nephron consists of the renal corpuscle (glomerulus capsule) connected to an elongated, tubular component composed of the proximal tubules, the thin limbs, and the distal convoluted tubules. The three major anatomical structures of the kidney are: (a) blood vessels, which handle 25% of the cardiac output, about one liter per minute; (b) the glomeruli, which filter the blood and concentrate the ultrafiltrate; (c) the tubules, which modify the filtrate; and (d) the interstitium, which concentrates the urine.

Glomerular diseases can be divided in two groups; the primary glomerular diseases and the secondary glomerular diseases, in which a systemic illness is affecting the glomeruli. Injury of the glomerulus can produce only limited responses. Immune mechanisms underlie the majority of the primary glomerular diseases, as well as some of the secondary ones. Many different syndromes can be distinguished in the kidney diseases, such as nephrotic syndrome, nephritic syndrome, asymptomatic hematuria proteinuria, acute and chronic renal failure, renal tubular defects, urinary tract infections, and nephrolithiasis.

Tumors of the kidney, the renal pelvis, ureters, and urinary bladder are not uncommon. Benign tumors of the urothelial lining at different levels are rare, and for papillary adenoma, a strict histological criteria must be followed. On benign renal cell tumors, we emphasize the oncocytomas, the angiomyolipoma, which has been associated in 25–50% of cases with tuberous sclerosis (TS). Among malignant neoplasms, renal cell carcinoma is the most frequent, and it comprises 80–90% of all malignant tumors of the kidney. These tumors can be sporadic or hereditary (although some are dominant) and seen in association with contributory factors as cigarette smoking, obesity, hypertension, unopposed estrogen therapy, and occupational exposure to petroleum products, and heavy metal or asbestos. The most common form of renal cell carcinoma is the clear cell type, to be followed by a papillary carcinoma and chromophobe carcinoma. Grading and staging of these tumors is very important for the prognosis.

Wilms' tumor (nephroblastoma) is the most common renal tumor in children, and it can be associated with WAGR syndrome (W–Wilms' tumor; A–*aniridia*; G–*genital* abnormalities; R–mental *retardation*).

The urinary bladder can exhibit pathology related to inflammation (cystitis) of different types of microorganisms that may be introduced into the urinary bladder, most commonly on the ascending route. The tumors of the urinary tract (renal caliceals, pelvis, ureters, bladder, and urethra), the most common being the transitional cell carcinoma of the urinary bladder. Cytogenic and molecular alterations of chromosome 9 deletion are often present. Different grades have been described with different grades of aggressiveness, from grade I to grade III.

Questions

DIRECTIONS (Questions 917 through 920): Each of the numbered items or incomplete statements in this section is followed by answers or by completions of the statement. Select the ONE lettered answer or completion that is BEST in each case.

917. Crescents are produced by which of the following?

(A) capillary loops
(B) endothelial cells
(C) mesangial cells
(D) parietal epithelial cells
(E) tubules

918. Where are immune complexes in early acute proliferative glomerulonephritis located?

(A) Bowman's capsule
(B) mesangium
(C) subendothelial
(D) subepithelial area "humps"
(E) tubular basement membrane

919. A 3-year-old girl developed generalized edema. A urine examination revealed heavy proteinuria (5 g/24 h). What is the most likely diagnosis?

(A) acute diffuse proliferative glomerulonephritis
(B) membranoproliferative glomerulonephritis
(C) membranous glomerulonephritis
(D) minimal change disease (lipoid nephrosis)
(E) rapidly progressive glomerulonephritis

920. What characterizes analgesic nephritis?

(A) acute tubular necrosis
(B) chronic interstitial inflammation with papillary necrosis
(C) diffuse and nodular glomerulosclerosis
(D) microabscesses
(E) proliferation of vascular endothelium

DIRECTIONS (Questions 921 through 930): The group of items in this section consists of a list of lettered options followed by a set of numbered words or phrases. For each numbered word or phrase, select the ONE lettered option that is most closely associated with it. Each lettered option may be selected once, more than once, or not at all.

Questions 921 through 925

(A) acute poststreptococcal glomerulonephritis
(B) chronic glomerulonephritis
(C) diabetic glomerulopathy
(D) membranous glomerulonephritis
(E) minimal change disease (lipoid nephrosis)

921. Spikes projecting from the glomerular basement membrane

922. Electrodense deposits or epithelial side of the membrane (humps)

923. Kimmelstiel–Wilson disease

924. Diffuse loss of foot processes

925. End-stage pool of glomerular disease from a number of glomerulonephritides

Questions 926 through 930

(A) acute pyelonephritis

(B) crescentic (rapidly progressive) glomerulonephritis

(C) membranous glomerulonephritis

(D) minimal change disease (lipoid nephrosis)

(E) poststreptococcal glomerulonephritis

926. Crescents are always present.

927. ASO (antistreptolysin-O) titers are elevated.

928. Normal glomeruli appear on light microscopy.

929. What is a disease affecting tubules, tubular interstitium, and renal pelvis?

930. What is the major cause of nephrotic syndrome in adults?

DIRECTIONS (Questions 931 through 941): Each of the numbered items or incomplete statements in this section is followed by answers or by completions of the statement. Select the ONE lettered answer or completion that is BEST in each case.

931. A person with extensive burns developed shock and acute renal failure. Which would be the most probable histologic changes in the kidney?

(A) crescents in most glomeruli

(B) fibrinoid necrosis of the arterioles and hyperplastic arteriolosclerosis

(C) multiple infarctions

(D) patchy necrosis of the proximal tubular epithelium

(E) pus within tubules and abscesses in the interstitium

932. What is the most common organism that causes chronic pyelonephritis?

(A) *Escherichia coli*

(B) hepatitis B virus

(C) human papilloma virus

(D) *Staphylococcus aureus*

(E) *Streptococcus pyogenes*

933. What is the most common malignant tumor associated with aniridia, genital anomalies, and mental retardation?

(A) embryonal rhabdomyosarcoma of the urinary bladder

(B) Ewing's tumor

(C) neuroblastoma

(D) sarcomatoid renal cell carcinoma

(E) Wilms's tumor

934. Patients with von Hippel–Lindau disease are at a higher risk to develop which of the following?

(A) hepatocellular carcinoma

(B) malignant melanoma

(C) renal cell carcinoma

(D) transitional cell carcinoma of the urinary bladder

(E) Wilms's tumor (nephroblastoma)

935. In IgA nephropathy (Berger's disease), electron dense deposits are found most prominently in which of the following?

(A) mesangium

(B) tubular basement membranes

(C) glomerular capillary basement membranes

(D) walls of the small veins

(E) walls of the arterioles and small arteries

936. Which is the most important prognostic factor for carcinoma of the urinary bladder?

(A) associated urothelial hyperplasia

(B) the depth of invasion

(C) the histologic type of cancer

(D) the location within the bladder

(E) the presence of urachal remnants

937. A-60-year old male developed painless hematuria, and the CT scan with contrast showed a 7-cm mass on the lower pole of the right kidney. What does this lesion most likely represent?

(A) medullary fibroma

(B) neuroblastoma

(C) renal cell carcinoma

(D) transitional cell carcinoma

(E) Wilms's tumor

938. Which of the following is the most common type of germ cell tumor?

(A) choriocarcinoma

(B) embryonal carcinoma

(C) polyembryoma

(D) seminoma

(E) yolk sac tumor

939. Which is a testicular tumor characterized by hemorrhage, necrosis, and composed of cytotrophoblastic and syncytiotrophoblastic cells?

(A) choriocarcinoma

(B) embryonal carcinoma

(C) seminoma

(D) teratoma

(E) yolk sac tumor

940. Which of the following tumors is more prevalent in infants and children?

(A) yolk sac tumor

(B) teratoma

(C) seminoma

(D) polyembryoma

(E) choriocarcinoma

941. Tumors that on histologic evaluation reveal more than one germ layer are which of the following?

(A) choriocarcinoma

(B) polyembryoma

(C) seminoma

(D) teratoma

(E) yolk sac tumor

DIRECTIONS (Questions 942 through 946): The group of items in this section consists of lettered options followed by a set of numbered words or phrases. For each numbered word or phrase, select the ONE lettered option that is most closely associated with it. Each lettered option may be selected once, more than once, or not at all.

(A) free PSA

(B) grading of prostatic carcinoma

(C) not considered a premalignant lesion

(D) osteoblastic metastasis

(E) presumptive precursor of prostatic carcinoma

942. Benign prostatic hyperplasia

943. Prostatic intraepithelial neoplasia (PIN)

944. Important in prognosis

945. Lower in men with prostatic cancer

946. Virtually diagnostic of prostate cancer

Answers and Explanations

917. **(D)** Crescents are a proliferation of parietal epithelial cells lining the Bowman's capsule in response to significant glomerular tuft injury allowing substances into the Bowman urinary space. This stimulates further proliferation of the cells. The biological behavior of the crescents allows the epithelial cell growth to proliferate over the course of days and obliterate the entire glomeruli. On rare occasions, it can resolve in a period of weeks or months, or the fibroepithelial structures may become fibrotic and hyalinized. *(Cotran et al., p. 943)*

918. **(D)** Acute proliferative glomerulonephritis, also so-called "post-streptococcal glomerulonephritis," is a disease characterized by antigen deposition of IgG and C3 in the subepithelial area of the basement membrane. These deposits are discrete and dense, and are called "humps." Although rare depositions of IgG and C3 are present in the subendothelial and mesangial area, they are not as frequent. *(Cotran et al., pp. 949–951)*

919. **(D)** In minimal change disease (lipoid nephrosis), classic clinical findings secondary to glomerular injury are massive proteinuria, hypoalbuminemia, peripheral edema, and hyperlipidemia. Lipoid nephrosis is of unknown etiology and pathogenesis. Epidemiologically, it is seen in children, most between the ages of 1–4 years. The clinical picture gives the pure nephrotic syndrome, which is selective proteinuria in over 90% of the cases (only albumin is lost in the urine). Blood pressure generally remains normal, and urine sediment is free of RBCs or WBCs. Of the other selections listed, membranous glomerulonephritis occurs in adults, and rapidly progressive glomerulonephritis and acute diffuse proliferative glomerulonephritis have different symptomatologies and clinical presentations. *(Cotran et al., pp. 954–956)*

920. **(B)** Analgesic abuse nephropathy is characterized histologically by chronic tubular interstitial nephritis accompanied by renal papillary necrosis. In general, such analgesics as acetaminophen and aspirin or in other forms are taken in combination. The consumption of one of them alone rarely produces analgesic abuse nephropathy. The papillary necrosis is induced by a combination of factors of toxic effect, as well as ischemic injury. Grossly, the papillae show extensive coagulation necrosis and occasional calcifications. Analgesic nephritis is not a suppurative process, therefore, it does not produce microabscesses or vascular endothelial proliferation. Acute tubular necrosis is an entirely different entity and is related to another cause, as is diffuse nodular sclerosis, which is basically a glomerulopathy. *(Cotran et al., pp. 978–980)*

921. **(D)** Membranous glomerulonephritis, which is the most common cause of nephrotic syndrome in adults, is histologically characterized by a diffuse thickening of the glomerular capillary wall. On electron microscopy studies, this diffuse thickening of the glomerular capillary wall is translated by irregular dense deposits between the basement membrane and the overlying epithelial cells. On light microscopy and with appropriate silver stains, it is possible to see the projections of the basement membrane forming characteristic spikes. *(Cotran et al., pp. 923–924, 949–964)*

922. (A) Characteristic changes in poststreptococcal glomerulonephritis show a rather enlarged, hypercellular glomeruli, and hypercellularity is secondary to inflammatory cells, endothelial and mesangial cell proliferation. On electron microscopic studies, this disease is characterized by large electron dense deposits on the subepithelial area. This deposit is called "humps." *(Cotran et al., pp. 923–924, 949–964)*

923. (C) Diabetic glomerulopathy includes histological such changes as capillary basement membrane thickening (diabetic microangiopathy). Diffuse glomerulosclerosis is an increase in mesangial matrix along with mesangial cell proliferation. Nodular glomerulosclerosis is described as nodular deposits of lamelated matrix within the mesangial core. This has been called Kimmelstiel–Wilson disease, which is characteristic but not pathognomonic of diabetic nephropathy. *(Cotran et al., pp. 923–924, 949–964)*

924. (E) In minimal change disease (lipoid nephrosis), the characteristic light microscopy is negative. On electron microscopy, however, a diffuse loss of foot processes is present with the cause or consequence proteinuria. *(Cotran et al., pp. 923–924, 949–964)*

925. (B) Chronic glomerulonephritis is considered a pathological entity in which many end-stage glomerular diseases are included. However, because there are cases of chronic glomerulonephritis in which no etiology could be found, this entity is still considered to be a separate entity. Such diseases as poststreptococcal glomerulonephritis, rapidly progressive glomerulonephritis, membranous glomerulonephritis, focal glomerulosclerosis, membranous proliferative glomerulonephritis, and IgA nephropathy are some of the most common contributors to the pool of chronic glomerulonephritis. *(Cotran et al., pp. 923–924, 949–964)*

926. (B) In rapidly progressive (crescentic) glomerulonephritis, light microscopy characterizes the presence of crescents in the majority of glomeruli. These crescents, which are formed by a proliferation of the parietal epithelial cells, line Bowman's capsule. The histology characteristic of these crescents that vary according to age, are rarely resolved, and frequently obliterate the whole glomeruli forming a hyaline structure. Sometimes they are accompanied by inflammatory cells. *(Cotran et al., pp. 949–956, 974–975)*

927. (E) Acute proliferative (streptococcal) glomerulonephritis appears in young children after 1–4 weeks of the streptococcal infection of the throat or another part of the body. This type of nephritis is typically an immunologically mediated disease in which the latent period between infection and development of nephritis is compatible with the build up of antibodies. Elevated titers of ASO are found in the blood of these individuals. *(Cotran et al., pp. 949–956, 974–975)*

928. (D) Minimal change disease (lipoid nephrosis) is the most frequent cause of nephrotic syndrome in children between the ages of 2–6 years of age. It is characterized by normal light microscopy. On electron microscopy, the findings are related with proteinuria, which is characterized by fusion of the foot processes. The disease dramatically responds to corticosteroid therapy, and the patient sometimes becomes corticosteroid dependent. Prognosis is excellent. *(Cotran et al., pp. 949–956, 974–975)*

929. (A) Acute pyelonephritis is the disease that affects the tubules, interstitium, and renal pelvis and is characterized by suppurative inflammation and occasional tubular necrosis. On light microscopy and in the early stage, there is an infiltration of polymorphonuclear cells, which is limited to interstitial tissue. This eventually will spread into the tubules as well as the renal pelvis. In most cases, it is an ascending infection, although hematogenous spread is also possible. Etiology in 95% of the cases is a single organism and usually a gram-negative bacilli (*E. coli*). In general, the hematogenous infection is by *Staphylococcus aureus, salmonella,* or *pseudomonas*. This disease is more commonly seen in females because of a short urethra, pregnancy, and obstructions or incomplete voiding for different anatomic or neurologic abnormalities. *(Cotran et al., pp. 949–956, 974–975)*

930. **(C)** Membranous glomerulonephritis is the most common cause of nephrotic syndrome in adults. On light microscopy, there is a diffuse thickening of the glomerular capillary wall that could more readily be appreciated with such special stains as PAS or silver stains. On electron microscopy, the glomerular basement membrane is irregularly thickened with spikes that protrude toward the uriniferous space. This irregular thickening is caused by deposition of electron-dense immune complexes. *(Cotran et al., pp. 949–956, 974–975)*

931. **(D)** Acute tubular necrosis (ATN) is a clinico-pathologic entity characterized morphologically by destruction of tubular epithelium and clinically by acute renal failure. ATN is the most common cause of acute renal failure. ATN could be divided into ischemic, in which the causes are shock, burns, and crush injury, and toxic tubular necrosis, caused by heavy metals, drugs, and organic solvents. The clinical course has an initial phase followed by a maintenance phase in which there is a decrease in urine output (oliguria) elevated BUN, hyperkalemia, and metabolic acidosis. This is followed by a recovery phase. *(Cotran et al., pp. 969–970)*

932. **(A)** Chronic pyelonephritis is damage of the pelvic calyces and tubules associated with scarring and secondary to inflammation caused by *Escherichia coli.* Histologically, there is interstitial fibrosis with or without accompanying chronic inflammation. In scar zones, some tubules disappear, and others are atrophic. Infiltrates, when present, contain lymphocyte macrophages and some plasma cells. The possibility of *Streptococcus pyogenes* or *Staphylococcus aureus* is much lower, and in general, hematogenous spread. Hepatitis B virus and human papilloma virus do not produce chronic pyelonephritis. *(Cotran et al., pp. 975–976)*

933. **(E)** Wilms' tumor is the most common renal tumor in children. Wilms' tumor can occur either sporadically or in children with congenital syndromes, and an increase in incidence is seen in WAGR syndrome (Wilms' tumor, *a*niridia, *g*enital anomalies, and mental *r*etardation). Ten percent of the cases show involvement of the opposite kidney. Microscopically, Wilms' tumor is composed of blastemic components, primitive glomeruli, tubules, and mesenchymal cells. Ewing's tumor occurs mostly in the bones. Neuroblastoma in the retroperitoneum and adrenal gland and sarcomatoid renal cell carcinoma, as well as embryonal rhabdomyosarcoma are rare. *(Cotran et al., pp. 487–489)*

934. **(C)** Renal cell carcinoma comprises 80–90% of all the malignant tumors of the kidney and 1–3% of all cancers in adults. Renal cell carcinoma occurs predominantly in the sixth to seventh decade of life. The epidemiologic factors, are: cigarette smoking, obesity, hypertension, and unopposed estrogen therapy; and occupational exposure to petroleum products, heavy metals, or asbestos. Most renal cell carcinomas are sporadic and usually solitary. There are three forms of hereditary renal cell carcinoma; one associated with Von Hippel–Lindau syndrome. The VHL gene in 80% of clear cell carcinomas shows loss of mutation or hypermethylation of the VHL gene. All other types of malignancies listed are not associated with Von Hippel–Lindau disease. *(Cotran et al., pp. 991–992)*

935. **(A)** IgA nephropathy was described in 1968 and is primarily characterized by mesangial proliferative changes seen in light microscopy as a diffuse mesangial deposit of IgA by immunofluorescence. It is the most common type of glomerulonephritis worldwide. On electron microscopy, it is possible to demonstrate mesangial deposits on all of the glomeruli, indicating that this lesion is diffuse, not focal. Occasionally, small subendothelial deposits may be found. The pattern of immunofluorescence parallels the distribution of deposits seen by electron microscopy. There is a strong diffuse mesangial reactivity to IgA that can be extended into the capillary loops. *(Cotran et al., pp. 961–962)*

936. (B) Tumors of the urinary bladder have a 2% incidence of all of malignant tumors, and 80% of the patients are between the ages of 50–80 years. The etiologic factors are occupational exposure to dye, rubber, leather, paint, organic chemicals, and cigarette smoking. Chromosome 9 deletions are frequently present in superficial urinary carcinomas. Many invasive urothelial carcinomas show deletion of 17p including the region of p53. Two microscopic patterns are described as flat and papillary. Different grades have been used for describing the degree of anaplasia. The most important and effective evaluation as a prognostic factor of the urinary bladder is the depth of invasion. *(Cotran et al., pp. 1003–1006)*

937. (C) The most important and frequent cause painless hematuria is renal cell carcinoma. This symptom is usually associated with palpable mass on the flank as well as the costovertebral pain. Occasionally, renal cell carcinomas are associated with paraneoplastic syndromes, which include polycythemia, hypercalcemia, hypertension, feminization or masculinization, Cushing's syndrome, and so forth. The other answers listed are mostly seen in children. Transitional cell carcinoma is more rare than renal cell carcinoma, and medullary fibroma is a benign tumor. *(Cotran et al., pp. 992–993)*

938. (D) Seminoma is the most common type of germ cell tumor and histologically can be divided into the spermatocytic type, the classic variant, and the anaplastic seminoma, the most common being the classic form up to 85%. On gross examination, the cross-section surface is classically homogenous and shows no evidence of necrosis or hemorrhage. Microscopically, the typical seminoma is characterized by large cells with distinct cell membranes and prominent nucleoli. These cells, which grow in a syncytial pattern, contain delicate connective tissue septae that can be infiltrated by a moderate amount of mature lymphocytes. The choriocarcinoma, although a highly malignant lesion, is rare—only 1%. The embryonal carcinoma is also an aggressive tumor, but the incidence is much lower. The

yolk sac tumor, as well as the polyembryoma are rare. *(Cotran et al., pp. 1019–2021)*

939. (A) Choriocarcinoma is a rare tumor of the testicles, but is characterized by hemorrhage and necrosis. This tumor, which is less than 1% of all of the germ cell tumors, is rarely seen in a pure form. In general, it is no larger than 5 cm in diameter, and HCG can be readily demonstrated in the blood. The cells seen in the hemorrhagic areas are cyto-, as well as syncytiotrophoblastic cells. *(Cotran et al., p. 1021)*

940. (A) Yolk sac tumors are more prevalent in infants and children up to 3 years of age. Sometimes it can be seen in adults, but usually it is a component of another germ cell tumor. On microscopic examination, the cells are cuboidal and thrown in pseudogranular structures, papillary formations, and solid cords. Moreover, as the name implies, in 50% of the tumors, there are structures that resemble primitive glomeruli. The presence of alphafetoprotein in the tumor cells is characteristic. *(Cotran et al., p. 1021)*

941. (D) Teratoma is a complex group of tumors derived from more than one layer of germ cells. These forms are fairly common in children and infants and is only secondary in frequence to yolk sac tumors. In adults, it can be associated with such other types as embryonal carcinomas in about 45% of the cases. Histologically, the mature teratomas are composed of heterogenous cells with organized structures. Layers of the mesodermal layer are represented by muscle islands, cartilage, and sometimes bone. The ectodermis shows differentiation into clusters of squamous epithelium as well as sebaceous glands. In immature teratomas, the cells are not completely differentiated or arranged in an organized fashion. A third type, which is called a teratoma with malignant transformation, shows a foci that may be a focus of squamous cell carcinoma or an adenocarcinoma in a mature teratoma. *(Cotran et al., pp. 1021–1022)*

942–946. (942-C, 943-E, 944-B, 945-A, 946-D) Prostatic hypertrophy is a benign enlargement of the prostatic tissue that is characterized by a nodular hyperplasia of the glandular and stromal elements of the prostate. It is as frequent as 70% at the age of 60 and 90% at the age of 70. In the etiology, there is little doubt that it is related to the action of androgens. A high percentage of tumors removed from the prostate also contain an in situ lesion called prostatic intraepithelial neoplasia (PIN). These lesions can be graded from I to III, depending upon the degree of the anaplasia of the cells or the pattern displayed. Tumors of the prostate are graded from I to V, depending on the anaplasia of the cells, as well as the pattern of the glandular formation. The Gleason score is obtained by adding the better differentiated areas with the poorly differentiated areas, which represents the Gleason score. Grading is very important in prostatic cancer, because the degree of differentiation of the glands correlates with prognosis. Measurement of the prostatic specific antigen (PSA), which is organ specific, has been carried out for many years as a screening procedure. Lately, further studies have revealed that the PSA can be measured in two different fractions, the free and the total. It has been proved that the lower the free PSA is found in men, the greater the possibility of its being a malignant tumor. Prostatic cancer spreads to the lymphatic system and also metastasizes early into the bones. The characteristic lesion in bone is osteoblastic metastasis. This is virtually diagnostic of the prostatic carcinoma in men. *(Cotran et al., pp. 1029–1033)*

REFERENCE

Cotran RS, Kumar V, Robbins SL. *Robbins Pathologic Basis of Disease,* 6th ed. Philadelphia: Saunders, 1999.

CHAPTER 13

Female Genital Tract and Breast

This chapter guides the reader into the different aspects and diseases of the female genital tract, as well as the breast. Most of the female genital tract is of mesodermal origin. The germ cells are of endodermal origin, and the vulva, as well as the epithelial lining of the vagina, are of ectodermal origin. In an adult female, measurement of the ovaries varies between 3–4 cm in the largest dimension. There are two parts of the ovaries; the cortex, which consists of spindle cells; and in the periphery, multiple follicles are present in various stages of maturation. The medulla of the ovary is made mostly of loosely arranged spindle cells with specialized epithelioid cells arranged in the hilus, which can produce steroids. In the ovary, it is also possible to find corpora luteum or corpora albicantia, depending on the patient's age and time of the cycle. The uterus weighs an average of 60–70 g, depending upon the patient's age and previous pregnancies. The uterus is composed of three different distinct regions; the cervix; the lower uterine segment; and the corpus of the uterus. The cervix is covered by squamous epithelium up to the squamocolumnar junction in which the mucosa changes for mucin-secreting single layer of cells. Internally, the lower uterine segment and corpus are lined by endometrial mucosa that is constantly changing, stimulated by hormones during the menstrual cycle. The cervix, which is the inferior portion of the uterus, interconnects the uterus with the vagina. Because of the location, it is exposed to trauma and infection. The exocervix is covered by nonkeratinizing squamous epithelium, and the endocervix is covered by a single layer of mucinous-secreting columnar cells. The endocervical canal connects with the exocervix, and at the transition of these two epithelial surfaces, called the squamocolumnar junction, which is considered the transformation zone.

The inflammatory changes in the cervix (cervicitis) can be specific or nonspecific and are commonly sexually transmitted. The cervix is also the site of benign, as well as malignant tumors, most frequently being the squamous cell carcinomas in which a progressive transition from the mild dysplasia to moderate and severe dysplasia can be seen as a precursor of squamous cell carcinoma.

The uterine corpus is, as previously mentioned, lined inside by endometrial mucosa that is surrounded by a thick layer of smooth muscle (myometrium). The myometrium is also the site of developing such benign tumors as leiomyomatas. Malignant tumors, although uncommon, can also occur, such as leiomyosarcoma.

BREAST

The breast, which embryologically develops from an ectodermal ridge that further extends into solid epithelial cords, deepens from the epidermis into the underlying mesenchymal tissue. It is the site of many pathological processes and is associated with benign, as well as malignant tumors. Lately, cancer of the breast has been found to be hereditary in some cases and mutations of the gene (BRCA1 and BRCA2) have been discovered in a low percentages of breast cancers. Because the breast epithelium is influenced by estrogen, as well as progesterone production, it undergoes changes cyclically, as well as with the patient's age, lactation, and pregnancy.

One of the most important benign pathological alterations of the breast are the fibrocystic changes. These fibrocystic changes encompass many epithelial changes ranging from cystic disease to hyperplasia of the ducts. These can be divided in proliferative and nonproliferative changes. The most important prognostic finding of the proliferative changes is the presence of atypical hyperplasia, which increases the risk for developing subsequent invasive carcinoma up to five times over the general population. Such benign tumors as fibroadenoma, the most common benign neoplasm of the breast, are generally found in the younger population.

Carcinoma of the breast has a variable histology and can be divided into two major categories; invasive carcinoma and carcinoma in situ. The origin of these cells can be either lobular or ductal. Lobular carcinoma can also be divided into different categories according to the histopathology; in the classic type, pleomorphic lobular carcinoma, and signet ring cell carcinoma. Ductal carcinoma can also be divided into different histologic types that include, medullary, metaplastic, tubular, colloid, papillary, adenocystic, and the classic infiltrating ductal carcinoma, the scirrhus type. Staging of the breast cancer is still the most important aspect of carcinoma of the breast in relation to the prognosis. Therefore, lymph node status is paramount. Presence of lymphatic invasion in the skin (inflammatory carcinoma of the breast) implies a serious prognosis. In a complete and comprehensive pathology report, there should be a statement of the presence of estrogen and progesterone receptors and HER-2/neu.

Questions

DIRECTIONS (Questions 947 through 956): Each group of items in this section consists of a list of lettered options followed by a set of numbered words or phrases. For each numbered word or phrase, select the ONE lettered option that is most closely associated with it. Each lettered option may be selected once, more than once or not at all.

Questions 947 through 951

(A) common ovarian neoplasm in the 3rd–6th decades; malignant forms associated with pseudomyxoma peritonei

(B) frequent between age 40–60; often bilateral, ovarian tumor

(C) tumor of the ovary that occurs in older women; not related to DES exposure

(D) uncommon ovarian tumor; age 40–70 resembles urinary tract epithelium

(E) 30% bilateral; may arise with endometriosis, second most common ovarian epithelial tumor

947. Serous neoplasm

948. Mucinous neoplasm

949. Endometrioid neoplasms

950. Clear cell neoplasm

951. Transitional (Brenner) cell neoplasm

Questions 952 though 956

(A) comprise 95% of germ cell tumors of the ovary (dermoid cyst)

(B) contains primitive embryonal tissue

(C) differentiating toward yolk sac structures, contain alpha-fetoprotein

(D) rare in ovary; usually represents a metastasis from a tumor in placenta, during pregnancy

(E) ovarian tumor is radiosensitive; 5-year survival rate 75–90%

952. Cystic teratomas

953. Dysgerminoma

954. Immature teratoma

955. Endodermal sinus tumor

956. Choriocarcinoma

DIRECTIONS (Questions 957 through 980): Each of the numbered items or incomplete statements in this section is followed by answers or by completions of the statement. Select the ONE lettered answer or completion that is BEST in each case.

957. State one of the most common characteristics of a serous cystadenocarcinoma of the ovary.

(A) It causes pseudomyxoma peritonea.

(B) It is composed of transitional epithelial cells.

(C) It is frequently bilateral.

(D) It is most common in children and young adults.

(E) It often metastasizes to the brain.

958. A mid-aged woman was found to have bilateral papillary carcinomas with stromal invasion. Which diagnosis is most likely

(A) Brenner tumor
(B) clear cell carcinoma
(C) endometrioid carcinoma
(D) mucinous cystadenocarcinoma
(E) serous cystadenocarcinoma

959. Of the neoplasms listed, which one is the most likely to cause endometrial hyperplasia?

(A) teratoma
(B) Brenner tumor
(C) mucinous adenoma
(D) serous cystadenocarcinoma
(E) granulosa cell tumor

960. A 28-year-old female shows clinical manifestations related to secretion of excess androgenic hormones, persistent anovulation. What is the most likely finding?

(A) endometriosis
(B) polycystic ovaries
(C) uterine leiomyoma
(D) endometrioid carcinoma of the ovary
(E) granulosa cell tumor of the ovary

961. What is the most useful laboratory test in evaluating the diagnosis or follow-up of choriocarcinoma?

(A) estriol
(B) alpha-fetoprotein
(C) CA-125
(D) carcinoembryonic antigen
(E) human chorionic gonadotropin, beta subunit

962. Which is the most common histological variant of endometrial adenocarcinoma?

(A) adenosquamous carcinoma
(B) clear cell carcinoma
(C) endometrioid carcinoma
(D) papillary serous cystadenocarcinoma
(E) squamous cell carcinoma

963. Which of the following neoplasms is typically functional and associated with estrogen secretions?

(A) serous cystadenocarcinoma
(B) Sertoli–Leydig cell tumor
(C) dysgerminoma
(D) granulosa-thecal cell tumor
(E) teratoma

964. What statement is correct in diagnosing leiomyosarcoma of the uterus?

(A) It is diagnosed by assessing mitotic activity and cytologic atypia.
(B) It is the most common uterine neoplasm.
(C) It has a 95% 5-year survival rate.
(D) It originates from endometrial stromal cells.
(E) It presents as multiple small, well-circumscribed nodules.

965. Out of the many causes of predisposition to ectopic tubal pregnancy, which is the most frequent?

(A) endometrial hyperplasia
(B) endometriosis
(C) multiparity
(D) ovarian neoplasms
(E) pelvic inflammatory disease

966. During the 10–18 weeks of gestation, a 28-year-old woman was exposed to DES (diethylstilbestrol). What is the most likely pathological process seen in the female baby?

(A) vaginal adenosis
(B) lichen sclerosis
(C) condyloma acuminatum
(D) Bowen's disease
(E) Bartholin duct cyst

967. A better control of the cervical carcinoma has been attributed to which of the following?

(A) early radical hysterectomy
(B) external beam radiation therapy
(C) treatment of precursor lesions after detection by cytologic screening
(D) the development of multiagent chemotherapeutic regimens

(E) public awareness of the risk factors for cervical cancer

968. Clinical and laboratory evidence suggests a strong association between which virus and cervical carcinoma?

(A) cytomegalovirus
(B) human papilloma virus
(C) HTLV-1
(D) provirus
(E) rotavirus

969. Which factor(s) is/are related to high risk of cervical dysplasia and carcinoma?

(A) high-risk male sexual partners
(B) large number of sexual partners
(C) low socioeconomic group
(D) young age at first intercourse
(E) all of the above

970. Which is the most important useful criterion for the differential diagnosis between borderline ovarian tumor and frank carcinoma?

(A) cytologic atypia
(B) mitotic activity
(C) serous differentiation
(D) stratified epithelial lining
(E) stromal invasion

971. How frequent is cancer of the breast in men for every 100 breast cancers in females?

(A) Fifty occur in men.
(B) Ninety occur in men.
(C) One occurs in men.
(D) Seventy occur in men.
(E) Twenty occur in men.

972. Which pathological changes carry the highest risk for developing breast carcinoma?

(A) apocrine metaplasia
(B) atypical ductal hyperplasia
(C) cystic dilation of duct
(D) squamous metaplasia
(E) stromal fibrosis

973. Of different histological types of carcinoma of the breast, which is the most likely to be bilateral?

(A) colloid carcinoma
(B) lobular carcinoma in situ
(C) medullary carcinoma
(D) papillary carcinoma
(E) tubular carcinoma

974. Of many different types of breast carcinoma, which is the one with the worst prognosis?

(A) colloid carcinoma
(B) phyllodes tumor, low grade
(C) infiltrating ductal scirrhous carcinoma
(D) papillary carcinoma
(E) tubular carcinoma

975. Which is the most common benign tumor of the breast?

(A) lipoma
(B) fibroadenoma
(C) hemangioma
(D) intraductal papilloma
(E) Phyllodes tumor, benign

976. What does carcinoma of the breast with abundant desmoplastic reaction (scirrhous carcinoma) indicate?

(A) mucin production by neoplastic cells
(B) elastic production by the neoplastic cells
(C) squamous metaplasia of the neoplastic cells
(D) stromal calcification
(E) stromal collagenization

977. In inflammatory carcinoma of the breast, what are the histological changes?

(A) carcinoma with a dense fibrous stroma
(B) carcinoma with a lymphocytic stroma
(C) groups of carcinoma cells filling dermal vascular channels
(D) neutrophils in the skin overlying the carcinoma
(E) single carcinoma cells infiltrating the dermis

978. Which of the following is the most important factor to predict breast cancer?

(A) the presence of carcinoma in situ
(B) lymph node metastasis (stage)
(C) mitotic activity
(D) cell type
(E) positive p53 (amplified)

979. Besides staging of breast cancer, what other factors may play a role in the prognosis?

(A) histologic grade
(B) estrogen receptors
(C) progesterone receptors
(D) oncogene expression (C-erb2, EGRF, p53)
(E) all of the above

980. Braca I and Braca II genes are related to pathogenesis of tumors of which of the following?

(A) ovarian cancer
(B) endometrial cancer
(C) breast and ovarian carcinomas
(D) melanoma
(E) lymphoma

Answers and Explanations

947. **(B)** Serous epithelial tumors of the ovary occur between the ages of 30–60 years. They frequently average 25 cm in diameter, and most of them are unilocular; 15% are bilateral. Histologically, they are lined by a single layer of columnar cells with no evidence of mucinous secretions, mitosis, or atypia. Occasional papillae could be found. *(Rubin and Farber, pp. 1005–1011)*

948. **(A)** Mucinous cystadenocarcinoma constitute up to 10% of all of ovarian cancers. The age group is similar to that of the serous tumors. In the malignant variety, there is evidence of stromal invasion of the ovary, and although the histologic picture can be variegated, it is mostly composed of mucin-secreting cells with different degrees of anaplasia. Pseudomyxoma peritonei is one of the complications of these tumors, which result in the accumulation of gelatinous mucinous material in the abdominal cavity. *(Rubin and Farber, pp. 1005–1011)*

949. **(E)** Endometrioid adenocarcinoma is an ovarian tumor histologically identical to those found in the endometrium. It accounts for 20–30% of the malignant tumors of the ovary and is second only to serous cystadenocarcinoma. One-third to one-half of the endometrioid carcinomas are bilateral. *(Rubin and Farber, pp. 1005–1011)*

950. **(C)** Clear cell carcinoma constitutes 5–10% of all of the ovarian cancers and usually occurs in the elderly group, after menopause. Forty percent of the cases are bilateral. Microscopically, the clear cell carcinoma is composed of cohesive cells with a polygonal shape and clear cytoplasm. When it creates lumens, the cells appear to protrude into the empty space in a hob-nail appearance. *(Rubin and Farber, pp. 1005–1011)*

951. **(D)** Brenner tumor is typically benign and occurs generally in women over 50 years of age. Histologically, the tumor is composed of solid nests of ovoid to spindloid cells in a dense fibrous stroma. The tumor cells, which are nonpleomorphic, resemble urothelial epithelium. *(Rubin and Farber, pp. 1005–1011)*

952. **(A)** The mature cystic teratoma (dermoid cyst) is the most common germ cell tumor of the ovary. On gross examination, it is cystic, contains yellowish, greasy material and in the solid areas, cartilage, bone, teeth, and microscopically we can find a variety of such tissues as skin, sweat glands, cartilage, brain, thyroid, and different kinds of mucinous secreting glands. *(Rubin and Farber, pp. 1010–1012)*

953. **(E)** Dysgerminoma, although it accounts for only 2% of all ovarian cancers, is frequent in females under 20 years of age. On examination, they are almost identical to their testicular counterpart of seminoma. Five-year survival in patients with this highly radiosensitive tumor is between 75–90%. *(Rubin and Farber, pp. 1011–1013)*

954. **(B)** The difference between mature and immature teratoma is that the immature teratoma, in addition to all of the components of the teratoma also contains immature embryonal tissues. Immature teratomas accounts for 20% of all of the malignant tumors in women under 20 years. Microscopically, they are composed of the same elements of the mature cystic teratomas plus embryonal elements. When metastasis occurs in the immature teratoma, they are composed of embryonal tissues. *(Rubin and Farber, pp. 1011–1013)*

955. **(C)** The yolk sac tumor is seen in young women under the age of 30 and histologically resembles the primitive yolk sac. Microscopically, the tumor is composed of spaces lined by cuboidal cells, some of them protruding in papillae, which has been called Schiller–Duval bodies. The cells that compose the yolk sac tumor secrete alpha-fetoprotein, which is measured in the peripheral blood and is useful for monitoring the effectiveness of the therapy. *(Rubin and Farber, pp. 1011–1013)*

956. **(D)** The choriocarcinoma of the ovary is a rare tumor, and it derives from ovarian germ cells. In women of reproductive age, choriocarcinoma could represent a metastasis from an intrauterine gestational tumor. Microscopically, it is composed of an admixture of malignant cyto- and syncytiotrophoblastic cells. The tumor cells secrete HCG, which are also useful for the diagnosis, as well as effectiveness of the tumor treatment. *(Rubin and Farber, pp. 1011–1013)*

957. **(C)** Serous cystadenocarcinoma of the ovary is the most common malignant ovarian tumor, and they are frequently bilateral. Microscopically, they show a variegated appearance with papillary patterns. Different degrees of anaplasia of the cuboidal to columnar cells that cover the papillae and occasional calcified concretions (psammoma bodies) are present. *(Rubin and Farber, p. 1007)*

958. **(E)** Refer to Answer 957. *(Rubin and Farber, p. 1007)*

959. **(E)** Granulosa cell tumor is an ovarian tumor frequently associated with secretion of estrogens. Because most of these tumors occur after menopause, they may produce endometrial hyperplasia, feminization, or rarely, hirsutism. *(Rubin and Farber, p. 1014)*

960. **(B)** Polycystic ovaries is a syndrome characterized by clinical manifestations related to the secretions of excess of androgenic hormones, persistent anovulation, and the ovaries contain many small peripheral cysts. *(Rubin and Farber, pp. 1003–1004)*

961. **(E)** Refer to Answer 956. *(Rubin and Farber, p. 1013)*

962. **(C)** Endometrial carcinoma is the most frequent cancer in U.S. women and the single most common gynecologic cancer. The pathogenesis of the endometrial cancer is linked to prolonged unopposed estrogen stimulation of the endometrium. The source of estrogen could be endogenous, as in cases of granulosa cell tumor, or exogenous. This tumor also occurs in association with a higher incidence of breast and ovarian cancers, which suggests a genetic predisposition. The most common histologic type is endometrioid. *(Rubin and Farber, pp. 993–995)*

963. **(D)** Granulosa cell tumors are derived from the follicular epithelium of the premordial follicules. These are most commonly seen in menopausal women, accounting for 2% of all ovarian neoplasms. Granulosa cell tumors typically secrete estrogen, which produces characteristic symptomatology. *(Rubin and Farber, pp. 993–995, 1014)*

964. **(A)** Leiomyosarcoma is a malignant neoplasm that originates in the smooth muscle of the myometrium. To differentiate this smooth muscle tumor from the benign leiomyomas, a careful count of the mitotic activity per 10 high-power fields should be done, as well as assessment of the nuclear atypia. *(Rubin and Farber, pp. 998–1000)*

965. **(E)** Ectopic tubal pregnancies occur in the fallopian tubes; Although, ectopic pregnancies could also occur in other parts of the female genitalia, including ovaries. Ectopic tubal pregnancy is the result of abnormal mucosal adhesions and irregularities in the lumen of the

tube secondary to chronic inflammatory disease. Rupture, which is the usual outcome if left alone, can lead to massive bleeding. *(Rubin and Farber, p. 1001)*

966. **(A)** Vaginal adenosis is described as the failure of the normal glandular epithelium that lines the embryonic vagina to be replaced during fetal life by squamous epithelium in the adult. These changes occur as a result of the use of diethylstilbestrol (DES) for high-risk pregnancies. *(Rubin and Farber, p. 974)*

967. **(C)** With the introduction of a screening test for cytologic evaluation of the cervical cells, a dramatic decrease in mortality for invasive cervical carcinoma has occurred. This has been accomplished because of the early detection of intraepithelial neoplasia, of different degrees, that may lead, if untreated, to carcinoma. Mild, moderate, and severe dysplasia can be diagnosed with regular Pap smears. In cases of high-grade dysplasia, further adequate treatment can be achieved early, before progressing into invasive carcinoma. *(Rubin and Farber, pp. 980–983)*

968. **(B)** The condyloma acuminatum, a verrucous growth of the cervical epithelium, is produced by human papilloma virus. Different types of virus are found, some of them with a highly increased risk of developing invasive carcinoma. Conversely, in 70% of invasive cancers, different types of HPV are found. *(Rubin and Farber, pp. 980–983)*

969. **(E)** All of the listed answers contain a high risk to develop cervical dysplasia and later carcinoma. Young age for first intercourse, the high-risk male sexual partners, large number of sexual partners, and low socioeconomic group are all contributory factors for developing cervical intraepithelial neoplasia. *(Rubin and Farber, pp. 980–983)*

970. **(E)** Malignant epithelial tumors of the ovary are characterized by cellular pleomorphism, different degrees of anaplasia of the cells, increasing mitotic activity, and the most important criteria would be the stromal invasion. Without the stromal invasion, the tumor could be considered only borderline. *(Rubin and Farber, pp. 1007–1008)*

971. **(C)** Cancer of the breast for males accounts for only 1% of the all breast cancers. The most common type is the infiltrating ductal carcinoma. Prognosis of these tumors is related to the staging, much as in females. BRCA2 gene is increased in the hereditary type of breast cancer. *(Rubin and Farber, pp. 1039–1040, 1046)*

972. **(B)** Atypical ductal hyperplasia is a proliferative lesion of the breast, which consists of an abnormal growth of cells into the ducts containing either cellular atypia or abnormal histologic pattern. The combination of both will be equal to carcinoma in situ of the breast, as long as it measures more than 2 mm in diameter. The risk of developing carcinoma of the breast in atypical hyperplasia is increased by four to five times that of the general population. *(Rubin and Farber, p. 1035)*

973. **(B)** Lobular carcinoma in situ is a proliferation of the lobular epithelium that fill and distend the ascini of the lobular unit. As long as the basement membrane is intact, there is no evidence of invasion. In general, it is not possible to palpate this lesion, which tends to be multifocal and bilateral. *(Rubin and Farber, pp. 1040–1042)*

974. **(C)** Colloid, papillary, phyllodes tumor, low-grade, and tubular, which is the best differentiated ductal carcinoma, are known to have better prognoses than infiltrating ductal scirrhous carcinoma. *(Rubin and Farber, pp. 1041–1045)*

975. **(B)** Fibroadenoma is the most common benign neoplasm of the breast and is composed of two elements: a mesenchymal element mostly composed of fibrous tissue; and the epithelial component, which consists of compressed and sometimes hyperplastic irregular ductal lumens. They are usually found in young women, and they may be hormonally reactive during pregnancy or menopause. *(Rubin and Farber, pp. 1035–1037)*

976. **(E)** Ductal carcinoma, which is the most common form of breast cancer, produces a marked stromal proliferation of fibrous tissue called *desmoplasia*. This fibrous tissue is infiltrated by the malignant cells. On gross examination, it presents as a hard fixed mass that is also easily detected on mammogram. For this clinical presentation, as well as the gross examination, on the surgical bench, it was named *scirrhous carcinoma*. *(Rubin and Farber, pp. 1041–1042)*

977. **(C)** When tumor of the breast invades the lymphatics, as well as the venules of the skin, it clinically produces a skin reaction that is reddish in color and for that reason is called inflammatory carcinoma of the breast. This dermolymphatic invasion correlates with the prognosis, which in this particular case is poor, despite the triple modality of therapy—radiation, chemotherapy, and surgery. *(Rubin and Farber, p. 1046)*

978. **(B)** Although the histological grade could be considered one of the factors relating to prognosis of the breast, the most important parameter is staging. This is correlated with the status of the lymph node metastasis. Despite multiple markers there is no better correlation than staging for prognosis of cancer of the breast. *(Rubin and Farber, pp. 1045–1046)*

979. **(E)** The histological grade, estrogen, and progesterone receptors, as well as C-erb2 are important factors for prognosis, as well as the prediction in the response to the treatment for breast cancer. *(Rubin and Farber, pp. 1045–1046)*

980. **(C)** The Braca I gene, which is located on chromosome 17, and the Braca II, which is located on chromosome 13, are both incriminated in the pathogenesis of hereditary breast and ovarian cancers. The most important changes here are the mutations, which seem to be responsible for less than 2% of the cases of breast cancer. *(Rubin and Farber, pp. 1039–1040)*

REFERENCE

Rubin E, Farber JL. *Pathology.* Philadelphia: Lippincott, 1999.

CHAPTER 14

Endocrine System

The endocrine system is composed of the major endocrine glands, modulated in their activity by the pituitary gland. This gland is the center of secretion of adenocorticotropic hormone (ACTH), follicular stimulant hormone (FSH), luteinizing hormone (LH), luteotropic hormone (LTH, prolactin), somatotropic (growth hormone, STH), and thyroid-stimulating hormone (TSH). All the endocrine glands secrete hormones, molecules that are directly poured to the blood and acting on target cells or organs at a distance. When the target is hit, there is a feedback mechanism of inhibitions, then regulating the activity of the gland. In general, diseases of the endocrine system are related to the under or overproduction of hormones that result in alterations of the homeostasis between various organs and systems of the body. All diseases of the endocrine system we discuss in this chapter are tumors, either benign or malignant, that may affect the production of hormones.

Hormones can also be produced in a variety of sites, either locally, or acting throughout the circulation. Many hormones can also extend their effects in the same tissues that are produced (autocrine mechanism).

Questions

DIRECTIONS (Question 981): The numbered item in this section is followed by answers. Select the ONE lettered answer that is BEST.

981. What will the pancreas of a patient with a long history of Type I insulin dependent diabetes mellitus histologically show?

   (A) almost complete absence of beta cells in most islets and lymphocytic infiltration
   (B) islet cell hyperplasia with abnormal islets budding from the ducts
   (C) normal structure
   (D) reduced numbers of beta cells and marked lymphocytic infiltrate in most islets
   (E) total replacement of the islets by amyloid

DIRECTIONS (Questions 982 through 984): For each numbered word or phrase, select the ONE lettered option that is most closely associated with it. Each lettered option may be selected once, more than once, or not at all.

   (A) abnormally small thyroid, elevated TSH, low T4
   (B) abnormally small thyroid, low TSH, elevated T4
   (C) enlarged thyroid, elevated TSH, T4
   (D) enlarged thyroid, low TSH, elevated T4
   (E) growth hormone excess

982. Grave's disease

983. Hashimoto's disease

984. Pituitary adenoma

DIRECTIONS (Questions 985 through 1001): Each of the numbered items or incomplete statements in this section is followed by answers or by completion of the statement. Select the ONE lettered answer or completion that is BEST in each case.

985. Which is the most common histologic features of the pancreatic islets in a patient with history of Type I diabetes mellitus?

   (A) no beta cells
   (B) hyperplastic beta cells
   (C) no beta cells with lymphocytic infiltration
   (D) normal and alpha cells
   (E) replaced by collagen

986. The histologic examination of thyroid reveals marked destruction of the thyroid parenchyma with lymphocytic infiltration, germinal centers, and Hurthle cell changes. These histologic features are consistent with which of the following?

   (A) Graves' disease
   (B) Hashimoto's disease
   (C) multinodular goiter
   (D) papillary thyroid carcinoma
   (E) subacute thyroiditis

987. Which is a pituitary adenoma most likely to cause?

   (A) decreased cortisol
   (B) decreased thyroxine
   (C) increased cortisol
   (D) increased prolactin
   (E) all of the above

988. Which is the most common type of a malignant thyroid tumor?

(A) follicular carcinoma

(B) lymphoma

(C) medullary carcinoma

(D) papillary carcinoma

(E) anaplastic carcinoma

989. A patient who is found to have increased cortisol levels and normal aldosterone most likely has which of the following?

(A) craniopharyngioma

(B) neoplasm of the adrenal cortex

(C) neoplasm of the adrenal medulla

(D) parathyroid adenoma

(E) pituitary adenoma

990. Deficiency of 21-hydroxylase causes an increase in which of the following?

(A) 17-hydroxyprogesterone

(B) aldosterone

(C) cortisol

(D) estriol

(E) norepinephrine

991. Diabetes insipidus occurs as a consequence of which of the following?

(A) anterior pituitary lesion

(B) posterior pituitary lesion

(C) pancreatic lesion

(D) adrenal hypertrophy

(E) parathyroid adenoma

992. Thyrotoxicosis is most likely present in which of the following?

(A) "cold" thyroid adenoma

(B) hyperfunctional multinodular goiter

(C) medullary thyroid carcinoma

(D) papillary thyroid carcinoma

(E) pituitary adenoma

993. In a patient with small cell anaplastic carcinoma of the lung, hypercalcemia could be secondary to which of the following?

(A) ACTH

(B) insulin-like growth factors

(C) parathyroid hormone

(D) parathyroid hormone-like peptide

(E) thyroid hormone

994. Which of the following neoplasm is most likely to produce aldosteronism?

(A) adenoma of the adrenal cortex

(B) lung carcinoma

(C) neoplasm of the adrenal medulla

(D) ovarian carcinoma

(E) pituitary adenoma

995. What is the most common neoplasm of childhood that arises in the adrenal medulla?

(A) craniopharyngioma

(B) medullary carcinoma

(C) neuroblastoma

(D) pheochromocytoma

(E) Wilms' tumor

996. The gross and microscopically appearance of the adrenal glands in a patient with small cell carcinoma of the lung and elevated cortisol levels would be which of the following?

(A) bilateral atrophy of the cortex

(B) bilateral hyperplasia of the cortex

(C) bilateral hyperplasia of the medulla

(D) neoplasm of the cortex with atrophy of the remaining cortex

(E) no pathologic changes

997. More than 60% of the cases of congenital adrenal hyperplasia represent an inborn deficiency of which of the following?

(A) 11-hydroxylase deficiency

(B) partial 21-hydroxylase deficiency

(C) multiple endocrine neoplasia, Type I

(D) multiple endocrine neoplasia, Type II

(E) Type 2 diabetes mellitus

998. Which is the most frequent cause of multi-nodular goiter?

(A) antithyroid antibodies
(B) ingestion of thyroid hormone
(C) iodine deficiency
(D) pituitary adenoma
(E) thyroid carcinoma

999. Craniopharyngioma may cause which of the following?

(A) pituitary hormonal deficiencies
(B) nerve compression
(C) growth retardation
(D) diabetes insipidus
(E) all of the above

1000. Which of the following is/are causes of hypoaldosteronism?

(A) 21-hydroxylase deficiency
(B) bilateral adrenalectomy for Cushing's syndrome
(C) idiopathic Addison's disease
(D) tuberculosis
(E) all of the above

1001. What are the most common morphological changes in Cushing's disease?

(A) an anterior pituitary adenoma and adrenal medullary hyperplasia
(B) an anterior pituitary adenoma and an adrenocortical adenoma
(C) an anterior pituitary adenoma and nodular adrenocortical hyperplasia
(D) anterior pituitary atrophy and adreno-cortical adenoma
(E) carcinomas of both the anterior pituitary and adrenal cortex

DIRECTIONS (Questions 1002 through 1009): Each group of items in this section consists of a list of lettered options followed by a set of numbered words or phrases. For each numbered word or phrase, select the ONE lettered option that is most closely associated with it. Each lettered option may be selected once, more than once, or not at all.

Questions 1002 through 1006

(A) ACTH deficiency
(B) aldosterone and cortisol deficiency
(C) calcitonin
(D) prolactin overproduction
(E) renin deficiency

1002. Primary Addison's disease

1003. Secondary Addison's disease

1004. 21-Hydroxylase deficiency

1005. Produced by parafollicular cells

1006. Galactorrhea, amenorrhea, infertility

Questions 1007 though 1009

(A) adenoma of all parathyroid glands
(B) adenoma of one parathyroid gland
(C) carcinoma of one parathyroid gland
(D) hyperplasia of all parathyroid glands
(E) hyperplasia of one parathyroid gland

1007. What is the most common finding in patients with primary hyperparathyroidism?

1008. What is the most common finding in patients with secondary hyperparathyroidism?

1009. What causes hyperparathyroidism in less than 5%?

DIRECTIONS (Question 1010): The numbered item in this section is followed by answers. Select the ONE lettered answer that is BEST.

1010. Which of the following agents is most likely to cause Type I diabetes mellitus in a suscep-tible individual?

(A) coxsackie B virus infection
(B) excess caloric intake
(C) glucagon ingestion
(D) iodine deficiency
(E) papilloma virus infection

Answers and Explanations

981. **(A)** Many lesions of the pancreas can be seen on histology, and they are more commonly associated with Type I than Type II diabetes. In Type I diabetes, there is reduction of the islets, with absence of beta cells and lymphocytic infiltration, which can be proved to be T cells with special immunoperoxidase staining. *(Cotran et al., pp. 920–922)*

982. **(D)** Over 95% of the cases with hyperthyroidism are caused by Grave's disease. This disease is produced by excessive hormonal production with an enlarged thyroid gland, decrease in TSH, and for most cases, elevated T4. *(Chandrasoma and Taylor, p. 842)*

983. **(C)** Hashimoto's thyroiditis is the most common cause of hypothyroidism worldwide. In this endemic area, it is because of the low iodine levels in the environment. It is autoimmune and results in destruction of the gland, which is diffusely enlarged and occasionally has some nodularity. Microscopic examination shows the destruction of the thyroid follicles, which is also associated with infiltration of the parenchyma by mononuclear inflammatory cells, mostly small lymphocytes with occasional well-developed germinal centers and plasma cells. Elevated TSH and T4 is usually found. *(Chandrasoma and Taylor, p. 846)*

984. **(E)** Pituitary adenomas are responsible for about 10% of the intracranial neoplasm. They may be nonfunctional or they can produce hypo- or hyperpituitarism. The effects of the parathyroid adenoma are related to mass effects by compression of the surrounding tissues, or by excessive hormonal secretion. Microscopically, the pituitary adenomas are pleomorphic and show different cell types. Only with the immunoperoxidase technique or with electron microscopy can the characteristics of the cells be defined. Excessive production of growth hormone affects the effector organs and causes increase in weight. Many patients with acromegaly also have evidence of decreased secretion of the pituitary hormones because of mass effect on the local area. *(Chandrasoma and Taylor, p. 835)*

985. **(C)** Refer to Answer 981. *(Cotran et al., pp. 920–921)*

986. **(B)** Hashimoto's thyroiditis is an autoimmune disease characterized by the presence of circulating antibodies to thyroid antigens. Hashimoto's thyroiditis is the most common cause of hypothyroidism in goiter. Gross examination of the thyroid gland in Hashimoto's thyroiditis shows that it is diffusely enlarged and sometimes slightly nodular. On cross section, it exhibits a nodular pattern with nodules of different sizes. Microscopically, the most important change is the lymphocytic infiltrates with well-developed germinal centers, Hurthle cell metaplasia, with follicular destruction, fibrosis, and occasional giant cells. *(Rubin and Farber, p. 1171)*

987. **(E)** Refer to Answer 984. *(Chandrasoma and Taylor, p. 835)*

988. **(D)** Papillary carcinoma is the most common type of cancer. It is three times more frequent in females than males. Microscopically, is characterized by papillary structures lined by cells with nuclear changes that are typical. Such changes include: intranuclear inclusions; grooves; and clear nuclei. Psammoma bodies are often present. *(Rubin and Farber, pp. 851–852)*

989. **(E)** Corticotropin adenomas secrete corticotropin. Cushing's disease develops when the corticotropin stimulates the adrenal cortex, inducing hypersecretion. The aldosterone is secreted in the zona glomerulosa of the adrenal gland. It is controlled by the renin-angiotensing mechanism that functions independent of the pituitary gland. *(Rubin and Farber, p. 1160)*

990. **(A)** More than 90% of the cases of congenital adrenal hyperplasia represent an inborn deficiency of the 21-hydroxylase. The gene of this inborn deficiency is located in chromosome 6. The enzymes that convert 17-hydroxyprogesterone to 11-dyoxycortisol do not occur, and the accumulated precursors are converted to antigens. Therefore, the 17-hydroxyprogesterone is increased. *(Rubin and Farber, p. 1184)*

991. **(B)** Diabetes insipidus occurs as a deficiency of antidiuretic hormone (ADH). Clinically, it is characterized by an increase in the volume of urine because of the kidney's inability to reabsorb water from the urine. The etiology of this process of the posterior pituitary gland includes head trauma, tumors, and inflammatory disorders, which can also involve the hypothymus. *(Cotran et al., p. 1129)*

992. **(B)** Thyrotoxicosis is secondary to elevated levels of T3 and T4. This hyperfunction of the thyroid tissue will produce a hypermetabolic state that is clinically characterized by nervousness, palpitations, muscle weakness, weight loss, diarrhea, heat intolerance, excessive perspiration, emotional liability, menstrual changes, and fine tremor of the hands, to mention only a few. Thyrotoxicosis can be caused by a variety of disorders that affect the thyroid gland, most importantly with the diffuse hyperplasia (Grave's disease), but is also seen in hyper-

function multinodular goiter and sometimes in hyperfunctional adenomas (toxic adenoma) thyroiditis, as well as the exogenous ingestion of thyroid hormones. *(Cotran et al., p. 1131)*

993. **(D)** Paraneoplastic syndromes are characterized by the secretion of hormones or hormone-like factors that elaborate different substances that are poured into the blood and cause variegated types of syndromes. Parathyroid hormone and its related peptide prostaglandin E are implicated in the hypercalcemia often seen in small cell anaplastic carcinoma of the lung. *(Cotran et al., p. 746)*

994. **(A)** Hyperaldosteronism is associated with adrenocortical adenoma. In general, the adenomas are small and tan-brown in color. The adrenals otherwise are normal. Aldosterone causes sodium retention resulting in hypertension and hypokalemic alkalosis. *(Chandrasoma and Taylor, p. 868)*

995. **(C)** Neuroblastoma is the most common childhood solid tumor, and generally, diagnosis is made before 1 year of age. Grossly, the tumor's size ranges from microscopically minute nodules to a mass larger than one kilogram. Smooth, encapsulated margins or infiltrative borders are seen surrounding the major vessels. Histologically, the tumors are composed of primitive appearing small cells with scant cytoplasm and characteristic rosette formation. Twenty-five to thirty percent of the neuroblastomas arise in the adrenal medulla. *(Cotran et al., pp. 485–487)*

996. **(A)** Adrenal cortical insufficiency (hypofunction) could be caused by either primary adrenal disease or increased stimulation of the adrenal glands (ACTH deficiency). The secondary type of adrenal cortical insufficiency is caused by disorders of the hypothymus and pituitary gland or metastatic cancer, infarction, or irradiation. In addition, prolonged administration of exogenous glucocorticoids suppresses the output of ACTH. In cases of small cell anaplastic carcinoma, secreting ACTH-like hormone can also produce atrophy of the cortex of the adrenal glands. *(Cotran et al., pp. 1161–1162)*

997. **(B)** It is the most common (60%) of the congenital adrenal hyperplasia. The main effects of partial 21-hydroxylase deficiency are: adrenal hyperplasia, high serum ACTH levels, and increased secretion of androgens. Because of the increase of androgens, clinically females show virilism, and precocious puberty is present in males. (*Chandrasoma and Taylor, p. 865*)

998. **(C)** Refer to Answer 992. (*Cotran et al., p. 1131*)

999. **(E)** Craniopharyngiomas are tumors derived from the vestigial remnants of the Rathke's pouch. These slow-growing tumors account for approximately 1–5% of intracranial tumors. Because of their location, in adults they can produce symptoms related to the encroachment on the optic chiasm and cranial nerves. In children, the growth produces such endocrine deficiencies as growth retardations, as well as other endocrine abnormalities. (*Cotran et al., p. 1129*)

1000. **(E)** On the adrenal cortex, the outermost layer, the zona glomerulosa, is the site of aldosterone secretion. It is stimulated by angiotensin and potassium and inhibits the atrial natriuretic peptide and somatostatin. All of the diseases listed act either by destruction, such as tuberculosis, or by such idiopathic reasons as Addison's disease can cause hypoaldosteronism. Also, 21-hydrolase deficiency, which represents an inborn deficiency of 21-hydroxylase, shows hypoaldosteronism for lack of production. Cushing's syndrome will also produce a decrease of aldosterone. (*Rubin and Farber, pp. 1183–1184*)

1001. **(C)** Cushing's syndrome is a disorder caused by a condition that produces an elevation of glucocorticoid levels. In clinical practice, most cases of Cushing's syndrome are induced by excessive administration of glucocorticosteroids. The other causes of Cushing's syndrome are primary hypothalamic–pituitary disease, which is a hypersecretion of ACTH. Most of these cases are produced by a pituitary gland adenoma. The secretion of ACTH leads to adrenocortical hyperplasia. (*Cotran et al., pp. 1152–1153*)

1002. **(B)** This is a primary chronic adrenocortical insufficiency, the etiologic factor seems to be secondary to an autoimmune disease. It results in progressive destruction of the adrenal cortex, and such clinical manifestations as adrenocortical insufficiency. Autoimmune adrenalitis accounts for 60–70% of the cases. (*Cotran et al., p. 1160*)

1003. **(A)** In the previous question, we speculated about the causes of primary adrenocortical insufficiency, and autoimmune adrenalitis was mentioned. Another cause of primary adrenocortical insufficiency is when the adrenal gland is replaced by metastatic carcinoma or destruction by infection, including tuberculosis. The secondary adrenocortical insufficiency may be caused by the deficiency by ACTH, which has many similarities to the previously described primary Addison's disease. (*Cotran et al., p. 1163*)

1004. **(B)** Refer to Answer 997. (*Rubin and Farber, p. 1184*)

1005. **(C)** The parafollicular cells or C cells are located in between the follicular epithelial cells of the thyroid gland. These cells are in charge of synthesizing the hormone calcitonin. The action of the calcitonin is to regulate the blood calcium by inhibiting the reabsorption of bone by osteoclasts. (*Cotran et al., p. 1131*)

1006. **(D)** The most frequent hyperfunctioning pituitary adenomas are the prolactinomas. They are recognized microscopically for weakly acidophilic cells or chromophobic cells. Prolactin can be demonstrated in the cytoplasm of the cells with immunoperoxidase techniques. Secretion of prolactin will lead to clinical pictures that can cause amenorrhea, galactorrhea, loss of libido, and infertility. (*Cotran et al., pp. 1125–1126*)

1007. **(B)** The causes of hyperparathyroidism are generally related to a neoplasm (adenoma). The most common neoplasm is a single adenoma in 75–80% cases. Primary hyperplasia of the glands accounts for 10–15%. Parathyroid carcinoma is less than 5%. Primary hyperparathyroidism is usually a disease of adults and is more common in females than males. *(Cotran et al., pp. 1148–1149)*

1008. **(D)** Secondary hyperparathyroidism is caused by a condition associated with a decrease in the level of serum calcium, which, in turn, leads to compensatory overactivity of the parathyroid glands. Renal failure is by far the most common cause of secondary hyperparathyroidism. *(Cotran et al., pp. 1150–1151)*

1009. **(C)** Parathyroid carcinoma is a rare disease. It accounts for less than 5% of hyperparathyroidism. Parathyroid carcinoma is usually a nonfunctioning tumor. Carcinomas of the parathyroid gland are usually larger than adenomas and appear to be firm, and not encapsulated masses that adhere to the surrounding soft tissues. *(Rubin and Farber, p. 1182)*

1010. **(A)** For a long time, is has been noted that epidemiologic studies suggest that the infection of coxsackieviruses of group B was associated with pancreatic diseases, which in susceptible persons would cause Type I diabetes. The way that this virus acts is producing an injury of the beta cells of the pancreatic islets and produces an immunologic reaction against the beta cells. *(Cotran et al., p. 917)*

REFERENCES

Chandrasoma P, Taylor CR. *Concise Pathology,* 3rd ed. Norwalk, CT: Appleton & Lange, 1998.

Cotran RS, Kumar V, Robbins SL. *Robbins Pathologic Basis of Disease,* 6th ed. Philadelphia: Saunders, 1999.

Rubin E, Farber JL. *Pathology.* Philadelphia: Lippincott, 1999.

CHAPTER 15

Hematopoietic System, Lymphopoietic System, and Skin

The myeloid cells in normal circumstances are located in the bone marrow spaces, and the stem cells located in this area produce, as a final product, erythrocytes, platelets, monocytes, and granulocytes. Reference is made to disorders of the red cells, including the morphology of the cells, as well as the results of autoantibody formation giving origin to the hemolytic anemias. Anemias affect the red cells either for lack of production, reduction of the volume secondary to blood loss, or destruction for different causes as a hemolytic anemia.

Disorders of the white cells, such as myeloid neoplasms (acute and chronic myeloid leukemias), are considered, as well as myelodysplastic and myeloproliferative syndromes. With respect to diseases that involve the lymph nodes and spleen, we especially emphasize the lymphomas, as well as reactive lymphadenopathy. B and T lymphocytes, as well as natural killer cells and mononuclear macrophages with their pathological process, are emphasized. Finally, on the diseases of the skin, we briefly consider the most common inflammatory changes in the skin, as well as the most common neoplasms.

Questions

DIRECTIONS (Question 1011): The numbered item in this section is followed by answers. Select the ONE lettered answer that is BEST.

1011. Mild to moderate normochromic or hypochromic anemia with poor utilization and increase in the marrow iron are characteristic of which of the following?

(A) anemia of chronic disease
(B) beta-thalassemia
(C) hereditary spherocytosis
(D) iron deficiency anemia
(E) megaloblastic anemia

DIRECTIONS (Questions 1012 through 1016): For each numbered word or phrase, select the ONE lettered option that is most closely associated with it. Each lettered option may be selected once, more than once, or not at all.

(A) anemia of chronic disease
(B) autoimmune hemolyte anemia
(C) folate deficiency
(D) iron deficiency
(E) Sickle cell disease

1012. Elevated mean corpuscular volume

1013. Decreased mean corpuscular volume

1014. Macrocytic anemia

1015. Microcytic hypochromic anemia

1016. Normochromic anemia without reticulocytosis

DIRECTIONS (Questions 1017 through 1019): Each of the numbered items in this section is followed by answers. Select the ONE lettered answer that is BEST in each case.

1017. The presence of leukoerythroblastosis in the peripheral smear suggests which of the following?

(A) alpha-thalassemia
(B) hemoglobin C disease
(C) hereditary spherocytosis
(D) iron deficiency anemia
(E) myelophthisic anemia

1018. Macrocytic anemia, hypersegmented neutrophils, antiparietal cell antibodies in a patient is most likely to have a deficiency of which of the following?

(A) niacin
(B) vitamin A
(C) vitamin B_1 (thiamine)
(D) vitamin B_{12} (cyanocobalamin)
(E) vitamin D

1019. The cell origin of most of the non-Hodgkin's lymphomas is which of the following?

(A) B-lymphocytes
(B) CD4+ T-lymphocytes
(C) CD8+ T-lymphocytes
(D) macrophages
(E) plasma cells

DIRECTIONS (Questions 1020 through 1023): For each numbered word or phrase, select the ONE lettered option that is most closely associated with it. Each lettered option may be selected once, more than once, or not at all.

(A) B-lymphocytes
(B) CD4+ T-lymphocyte
(C) CD8+ T-lymphocyte
(D) histiocytes/monocyte
(E) plasma cells

1020. Non-Hodgkin's lymphoma

1021. Mycosis fungoides/Sezary syndrome

1022. Multiple myeloma

1023. True histiocytic lymphoma

DIRECTIONS (Questions 1024 through 1027): Each of the numbered items in this section is followed by answers. Select the ONE lettered answer that is BEST in each case.

1024. A B-cell neoplasm, with 11,14 translocation and BCL1 rearrangement is most likely which of the following?

(A) follicular lymphoma
(B) mantle cell lymphoma
(C) mycosis fungoides
(D) marginal lymphoma
(E) large cell lymphoma

1025. Fever, sore throat, generalized lymph node enlargement and lymphocytosis with atypical lymphocytes are characteristic of which of the following?

(A) chronic lymphocytic leukemia
(B) infection with Epstein–Barr virus
(C) infection with *Streptococcus pyogenes*
(D) drug reaction
(E) miliary tuberculosis

1026. Which is most common in middle-aged patients, with tumor cells that are CD10+, BCL2+ and frequent 14,18 translocation?

(A) Hodgkin's disease
(B) small lymphocytic lymphoma

(C) multiple myeloma
(D) T cell lymphoma
(E) follicular lymphoma

1027. The identification of Auer rods in the cytoplasm of leukemic cells advocates for the diagnosis of which of the following?

(A) acute lymphocytic leukemia
(B) acute myelogenous leukemia
(C) chronic lymphocytic leukemia
(D) chronic myelogenous leukemia
(E) hairy cell leukemia

DIRECTIONS (Questions 1028 through 1031): For each numbered word or phrase, select the ONE lettered option that is most closely associated with it. Each lettered option may be selected once, more than once, or not at all.

(A) (8,14) chromosome translocation
(B) (9,22) chromosome translocation
(C) (11,14) chromosome translocation
(D) (14,18) chromosome translocation
(E) (15,17) chromosome translocation

1028. Burkitt's lymphoma

1029. Mantle cell lymphoma

1030. Follicular lymphoma

1031. Promyelocytic leukemia

DIRECTIONS (Questions 1032 through 1037): Each of the numbered items in this section is followed by answers. Select the ONE lettered answer that is BEST in each case.

1032. In follicular hyperplasia of lymph nodes, there is stimulation of which of the following?

(A) B cells
(B) T cells
(C) endothelial cells
(D) fibroblasts
(E) macrophages

1033. Myeloid metaplasia with myelofibrosis is most likely seen in which of the following pathological processes?

   (A) chronic lymphocytic leukemia
   (B) Hodgkin's disease, nodular sclerosis
   (C) megaloblastic anemia
   (D) polycythemia vera
   (E) refractory anemia

1034. Which type of Hodgkin's disease is known to have a better prognosis?

   (A) immunoblast predominance
   (B) lymphocyte depletion
   (C) lymphocyte predominance
   (D) mixed cellularity
   (E) nodular sclerosis

1035. In which portion of the lymph node is it possible to see a proliferating B cell lymphocyte?

   (A) B cells do not occur in lymph nodes.
   (B) They can be seen in germinal centers.
   (C) They can be seen in the paracortex.
   (D) They can be seen in the postcapillary venules.
   (E) They can be seen in the subcapsular sinus.

1036. Which is/are indicator(s) used for the prognosis in Hodgkin's disease?

   (A) age
   (B) stage
   (C) histologic subtype
   (D) B symptoms
   (E) all of the above

1037. Which is the most common pathological finding in lymph nodes that are close to a malignant neoplasm?

   (A) acute lymphadenitis
   (B) follicular hyperplasia
   (C) granulomatous inflammation
   (D) paracortical hyperplasia
   (E) sinus histiocytosis

DIRECTIONS (Questions 1038 and 1039): For each numbered word or phrase, select the ONE lettered option that is most closely associated with it. Each lettered option may be selected once, more than once, or not at all.

   (A) B cell stimulation
   (B) T cell stimulation
   (C) fibroblast stimulation
   (D) macrophage stimulation
   (E) CD14 markers

1038. Sinus histiocytosis of lymph nodes

1039. Paracortical hyperplasia of lymph nodes

DIRECTIONS (Questions 1040 through 1049): Each of the numbered items in this section is followed by answers. Select the ONE lettered answer that is BEST in each case.

1040. What type of cell is necessary to make the diagnosis of Hodgkin's disease

   (A) eosinophil
   (B) lacunar cell
   (C) Lukes–Collins cell
   (D) plasma cell
   (E) Reed–Sternberg cell

1041. Which type of Hodgkin's disease has the worst prognosis?

   (A) the lymphocytic depletion type
   (B) the lymphocytic predominance type
   (C) the mixed cellularity type
   (D) there is no difference
   (E) the nodular sclerosing type

1042. In Hodgkin's disease, which is the type characterized by the fewest number of Reed–Sternberg cells?

   (A) lymphocyte depleted
   (B) lymphocyte predominant
   (C) mixed cellularity
   (D) nodular sclerosis
   (E) Reed–Sternberg abundant in all

1043. Which type of lymphoma is characterized by the following follicular pattern?

(A) follicular center cell lymphoma

(B) lymphoblastic lymphoma

(C) small (well differentiated) lymphocytic lymphoma

(D) B cell immunoblastic lymphoma

(E) T cell immunoblastic lymphoma

1044. What is the etiological agent of Burkitt's lymphoma?

(A) cytomegalovirus

(B) Epstein–Barr virus

(C) measles virus

(D) papillomavirus

(E) slow virus agent

1045. In mycosis fungoides, the cell origin is which of the following?

(A) B cell disorder

(B) disease of histiocytes

(C) disease of macrophages

(D) disease of myelocytes

(E) disease of CD4+ T cell lymphocytes

1046. Of the following lymphomas, which is the low-grade type?

(A) Burkitt's lymphoma

(B) diffuse, small cleaved cell lymphoma

(C) large-cell immunoblastic lymphoma

(D) lymphoblastic lymphoma

(E) small lymphocytic lymphoma

1047. Which malignant neoplasm of the skin has the worst prognosis?

(A) acral–lentigenous melanoma

(B) basal cell carcinoma

(C) lentigo maligna melanoma

(D) nodular melanoma

(E) squamous cell carcinoma

1048. Merkel cell carcinoma is a malignant neoplasm in which the cell origin is which of the following?

(A) melanocyte

(B) neuralcrest derivative

(C) cell of hair follicle

(D) cell of sebaceous gland

(E) cell of sweat gland

1049. Which is the most likely precursor of squamous cell carcinoma?

(A) drug-induced dermatitis

(B) dysplastic nevus

(C) parakeratosis

(D) seborrheic keratosis

(E) solar (actinic) keratosis

DIRECTIONS (Questions 1050 through 1055): The group of items in this section consists of a list of lettered options followed by a set of numbered words or phrases. For each numbered word or phrase, select the ONE lettered option that is most closely associated with it. Each lettered option may be selected once, more than once, or not at all.

Questions 1050 and 1051

(A) Candida infection

(B) contact dermatitis

(C) drug reaction

(D) herpes virus infection

(E) poxvirus infection

1050. Poison ivy

1051. Shingles

Questions 1052 through 1055

(A) epidermal hyperplasia and parakeratosis

(B) infiltrate at dermal/epidermal junction

(C) inflammation of subcutaneous fat lobules or interlobular septae

(D) intraepidermal vesicles and spongiosis

(E) leukocytoclastic vasculitis

1052. Psoriasis

1053. Contact dermatitis

1054. Lichen planus

1055. Erythema nodosum

DIRECTIONS (Questions 1056 through 1058): Each of the numbered items in this section is followed by answers. Select the ONE lettered answer that is BEST in each case.

1056. What is the most common skin malignant neoplasm in the United States?

(A) basal cell carcinoma

(B) malignant melanoma

(C) Merkel cell tumor (carcinoma)

(D) squamous cell carcinoma

(E) sweat gland carcinoma

1057. What is the most important differential diagnosis in keratoacanthoma?

(A) basal cell carcinoma

(B) malignant melanoma

(C) Merkel cell carcinoma

(D) seborrheic keratosis

(E) squamous cell carcinoma

1058. Linear distribution of IgG, IgM, and C3 along the basement membrane of the epidermis is most typical of which of the following?

(A) psoriasis

(B) atopic dermatitis

(C) dermatitis herpetiformis

(D) lupus erythematosis

(E) erythema nodosum

DIRECTIONS (Questions 1059 through 1071): The group of items in this section consists of a list of lettered options followed by a set of numbered words or phrases. For each numbered word or phrase, select the ONE lettered option that is most closely associated with it. Each lettered option may be selected once, more than once, or not at all.

Questions 1059 through 1061

(A) herpes

(B) ringworm

(C) Rocky Mountain spotted fever

(D) sarcoidosis

(E) scrofula

1059. Tzanck smear

1060. potassium hydroxide preparation

1061. subcutaneous nodules, erythematous plaque

Questions 1062 through 1066

(A) substitution—valine for glutamic acid

(B) hereditary spherocytosis

(C) impaired beta globin synthesis

(D) failure of myeloid stem cell

(E) most common form of hemolytic anemia

1062. Spectrin deficiency

1063. Sickle cell disease

1064. Aplastic anemia

1065. Warm antibody hemolytic anemia

1066. Beta-thalassemias

Questions 1067 through 1071

(A) fibrous obliteration of marrow

(B) symptoms related to an increase in red cell mass

(C) ringed sideroblasts

(D) Philadelphia chromosome

(E) polycythemia

1067. Myeloproliferative syndrome

1068. Myelodysplastic syndrome

1069. Polycythemia vera

1070. Myelofibrosis with myeloid metaplasia

1071. Chronic myelogenous leukemia

Answers and Explanations

1011. **(A)** Anemia of chronic disease is common in chronic infections, as well as such other inflammatory chronic processes as rheumatoid arthritis and systemic lupus erythematosis. Renal diseases are also frequently accompanied by this type of anemia. In general, it is normocytic normochromic, but it could be hypochromic. Ferritin levels are either normal or high. It is believed that this type of anemia is caused by shortening of the erythrocytes length of life and poor utilization of iron. The other anemias listed do not have these characteristics. *(Rubin and Farber, p. 1073)*

1012. **(C)** Anemia secondary to deficiency of B_{12} and folate are characterized by defective synthesis of DNA. The cells that can be studied on the bone marrow smears show a characteristic change in the morphology, such as abnormally large cells, which leads to an increase in mean corpuscular volumes. Other changes that can be seen in megaloblastic anemia are hypersegmentation of the polymorphonuclear cells and changes in the erythroid precursors in which the nucleus and the cytoplasm have a disassociation with respect to maturation. *(Cotran et al., pp. 621–623)*

1013. **(D)** Anemia produced by iron deficiency is one of the most common causes of a decrease in red cell volume. Approximately 80% of the total iron found in the body is present in the hemoglobin, myoglobin, and iron-containing enzymes. The storage of iron is in the form of ferritin or hemosiderin. One milligram of iron is required to maintain normal iron stores to cover the needs of metabolism. This should be absorbed from the diet on a daily basis. When there is not enough iron, either by diet deficiency or problems with reabsorption, increased requirements, or blood loss, it leads to hypochromic microcytic anemia. This depletion of iron-containing enzymes is reflected better in the morphology than can be seen in the bone marrow smears. Also, an increase in the number of normoblasts is noted, with no evidence of iron staining in the cells. On examination of the peripheral blood, the red cells are smaller and with less chromatin (hypochromic). The small size of the red cells leads to a decrease in corpuscular volume. *(Cotran et al., pp. 627–630)*

1014. **(C)** Refer to Answer 1013.

1015. **(D)** Refer to Answer 1013.

1016. **(A)** Refer to Answer 1011.

1017. **(E)** In diseases in which the marrow is destroyed or replaced in large amounts, a form of marrow failure is produced and is known as myelophthisic anemia. To compensate for daily requirements, the marrow release on the peripheral blood immature forms of the red cells, as well as the white cells, which are known as leukoerythroblastosis. In addition, release of these immature cells in the peripheral blood is thought to be secondary to the destruction of the microenvironment of the marrow. Myelophthisic anemia can occur in any kind of metastatic tumor that replaces, in large portion, as well as the marrow in multiple myeloma, leukemia, myelofibrosis, and so forth. *(Cotran et al., p. 632)*

1018. **(D)** A major form of megaloblastic anemia is attributable to deficiency of B_{12}. In this type of anemia, there is an impaired synthesis of DNA, which leads to distinctly morphological features of the peripheral blood characterized by elevated mean corpuscular volume, as well as morphological changes of the marrow elements, which have been explained in question 2. The daily requirement for vitamin B_{12} is 2–3 mg and is not present in plants and vegetables. Absorption requires intrinsic factors that are secreted by the parietal cells of the gastric mucosa. Vitamin B_{12} deficiency can be produced by inadequate intake, problems with the absorption by impaired gastric mucosa, exocrine pancreatic function, parasitic infestation, and other diseases. Vitamin B_{12} deficiency is also very close in correlation with the folic acid, because the administration of folic acid improves the B_{12} deficiency anemia. *(Cotran et al., pp. 621–626)*

1019. **(A)** The lymphomas that originate in the B cells are the most common type of lymphomas. The B lymphocytes constitute approximately 15–20% of the circulating peripheral lymphocytes. They are also present in the lymph nodes, spleen, tonsils, and bone marrow. In the lymph nodes, they are mainly seen in the germinal centers and in the white pulp in the spleen. B cells, which are in charge of the humoral immunity upon stimulation from the T cells, mature into plasma cells that secrete immunoglobulins. *(Chandrasoma and Taylor, pp. 449–453)*

1020. **(A)** Refer to Answer 1019. *(Chandrasoma and Taylor, pp. 449–453)*

1021. **(B)** Mycosis fungoides and Sezary syndrome seem to be a manifestation of a single process characterized by neoplastic transformation of T lymphocytes, which are CD4+. In mycosis fungoides, different stages of the disease have been described with a premycotic phase that progresses to a plaque phase and finally to the tumorstage. Sezary syndrome is a variant characterized by generalized exfoliative erythroderma. This skin manifestation is usually associated with leukemia cells in the peripheral blood. These peripheral T cell neoplasms are of indolent clinical behavior with a long-term survival. *(Chandrasoma and Taylor, pp. 453–454)*

1022. **(E)** The neoplasm that originates in the plasma cells is referred to as plasma cell dyscrasias. The B cells have, after stimulation, a differentiation into plasma cells that secrete immunoglobulins for the humoral immunity. The production of immunoglobulin, coupled with the heavy and light chains, is always well balanced. When a neoplasm on the plasma cells occurs, this balance is broken, which leads to an overproduction of light or heavy chains. This is manifested in the serum by monoclonal gammopathies, dysproteinemia, and paraproteinemia. Multiple myeloma is the most important and most common disorder of the neoplastic transformation of the plasma cells. Clinically, it is characterized by neoplastic replacement of the bone marrow throughout the entire skeletal system. *(Cotran et al., pp. 663–666)*

1023. **(D)** Tumors that originate in these cells (histiocytes and monocytes) are exceedingly rare. The cell type must be done with specific markers, for such monocytes/histiocytes antibodies as CD68, CD11. Clinically, histiocytic lymphomas are aggressive and refractory to treatment. Morphologically, the neoplastic cells exhibit an enlarged nucleus with prominent nucleoli and clump chromatin distribution. The cytoplasm is scanty, granular, and eosinophilic. *(Chandrasoma and Taylor, p. 460)*

1024. **(B)** Mantle cell lymphoma is a rare type of B cell lymphoma that accounts for 3–5% of all non-Hodgkin's lymphomas. The origin of these tumor cells is located on the mantle area of the germinal centers and contains characteristic molecular abnormalities. The morphology of the lymphoma could be nodular or diffuse pattern. The cells are rather monotonous, small with irregular nuclear membrane. On the peripheral blood in up to 40% of the cases, we can see lymphoma cells circulating. Mantle cell lymphoma frequently shows 11:14 translocation. This alteration is known as a

BCL1, and is detected in about 70% of the cases. BCL1 encodes cyclin D₁, which is a protein involved in the regulation of the G1 to S phase. The prognosis of mantle cell lymphoma is rather poor, with a median survival of 3–4 years. (*Cotran et al., pp. 667–668*)

1025. **(B)** Infection with EB virus is transmitted by close human contact. The clinical picture of infectious mononucleosis is that of a disease that is characterized by fever, generalized lymphadenopathy, sore throat, and splenomegaly. On examination of the peripheral blood, there is a lymphocytosis with atypical lymphocytes. These cells are proved to be activated T cells. The virus attacks the epithelial cells as well as the B lymphocytes. On examination of the peripheral blood, the atypical lymphocytes represent suppressor T lymphocytes, characteristic of this disease. Such lymphoid organs spleen and lymph nodes are enlarged and for the most part, the architecture is usually preserved, but occasional cells resembling Reed–Sternberg cells can be found. Focal areas of necrosis can also be present. The final diagnosis of this disease is over specific findings such as lymphocytosis with the atypical lymphoid cells previously described, a positive heterophil reaction (monospot test), and specific antibodies for EBV antigens. (*Cotran et al., pp. 371–372*)

1026. **(E)** Follicular lymphoma is the most common form of non-Hodgkin's lymphoma in the United States. It affects men and women equally and is less common in Europe and rare in Asia. The cell origin of this tumor resembles the cells of the germinal centers. Morphologically, we observe small and larger cells. These contain cleaved nucleus (indentations of the nuclear membrane) and protrusions. They cytoplasm is scant, and the nucleoli is not prominent. Immunologically these cells, typed as B cells with markers express CD19, CD20, and CD10. In contrast with Mantle cell lymphoma and small lymphocytic neoplasms of B cell origin, CD5 is not expressed. BCL2, which is a protein that is negative in the normal follicular center, is expressed in follicular neoplasms. There is a characteristic 14:18 translocation, and this translocation leads to an overexpression of BCL2 protein. On clinical aspect, the overall median survival of this tumor is 7–9 years. (*Cotran et al., pp. 659–661*)

1027. **(B)** Auer rods, which represent abnormal azurophilic granules, aggregate to form rod-like structures in the cytoplasm of the leukemic cells of a bright red color. With special stains, Auer rods are intensely positive for peroxidase. The presence of Auer rods in the cytoplasm of the leukemic has been considered evidence of myeloid differentiation. (*Rubin and Farber, pp. 1117–1119*)

1028. **(A)** Burkitt's lymphoma is a B cell neoplasm composed of small, noncleaved cells. These tumors are considered high grade, and they present as rapidly progressive neoplasms. Morphologically, the tumor cells show a round nucleus with a blue cytoplasm. In many areas of the tumor, we can see interspace on the tumor cells, benign macrophages with phagocytized material. This gives the appearance is of the "starry sky" pattern. The lymphocytes stain for B cell markers and also contain a characteristic chromosomal abnormality—the translocation of the proto-oncogene C-myc on chromosome 8 to chromosome 14. Two forms of Burkitt's lymphoma have been described: the endemic type seen in Africa and parts of New Guinea, in which EB virus is identified in 95% of the cases; and the sporadic Burkitt's lymphoma or American Burkitt's lymphoma, in which only 15% are positive for EB virus. (*Rubin and Farber, pp. 1138–1139*)

1029. **(C)** Refer to Answer 1024. (*Cotran et al., pp. 667–668*)

1030. **(D)** Refer to Answer 1019. (*Cotran et al., pp. 1135–1136*)

1031. **(E)** Promyelocytic leukemia (M3) morphologically shows the leukemia cells having abundant eosinophilic cytoplasm with numerous Auer rods. Clinically, this leukemia may develop disseminated intravascular coagulation, secondary to the release of cytoplasmic granules or Auer rods. Another characteristic of this leukemia is that it often shows the translocation 15,17, which disrupts the retinoic acid receptor genes. This leukemia is treated with all-transretinal acid, which causes the promyelocytes to be differentiated into neutrophils. Other recent modalities of treatment have been the use of arsenic trioxide. *(Rubin and Farber, p. 1119)*

1032. **(A)** Chronic reactive nonspecific lymphadenitis is characterized for changes that can be related to the different compartments. These include, follicular hyperplasia, paracortical lymphoid hyperplasia, or sinus histiocytosis. When we have follicular hyperplasia, the etiologic factor could be an inflammatory bacterial process that stimulates the B cells. The nuclear and cytoplasmic structures in these stimulated cells change from small resting B lymphocytes to larger and more active cells. In addition to bacterial infections, other diseases can stimulate the follicular centers. Such systemic diseases as rheumatoid arthritis, toxoplasmosis, and HIV infections can produce similar reactions. It is important to distinguish between follicular hyperplasia and follicular lymphoma. *(Cotran et al., pp. 649–650)*

1033. **(D)** Refer to Answer 1068. *(Cotran et al., pp. 682–683)*

1034. **(C)** Hodgkin's disease is a malignant neoplasm characterized by the presence of large binucleated cells called Reed–Sternberg cells in an appropriate cellular setting in the background. It primarily affects the lymph nodes, but also extralymphoid Hodgkin's disease could occur. The classic classification of Hodgkin's disease has been into four different types; lymphocytic predominance, mixed cellularity, lymphocytic depletion, and nodular sclerosis. The lymphocytic predominance of Hodgkin's disease morphologically is presented by an abundance of lymphocytes accompanied by a variants of Reed–Sternberg cells, which have been called LH (lymphocytic and histiocytic) cells. These cells express B cell markers, which is unique to this variant of Hodgkin's disease and positive

for CD45 (leukocytic antigen). They are usually negative for such Hodgkin's disease classic markers such CD15 (Leu-M1) and CD30 (Ki-1). Classically, this disease is predominant in young males, and the most common areas affected are in the cervical lymph nodes, as well as in other locations, symptoms are usually absent. Prognosis of lymphocytic predominant Hodgkin's disease is the best of the four. *(Rubin and Farber, p. 1146)*

1035. **(B)** Refer to Answer 1032. *(Cotran et al., pp. 649–650)*

1036. **(E)** Staging of Hodgkin's disease seems to be one of the most important factors for prognosis of this disease. Classically, the 5-year survival rate in stages I and IIA is close to 90%. Other important parameter in the prognosis are the histological subtype in which lymphocytic depletion seems to be the worst, and age, which is very closely related to the histologic subtype, because the worse prognosis of Hodgkin's disease is seen in the second pick of the age incidence and is also related to the B symptoms that appear in the presentation of the disease. *(Cotran et al., pp. 670–673)*

1037. **(E)** Sinus histiocytosis is hyperplasia of the endothelial lining of the sinusoids that become dilated and contain many histiocytes. This reaction, which is also called reticular hyperplasia, has become very prominent in lymph nodes when in draining cancerous process. This is particularly common in the axillary nodes when cancer of the breast has been detected. It is thought to represent a reaction or an immune response to the host against the tumor products. *(Cotran at al., p. 650)*

1038. **(D)** Refer to Answer 1036. *(Cotran et al., p. 650)*

1039. **(B)** In normal lymph nodes, the paracortical area is predominantly composed of T cells. When there is a reaction in these regions, the paracortical area becomes enlarged, and it encroaches upon the B cell of the follicular areas. When these T cells become activated, the nucleus enlarges, shows a prominent nucleoli, and the cytoplasm is abundant. These are called immunoblasts. Changes of these types are encountered in immunological reactions produced by drugs, viral infections, or cases of infectious mononucleosis. *(Cotran et al., p. 650)*

1040. **(E)** The Reed–Sternberg cells can be classified as the classic type, the mononuclear variants, the lymphocytic histiocytic variant, lacunar, and pleomorphic variant. The classic Reed–Sternberg cell is a binucleated cell that contains an ovoid-shaped nucleus with regular contours and prominent eosinophilic nucleoli. The cytoplasm is abundant and eosinophilic. On cytogenetic studies, the Reed–Sternberg cells are either aneuploid or frequently hypertetraploid. The classic Reed–Sternberg cell is thought to be an end-stage cell that does not divide. The mononuclear variants of the Reed–Sternberg cell so-called "Hodgkin's cell" could be identified in any subtype of Hodgkin's disease, but they are not diagnostic of Hodgkin's. The histological appearance is similar to the Reed–Sternberg cell, but with only one nucleus. In the lymphocytic predominance variant of Hodgkin's disease, the Reed–Sternberg cell shows a multilobed nucleus (popcorn nucleus) with inconspicuous nucleoli. These cells, on immunoperoxidase staining, are different from the classic Reed–Sternberg cells, in that they contain B cell markers. The lacunar variants of the nodular sclerosing type of Hodgkin's disease is confined into a clear space (lacuna). The cell inside of the lacuna could be mononuclear or typical binucleated Reed–Sternberg cell. On the pleomorphic variant, the cells exhibit a multiple nucleus with prominent eosinophilic nucleoli. *(Rubin and Farber, p. 1142)*

1041. **(A)** Clinically, these represent the most aggressive form of Hodgkin's disease. In general, it is present in middle age to elderly men. At the time of diagnosis, it is usually at an advanced stage (III or IV) with "B" symptoms. The overall cure rate for lymphocytic

depleted Hodgkin's disease is approximately 40–50%. Morphologically, it is characterized by an abundance of Reed–Sternberg cells; whereas, the lymphocytes are very scattered and sparse. *(Rubin and Farber, p. 1146)*

1042. **(B)** Lymphocytic predominant Hodgkin's disease, which has been subdivided into nodular and diffuse subtypes, is the most indolent and better prognosis of Hodgkin's diseases. The Reed–Sternberg cells are very rare and sometimes require multiple sections to find the classic Reed–Sternberg cell. Variants of Reed–Sternberg cells generally show markers of B cell, with a positive marker for CD19, 20, and 23. In addition, they show markers for CD45 (leukocytic common antigen). For this reason and the fact that they are negative for the traditional markers of Hodgkin's disease such as CD15 and CD30, this category of Hodgkin's disease is considered separate. *(Rubin and Farber, p. 1142)*

1043. **(A)** Refer to Answer 1026. *(Rubin and Farber, pp., 1135–1136)*

1044. **(B)** Refer to Answer 1028. *(Rubin and Farber, pp. 1138–1139)*

1045. **(E)** Refer to Answer 1021. *(Chandrasoma and Taylor, pp. 453–454)*

1046. **(E)** Small lymphocytic lymphoma is a neoplastic proliferation of the small lymphocytes that morphologically and phenotypically are indistinguishable from chronic lymphocytic leukemia. The morphology of this process is a replacement of the normal lymph node architecture by a diffuse proliferation of the small lymphocytes with very condensed chromatin pattern and indiscernible cytoplasm. Occasionally, we may see areas wherein the cells become slightly enlarged, and these are called proliferation centers. The clinical features show that most of the patients are elderly and have been asymptomatic for a long time; they generally present with lymphadenopathy, as well as splenomegaly. The prognosis of this neoplasm is variable, but patients that present with small tumor burden may survive for more than 10 years. Transformation of this process into a more aggressive B cell lymphoma is seen in about 10% of patients. *(Rubin and Farber, p. 1135)*

1047. **(D)** Malignant melanoma, which is a neoplasm of the skin and could also originate in other internal organs, is most commonly seen in areas exposed to sunlight. Although asymptomatic in the very early stages, it exhibits gross subtle changes that may sound an alert for early diagnosis, such as uneven discoloration, borders, size, and symmetry. The growth pattern of the malignant melanoma is also important in the diagnosis. Those with nodular-type with vertical growth are the worst prognosis. Different levels of infiltration of the epidermis is also very important when considering therapy, as well as prognosis. *(Cotran et al., pp. 1178–1179)*

1048. **(B)** Merkel cell carcinoma originates in the neuroendocrine cells of the skin situated in the basal epidermis. It usually occurs in patients over the age of 60 and histologically is composed of small cells with scant cytoplasm. The nucleus contains a chromatin with inconspicuous nucleoli. The cells are slightly ovoid, and they grow in nests and may infiltrate in individual cells. Histologically, they resemble the small cell anaplastic carcinoma of the lung. The confirmation of a Merkel cell carcinoma of the skin is with the finding of neurosecretory granules in the cytoplasm either by electron microscopy or immunoperoxidase markers such as neuron special enolase or chromogranin. *(Chandrasoma and Taylor, p. 894)*

1049. **(E)** Squamous cell carcinoma, which is the most common tumor arising on sun exposed areas in elderly patients, has a higher incidence in men than in women. The predisposing factors for this lesion in addition to sunlight are industrial carcinogens, chronic ulcerations, burns, scars, and ionizing radiation. However, the most accepted exogenous cause of squamous cell carcinoma is exposure to ultraviolet light with subsequent DNA damage and is associated with chromosomal mutations. *(Cotran et al., p. 1184)*

1050. **(B)** Poison ivy is an allergic contact dermatitis to a cell-mediated hypersensitivity reaction in the skin. This is the most common cause of contact dermatitis caused by exposure to various plants. Morphological changes show that the epidermal keratinocytes are separated from the subjacent corneum creating a sponge-like appearance. The stratum corneum contains coagulated proteins. Numerous inflammatory cells and, most prominently, eosinophils are present. The vesicles contain lymphocytes and macrophages. *(Rubin and Farber, p. 1271)*

1051. **(D)** Herpes infections are produced by a DNA virus that encompasses a few distinct diseases. Varicella-zoster virus produces two distinct diseases: chicken pox and herpes zoster. These are restricted to humans and spread from person-to-person primarily by the respiratory route. Pathologically, skin lesions of shingles (zoster) are indistinguishable from the chicken pox lesions. They form a vesicle that is filled with neutrophils and further erodes to become an ulceration. Multinucleated giant cells and nuclear inclusions are present. *(Rubin and Farber, pp. 366–367)*

1052. **(A)** Psoriasis is a chronic inflammatory disease of the skin (dermatosis) that affects 1–2% of the population of the United States. Clinically, it most frequently affects the skin on the elbows, knees, skull, and lumbosacral areas. Morphologically, it shows an atypical lesion that is well demarcated, pink, and covered by loosely adherent scales of a silver-white color. The histological sections demonstrate epidermal hyperplasia, parakeratotic scales, and minute microabscesses of neutrophils. A chronic inflammatory cell infiltration is present in the papillary dermis. *(Cotran et al., pp. 1198–1199)*

1053. **(D)** Refer to Answer 1049. *(Rubin and Farber, p. 1271)*

1054. **(B)** Lichen planus is a self-limited lesion and generally resolves spontaneously in 1 or 2 years after onset. It affects the skin as well as the mucous membranes. Cutaneous lesions are usually itchy and violaceous in color. On histological sections, it is characterized by an infiltrate of lymphocytes along the dermal–epidermal junction. These lymphocytes show a very close relationship to the basal cells, which undergo necrosis, and these necrotic cells are carried up from the basal layer to the inflammatory papillary dermis are referred to as colloid or Civatte bodies. *(Cotran et al., pp. 1199–1200)*

1055. **(C)** Erythema nodosum is a panniculitis that is an inflammatory reaction of the subcutaneous fat and connective tissue septa. Erythema nodosum is the most common form of panniculitis. The histological sections of erythema nodosum are distinctive. The connective tissue septa that divides the adipose tissue is edematous, widened, and neutrophil infiltration is present. Later in the disease, the infiltration changes for lymphocytes, histiocytes, and multinucleated giant cells. Occasional eosinophils may be seen. Vasculitis is not present. *(Cotran et al., pp. 1207–1208)*

1056. **(A)** Basal cell carcinoma is the most common cancer of the skin in the United States. This neoplasm also occurs on sun-exposed areas in light pigmented people. The clinical presentation is variable from pearly white papules to pigmented lesions and telangiectatic nodules. On microscopic examination, they are formed by cells that resemble the basal layer of the epidermis. They are arranged in clusters and irregular nests with peripheral palisading. These nests are separated by delicate bands of fibrous tissue with discreet chronic inflammatory infiltrate. This tumor is characterized by having a local aggressive behavior, which recurs if it is not completely excised. Metastasis are rare. *(Cotran et al., p. 1186)*

1057. **(E)** Keratoacanthoma is a rapidly developing neoplasm that is circumscribed and histologically resembles well-differentiated kera-tinizing squamous cell carcinoma. A characteristic of this lesion is, if left alone, it will heal spontaneously. On gross examination, it appears to be flesh colored and dome-shaped with a central area of keratin-filled plugs. On microscopic examination, it is characterized by a central keratin-filled crater surrounded by epidermis that extends to the side, forming a collarette. The epithelium is composed of large keratinocytes with abundant keratinization of the cytoplasm and characteristic glassy appearance. The tumor appears to be infiltrating in the superficial layers of the collagen and elastic fibers. In the beginning, the lesion is devoid of inflammatory cells; however, as the lesion ages, it becomes surrounded by inflammatory cells, mostly lymphocytes. *(Cotran et al., pp. 1181)*

1058. **(D)** One of the manifestations of systemic lupus erythematosus is the involvement of the skin. This type of lupus is called discoid lupus erythematosus, characterized by scaly, circumscribed lesions with zones of hypopigmentation or hyperpigmentation. On histological findings, the lesion is characterized by a perivascular and periappengeal infiltrates mostly composed of lymphocytes and extending to the dermal–epidermal junction. Hyperkeratosis is present, involving the hair follicles. Characteristics on direct immunofluorescence show a granular band of immunoglobulin for IgG, IgM, and C3. It is seen in the dermal–epidermal and follicular junctions. *(Cotran et al., pp. 1200–1201)*

1059. **(A)** Herpes infections can be diagnosed with the Tzanck test, which is a microscopic examination of the vesicular fluid. The vesicles and shallow ulcerations contain the virus, and in a touch prep made on a glass slide and properly stained, will demonstrate the multinucleated giant cells of the paracytized cells by the virus. These intranuclear inclusions could be seen not only on the multinucleated giant cells, but also in single cells with a ground glass appearance of the nucleus. *(Cotran et al., p. 757)*

1060. **(B)** In dermatophyte infections, tinea (ringworm) are a group of fungi that infect the keratin of a stratum corneum of the hair and nails. They do not penetrate deeper parts of the skin. Clinically, the lesion is characterized by circular and elevated red scaly lesions that may exudate fluid. They may affect different parts of the body (tinea corporis), the groin (tinea cruris), or the feet (tinea pedis). The diagnosis is confirmed by scraping one of the infected areas and, mounted under a cover slip, adding potassium hydroxide, which dissolves the keratin. Then, the mycelial fungi can be seen. *(Chandrasoma and Taylor, p. 882)*

1061. **(D)** Sarcoidosis is a systemic granulomatous disease of unknown etiology. Because it is a systemic disease, almost any organ of the body can be affected; most prominently the lungs, lymph nodes, and skin. The skin lesions are seen in one-third to one-half of the cases. When sarcoidosis is present in the skin, it shows different microscopic appearances, such as discrete subcutaneous nodules elevated erythematous plaques, as well as flat lesions. These lesions may also appear in the mucous membranes in the oral cavity. On histologic sections, the characteristics of non-caseating granulomas are present. *(Cotran et al., pp. 734–725)*

1062. **(B)** This disorder is characterized by an intrinsic defect of the red cell membrane that, in turn, makes the red cells become spheroidal. This deformation of the membrane makes it vulnerable to sequestration and destruction in the spleen. The changes that occur in the red cells that make the change from flat to spheroidal are the deficiency of spectrin which is a protein that acts in the membrane of the cytoskeleton of the red cells. *(Cotran et al., p. 607)*

1063. **(A)** Sickle cell disease is a hereditary hemoglobinopathy characterized by deformity of the red cells, secondary to structural changes of the hemoglobin. Because of a lack of oxygen in this type of hemoglobin, molecules undergo aggregation and polymerization. This changes the hemoglobin from a free-flowing liquid to a viscous gel, leading to deformity of the red cells. The facts are sec-

ondary to a substitution of valine for glutamic acid on the sixth position of the beta-globulin chain. *(Cotran et al., p. 611)*

1064. **(D)** The basis of the aplastic anemia is a failure of the multipotent myeloid stem cells in the production of differentiated cell lines. It could be acquired or inherited. A long list of the major causes of aplastic anemia include, idiopathic, chemical agents, physical agents, viral infections, and miscellaneous others. Morphology of the bone marrow in aplastic anemia is markedly hypocellular, and the marrow spaces are replaced by adipose tissue; although, a few marrow elements can still be identified, accompanied by a few lymphocytes and mature plasma cells. The prognosis of aplastic anemia is related to the etiologic factor. *(Cotran et al., p. 630)*

1065. **(E)** Hemolytic anemias are characterized by a shortening of the normal red cell life span, accumulation of the products of the hemoglobin catabolism, and a marked increase in erythropoiesis within the bone marrow, to compensate for the loss of red cells. Warm antibody hemolytic anemia is the most common form of hemolytic anemia. In about 50% of patients, the etiology is unknown, and in the other 50%, an etiology factor can be identified, creating an antibody that binds to the red cells. The red cells are taken and destroyed by splenic macrophages. Because the spleen becomes very active in this disease, generally there is moderate splenomegaly. *(Cotran et al., p. 620)*

1066. **(C)** In beta-thalassemias, a marked reduction of normal beta-globin chains is present. There are no abnormalities on the synthesis of alpha-chains. The beta-thalassemias can then be divided into two different groups: one that has a total absence of beta-globin, and another has a markedly reduced beta-globin. Impaired synthesis of the beta-globin produces anemia by two different mechanisms, lack of adequate HbA formation and, therefore, the concentration of hemoglobin in the cells is lower, and the morphology is that of a hypochromic red cell. In addition, the red cells can be affected on their survival span, as well as their precursors. The mechanism is secondary to the accumulation of alpha-globin chains accumulated in the cytoplasm of the red cells, as well as red cell precursors because of the lack of normal Beta chains to bind to. These inclusions damage the cell membranes and reduce their plasticity. In this form, the cells undergo apoptosis in the bone marrow and phagocytosis in the spleen. (Cotran et al., pp. 615–616)

1067.   (E) There are four disorders known as myeloproliferative disorders. These are chronic myelogenous leukemia, polycythemia vera, essential thrombocytosis, and myelofibrosis with myeloid metaplasia. Polycythemia vera is a neoplasm that originates in a multipotent myeloid stem cell. The characteristic of this syndrome is overproduction of erythroid, granulocytic, and megakaryocytic elements. This is also seen in the peripheral blood as an increase of all of the elements mentioned. Although the cause of polycythemia vera has not been established, it is believed that many growth factors affect the hemopoietic stem cells in different pathways, rendering them hyperactive. The erythropoietin levels in polycythemia vera are not elevated. The morphology of the bone marrow is hypercellular with an increase in erythroid series, but there is also an increase in the precursors of the granulocytic series and megakaryocytes. If the disease progresses, an increase in fibrous tissue of the marrow is present, at which time the development of extramedullary hematopoiesis increases, in the spleen, liver, and lymph nodes. On the clinical course, the most important symptoms are related to the expansion of the red cells. (Cotran et al., p. 679)

1068.   (C) Myelodysplastic syndrome is a group of bone marrow stem cell disorders characterized by maturation defects and results in ineffective hematopoiesis. In myelodysplastic syndrome, there is a high risk of transformation into acute myelogenous leukemia. Many different types of myelodysplastic syndromes have been defined, and these are related to the count of the immature cells in the bone marrow. Many abnormalities in the

blood are present that include ringed sideroblasts. These elements are erythroid precursors containing iron in the mitochondria that is visible with special stains as a perinuclear aggregate. Other changes that can be seen in the bone marrow biopsy are pseudo-Pelger–Huet anomaly. These are polymorphonuclear cells with only two nuclear lobes. The white cells show a hypo- or hypergranularity with giant forms. The red precursors could be bilobed or with deformities of the nuclear membranes. The megakaryocytes show either mononuclear forms, micro forms, or abnormal polylobed forms. (Cotran et al., p. 678)

1069.   (B) Refer to Answer 1066. The changes are related to the high hematocrit that is seen in the peripheral blood with decrease of the blood flow, vascular distention, congestion, and stasis. A high percentage of the patients are hypertensive, with headaches, dizziness, and gastrointestinal symptoms. The abnormal blood flow previously mentioned, produces an increased risk of bleeding and thrombotic episodes. (Cotran et al., p. 682)

1070.   (A) Myelofibrosis by definition is a myeloproliferative syndrome that is histologically characterized by an increase in fibrous tissue and obliteration of the marrow spaces, with a decrease in the amount of myeloid cells. The replacement of the marrow spaces by fibrous tissue is thought to be secondary to two factors that are derived from the platelets. These are the platelet derivative growth factor and the transforming growth factor-beta. These proteins, which are synthesized by the megakaryocytes, stimulate the fibrosed tissue and cause angiogenesis. Once the myelofibrosis process is established, a myeloid metaplasia is seen in the spleen, as well as such other potential hematopoietic elements as liver and extramedullary hematopoiesis of the lymph nodes. (Cotran et al., pp. 683–684)

1071.   (D) This leukemia is characterized by the presence of a molecular abnormality that is the translocation involving the BCR gene of chromosome 9 and the ABL gene on chromosome 22. The Philadelphia chromosome is characteristic of this type of leukemia, which can be demonstrated in more than 90% of the cases. On the molecular level, this represents a balance and reciprocal translocation. With this translocation, a hybrid gene is formed that encodes a unique protein that enhances thymosin kinase activity. A new and exciting report of therapeutic agents (Glevax) has been on trial for 3 years with more than amazing results. *(Cotran et al., p. 680)*

REFERENCES

Chandrasoma P, Taylor CR. *Concise Pathology,* 3rd ed. Norwalk, CT: Appleton & Lange, 1998.

Cotran RS, Kumar V, Robbins SL. *Robbins Pathologic Basis of Disease,* 6th ed. Philadelphia: Saunders, 1999.

Rubin E, Farber JL. *Pathology.* Philadelphia: Lippincott, 1999.

CHAPTER 16

Bone, Joints, and Soft Tissue

The 206 bones that compose the normal skeleton serve different functions in the body: mechanical support, protection of internal structures, and harboring the hematopoietic elements for normal production of the cellular elements of the blood. Moreover, it plays a very important role in the metabolism, particularly minerals, for the control of the calcium, phosphorous, and minerals. The bones can be divided by form, as well as their embryologic origin. The composition is of a heavy mineralized matrix, which is mostly composed of collagen type I, and for three types of cells that originate in the pluripotential osteal progenitor cell. These cells are the osteoblasts responsible for production of the collagen type I and the formation of osteoid that will eventually mineralize and form the lamellar bone. Osteocytes are the cells that mature and remain embedded in the mineralized collagen, but maintain their connection with "neighbor" cells by a dendritic process through system of canniculae. Finally, the osteoclasts are multinucleated cells, whose basic function is bone reabsorption. Throughout their entire life, the bones undergo remodeling with reabsorption and production of new bone. The questions in this chapter related to bone will be of the most common processes that affect the skeletal system, such as inflammatory process, metabolic process, and benign and malignant neoplasms. Furthermore, we emphasize pathologic changes in the joints, which will include the synovium and the most important processes that affect the capsule, the synovium, and articular cartilage, which include crystal depositions, inflammatory process, neoplasms, and degenerative processes.

For the soft tissues, we especially consider tumors and tumor-like lesions. Because these are mesenchymal derivatives, the proliferations occur elsewhere in the body, as well as in the internal viscera. Their benign and malignant counterparts try to recopilate the adipose tissue, fibrous tissue, skeletal muscle, smooth muscle, nerves, and vessels. Sarcomas, the malignant neoplasms of the soft tissue, contain general features that make them distinct from their epithelial counterparts.

Questions

DIRECTIONS (Questions 1072 and 1073): Each of the numbered items in this section is followed by answers. Select the ONE lettered answer that is BEST in each case.

1072. The major pathologic change in degenerative joint disease occurs in which of the following?

   (A) articular bone
   (B) articular cartilage
   (C) capsule
   (D) synovium
   (E) tendon

1073. Subcutaneous nodules in and around the joints are most characteristic of patients with which of the following?

   (A) bacterial arthritis
   (B) degenerative joint disease (osteoarthritis)
   (C) psoriasis
   (D) rheumatoid arthritis
   (E) tuberculous arthritis

DIRECTIONS (Questions 1074 through 1076): For each numbered word or phrase, select the ONE lettered option that is most closely associated with it. Each lettered option may be selected once, more than once, or not at all.

   (A) degenerative joint disease (osteoarthritis)
   (B) gout
   (C) infectious arthritis
   (D) rheumatoid arthritis
   (E) viral arthritis

1074. Commonly affects the knee joint

1075. Pannus

1076. Most common joint disease

DIRECTIONS (Questions 1077 through 1094): Each of the numbered items in this section is followed by answers. Select the ONE lettered answer that is BEST in each case.

1077. A child develops chills, temperature of 102°, and a painful swollen knee. What test will you order to resolve this clinical problem?

   (A) culture of joint fluid from the affected knee
   (B) Lyme disease test
   (C) magnetic resonance imaging
   (D) serum protein electrophoresis
   (E) study the crystals in synovial fluid

1078. Most commonly osteosarcomas metastasize hematogenously to which of the following?

   (A) brain
   (B) liver
   (C) lungs
   (D) regional nodes
   (E) spleen

1079. Chondromas are tumors composed most of which of the following?

   (A) cortical bone
   (B) periosteum
   (C) fibrous tissues
   (D) cartilage
   (E) nonmineralized bone matrix

1080. Osteonecrosis (avascular necrosis) results from which of the following?

(A) fracture
(B) corticosteroids
(C) thrombosis and embolism
(D) venous hypertension
(E) all of the above

1081. What age group is more affected by osteosarcoma?

(A) 5- to 10-year-old females
(B) 10- to 20-year-old males
(C) 40- to 60-year-old females
(D) males 75 years old or older
(E) anyone regardless of age or sex

1082. Multiple myeloma is a neoplastic proliferation of which of the following?

(A) endothelial cells
(B) plasma cells
(C) T-lymphocytes
(D) NK cells
(E) epithelial cells

1083. Periosteal elevation in osteosarcoma is radiologically identified as which of the following?

(A) O ring sign
(B) exostosis
(C) nidus
(D) Codman's triangle
(E) sequestrum

1084. Where do 60% of osteogenic sarcomas arise?

(A) sternum
(B) skull
(C) spine
(D) pelvic bones
(E) metaphyseal ends of distal femur and proximal tibia

1085. A benign bone tumor that arises on subperiosteal or endosteal surfaces is which of the following?

(A) osteoma
(B) osteoid osteoma
(C) osteoblastoma
(D) chondroma
(E) Ewing's tumor

1086. Radiologically, "onion skin" is a radiologic term used for which of the following?

(A) lymphoma of bone
(B) metastatic carcinoma
(C) chondrosarcoma
(D) osteoblastoma
(E) Ewing's sarcoma

1087. The bone neoplasm that causes nocturnal pain and is dramatically relieved by aspirin is which of the following?

(A) osteochondroma
(B) osteoid osteoma
(C) osteosarcoma
(D) metastatic carcinoma
(E) multiple myeloma

1088. Approximately 85% of which of the following tumors show a translocation of chromosomes 11 and 22?

(A) Ewing's sarcoma
(B) osteosarcoma
(C) osteoblastoma
(D) metastatic carcinoma
(E) multiple myeloma

1089. Which bone neoplasm is least likely to produce bone?

(A) chondrosarcoma
(B) giant cell tumor
(C) osteosarcoma
(D) osteochondroma
(E) osteoid osteoma

1090. Of the following benign soft-tissue tumors, which is considered more aggressive?

   (A) ganglion cyst
   (B) deep-seated fibromatosis
   (C) fibrous histiocytoma
   (D) leiomyoma
   (E) lipoma

1091. More than 50% of which tumors are associated with neurofibromatosis?

   (A) angiosarcoma
   (B) dermatofibrosarcoma protuberans
   (C) fibrosarcoma
   (D) malignant schwannoma
   (E) Kaposi's sarcoma

1092. The most common sarcoma in children is which of the following?

   (A) embryonal rhabdomyosarcoma
   (B) fibrosarcoma
   (C) malignant fibrous histiocytoma
   (D) leiomyosarcoma
   (E) liposarcoma

1093. Osteoporosis is secondary to which of the following?

   (A) age
   (B) reduced physical activity
   (C) genetic factors
   (D) hormonal influence
   (E) all of the above

1094. Paget's disease may be which of the following?

   (A) monostotic
   (B) have different histology in different stages
   (C) mosaic pattern is characteristic
   (D) a variety of tumors may develop
   (E) all of the above

DIRECTIONS (Questions 1095 through 1101): Each group of items in this section consists of a list of lettered options followed by a set of numbered words or phrases. For each numbered word or phrase, select the ONE lettered heading that is most closely associated with it. Each lettered heading may be selected once, more than once, or not at all.

Questions 1095 through 1098

   (A) pseudogout
   (B) pyogenic osteomyelitis
   (C) metastatic disease
   (D) chondrosarcoma
   (E) osteochondroma

1095. Most common form of skeletal malignancy

1096. Commonly arises in pelvis, shoulder, and hips

1097. Almost always caused by bacteria

1098. Calcium pyrophosphate crystal deposition

Questions 1099 through 1101

   (A) synovial sarcoma
   (B) malignant fibrous histiocytoma
   (C) rhabdomyosarcoma
   (D) fibrosarcoma
   (E) chondrosarcoma

1099. Most common soft tissue sarcoma in childhood

1100. Biphasic morphology

1101. Most common malignant mesenchymal tumor in adults

DIRECTIONS (Question 1102): The numbered item in this section is followed by answers. Select the ONE lettered answer that is BEST.

1102. In hyperparathyroidism, the parathyroid hormone acts over

   (A) osteoclasts
   (B) osteocytes
   (C) osteoblasts
   (D) periosteal cells
   (E) endothelial cells

Answers and Explanations

1072. **(B)** Degenerative joint disease, also called osteoarthritis, is a process characterized by the progressive destruction of the articular cartilage. Although inflammatory changes are present in the articular joint with osteoarthritis, it is considered a reaction to the destruction of the cartilage. Osteoarthritis can be divided into primary, which is considered "wear and tear" arthritis, and secondary, which is a progressive, degenerative process of the cartilage and subchondral bone. The articular changes in secondary osteoarthritis are responding to such other causes as, trauma, crystal deposition, infection, or osteonecrosis. *(Rubin and Farber, p. 1392)*

1073. **(D)** Rheumatoid arthritis is a systemic disease that affects the joints. The initial insult seems to be in the synovium, which leads to an exuberant growth of connective tissue, penetrating the bone, leading to deep morphological alterations of the articular cartilage and surrounding tissue. On the skin, the most characteristic change is rheumatoid nodules that are seen in approximately 25% of the cases. The rheumatoid nodules, which are grossly nontender, subcutaneous masses, microscopically show a central area of fibrinoid necrosis surrounded by palisading epithelioid histiocytes. *(Cotran et al., pp. 1248–1251)*

1074. **(C)** The infection of a joint can be originated in the focus of infection in the vicinity, such as osteomyelitis or an abscess of the soft tissue or secondary to hematogenous dissemination. The most common organisms are gonococcus, *Staphylococcus*, *Streptococcus*, and *Haemophilus influenzae*. The classic clinical presentation is a sudden onset of acute joint pain with restricted motion. This is accompanied by systemic findings of fever and leukocytosis. In 90% of the cases of nongonococcal arthritis, it involved only a single joint. The most common affected joint is the knee, followed by the hip and shoulder. *(Cotran et al., p. 1253)*

1075. **(D)** Rheumatoid arthritis, which is a chronic systemic inflammatory disorder that affects many organs in the body, also produces destruction of the joints by proliferation of the synovium with granulation tissue, fibroblasts, and new vessel formation with acute and chronic inflammatory cell infiltrate. This exuberant growth of granulation tissue is called pannus synoviales. The progressive growth of this tissue erodes the cartilage and bone and bridges the two bone ends producing fibrous ankylosis, which can progress to bony ankylosis. *(Cotran et al., pp. 1248–1251)*

1076. **(A)** Refer to Answer 1072. *(Cotran et al., pp. 1246–1249)*

1077. **(A)** Because we suspect that this patient has a suppurative arthritis, the test to order would be a culture of the joint fluid from the affected knee to ascertain which organism is involved and, with further culture and sensitivity, to determine which is the antibiotic of choice. It would also be important to determine whether this is a hematogenous spread or a process secondary to osteomyelitis or contamination of the joint by a wound. *(Cotran et al., p. 1253)*

1078. **(C)** Osteosarcoma, malignant tumor of the bone, originates in the osteoblasts. Although it has a bimodal distribution, most of the patients are under 20 years of age. The type of osteosarcoma identified as the hereditary form in which mutations of the retinoblastoma gene produces a greater risk of developing osteosarcoma, and the sporadic type in which no mutations can be seen. Different classifications of osteosarcomas can be made according to the anatomic position in the bone, the degree of differentiation, and histologic variants. The neoplastic cell, for the most part, forms bone, and this neoplastic bone is composed of irregular, poorly formed spicules surrounded by neoplastic cells. Characteristic of this tumor is the high incidence of lung metastasis seen through the bloodstream. *(Cotran et al., pp. 1236–1237)*

1079. **(D)** Chondromas are benign tumors mostly composed of hyaline cartilage. According to the position if they are encountered in the medullary canal, they are called chondromas. If they are present in the surface of the bone, they are called subperiosteal or juxtacortical. Ollier disease is a syndrome in which multiple enchondromas are found, and when associated with hemangiomas, the disorder is called *Maffucci syndrome. (Cotran et al., pp. 1238–1239)*

1080. **(E)** Infarction (avascular necrosis) of the bone occurs as a result of ischemia by different mechanisms. That could include vascular interruption secondary to a fracture, corticosteroids, thrombosis and embolism, increased intraosseous pressure with vascular compression and venous hypertension. Moreover, cases of idiopathic necrosis of the bone can be seen. The necrosis seen secondary to steroid administration generally follows a high dose of this medication for a short period of time. Morphologically, there is extensive necrosis of the bone marrow, and the bone spicules show disappearance of the osteocytes and osteoblasts. Although the cartilage in the joint remains viable, with time it becomes detached and undergoes necrosis. *(Cotran et al., p. 1231)*

1081. **(B)** Osteosarcoma most commonly occurs in this age group, and 75% of the patients are under 20 years of age. There is a second peak in the elderly, but this is generally associated with such other diseases as Paget's disease, bone infarcts, or previous radiation. Almost 50% of the osteosarcomas occur above the knee. *(Cotran et al., pp. 1236–1237)*

1082. **(B)** Multiple myeloma is a neoplasm characterized by a malignant proliferation of terminally differentiated B lymphocytes, the plasma cells. The neoplastic cells seem to be originate in a B-differentiated cell that can be recovered in some of the patients in the peripheral blood and have the identical characteristic to the neoplastic plasma cells. Multiple myeloma is characterized by a multifocal infiltration of the bone marrow by malignant plasma-like cells. This proliferation leads to the destruction of the bone and pathological fractures. These tumors can secrete different kinds of light chains and heavy chain proteins that can be studied with the appropriate clinical laboratory test. In addition, nonsecretory myelomas can be found, as well as biclonal. On histological evaluation of the bone marrow biopsy, the spaces are largely replaced by a malignant proliferation of plasma cell, growing in sheets and sometimes intermingling with the hematopoietic elements. *(Cotran et al., pp. 664–666)*

1083. **(D)** Osteosarcoma that originates into the intramedullary canal generally breaks through the cortex into the soft tissue and the epiphyses. Often, the periosteum in this area becomes elevated and on radiographic studies, shows a characteristic triangular-shaped area of periosteal elevation called *Codman's triangle.* The O ring sign is a radiologic term used for the diagnosis of enchondromas that show characteristic nodules of cartilage that are well circumscribed, producing oval lucencies. *Exostosis* is another term for osteochondromas that is a benign cartilage cap outgrowth, attached to the skeleton by bony stock. Nidus is the center of osteoid osteoma, which are circumscribed lesions composed of interconnecting small bone trabecules of woven bone. The center of the lesion elicits a great amount of reactive bone that encircles the lesion. The actual tumor located in the center is known as the nidus and is seen radiologically as a round lucency that could be focally calcified. Sequestrum refers to the center of the dead bone in pyogenic osteomyelitis, surrounded by reactive new bone formation. *(Cotran et al., pp. 1237–1238)*

1084. **(E)** Refer to Answer 1081. *(Cotran et al., pp. 1236–1238)*

1085. **(A)** Osteomas are sessile tumors that project into the subperiosteal or endosteal surfaces of the cortex. They are most commonly seen in the scalp or the facial bones. Although they are generally slow-growing tumors of little clinical significance, they appear symptomatic when they impinge into such nearby structures as brain or eyes. *(Cotran et al., p. 1235)*

1086. **(E)** Onion skin is a radiologic term used for a characteristic of periosteal reaction that produces multiple layers of reactive bone. This is commonly seen in Ewing's sarcoma; however, there could be another process in the bone, such as pyogenic osteomyelitis that can also produce the onion skin phenomenon. This is not diagnostic of Ewing's sarcoma. *(Cotran et al., p. 1244)*

1087. **(B)** Osteoid osteomas are benign tumors, no more than 2 cm in diameter, that tend to occur in the younger population, with 75% under 25 years of age. They have a predilection for the femur or tibia occupying the cortex and less frequently the medullary cavity. They are painful lesions, and the pain is caused by excess prostaglandin E_2 production. This pain is characteristically nocturnal and is relieved by aspirin. *(Cotran et al., 1235)*

1088. **(A)** Ewing's sarcoma is a malignant bone neoplasm that originates in the medullary canal and is composed of small uniform round cells. This tumor belongs to the primitive neuroectodermal tumors (PNET) of childhood. Approximately 85% of these tumors show the *c-myc* oncogene expression.

In approximately 85% of the Ewing's sarcoma and PNETs, there is a reciprocal translocation of chromosomes 11 and 22. *(Cotran et al., p. 1244)*

1089. **(B)** Giant cell tumors contain abundant multinucleated giant cells of the osteoclastic type. Another name for this tumor is *osteoclastoma*. It is a benign, locally aggressive neoplasm that is postulated to have a monocyte–macrophage lineage. Grossly, they are red-brown in color and undergo cystic degeneration. These lesions do not produce bone. It was thought that these tumors are always benign, recently a more aggressive type has been described in which up to 4% of these tumors metastasize to the lung. The other lesions mentioned, such as chondrosarcoma may contain areas of bone formation with calcification. Osteochondroma has a base formed by bone. In addition, osteosarcoma, particularly the well differentiated variety, contains extensive areas of bone formation and mineralization, and the osteoid osteoma also produces bone spicules. *(Cotran et al., pp. 1244–1245)*

1090. **(B)** Deep-seated fibromatosis, also known as desmoid tumors, are composed of exuberant proliferation of fibrous tissue that borderlines low-grade fibrosarcomas. Most commonly seen in the anterior portion of the abdominal wall and in the young population. Desmoid tumors are divided into extra and intra-abdominal. The extra-abdominal are related to the anterior abdominal wall in pregnant women. It is located in the mesenteric fat or pelvic walls. Morphologically, they are composed of fibroblasts that show extensive areas of collagenization in the center. In the periphery, the fibroblasts appear to have more atypical and mitotic figures are infrequent. They can recur after excision, and they are locally aggressive. Some of these tumors respond well to treatment with tamoxifen. *(Cotran et al., pp. 1262–1263)*

1091. **(D)** Malignant peripheral nerve sheath tumors (malignant schwannoma) are highly malignant neoplasms that are locally invasive and eventually metastasize. These tumors are associated in more than 50% with the neurofibromatosis type I. These tumors have also been described following radiation therapy. Histologically, these lesions are not encapsulated and show extensive invasion to the adjacent tissue. Pleomorphic spindle cells, reminiscent of a fibrosarcoma or a malignant fibrous histiocytoma may be found. Mitoses, necrosis, and extensive areas of hemorrhage can be seen. With immunoperoxidase technique, it can be reactive for S-100 protein. When these tumors undergo such diverse histologic changes skeletal muscle or epithelial structures, they have been termed *Triton tumors*. Cartilage and bone can also be found. *(Cotran et al., pp. 1353–1354)*

1092. **(A)** Refer to Answer 1101. *(Cotran et al., p. 1265)*

1093. **(E)** Osteoporosis is a term that indicates the decrease in bone mass associated with changes in the structure of the bone that leads to fractures. It could be localized to a limb or generalized. Multiple factors have been incriminated in the origin of osteoporosis, which are more commonly associated with age-related bone loss as in senile osteoporosis and secondary to endocrine disorders, neoplasia, gastrointestinal factors, and drugs. Some of the most important related factors to osteoporosis are reduced physical activity, genetic factors, nutritional state, and hormonal influences. *(Cotran et al., pp. 1222–1223)*

1094. **(E)** Paget's disease is a skeletal disease characterized by osteoblastic bone formation and osteoclastic reabsorption. The disease can be seen in different histologic pictures, according with the stage. In the initial phase, the osteolytic process is more prominent than the bone formation. This is followed by a stage in which the osteolytic osteoclastic state balances out, with a predominance of osteoblastic activity formation. Finally, there is a burnt-out quiescent osteosclerotic stage. Histologically, the bones are dense, and show a characteristic mosaic pattern of lamellar bone. This is produced by prominent cement lines in which there is no perfect alignment of the different units of the lamellar bone. The bone marrow close to the areas of activity suffers fibrosis and replacement of the marrow elements by fibroblasts. A variety of benign and malignant tumors may develop in Paget's disease, such as giant cell tumors, osteosarcomas, malignant fibrohistiocytomas, or chondrosarcomas. *(Cotran et al., p. 1227)*

1095. **(C)** Metastases of the bones is the most frequent tumor of the skeleton. The most common root of dissemination of a malignant neoplasm into the bone is the hematogenous spread. The overwhelming majority of the tumors that metastasize in men to the bones are the prostate, in female the breast, followed by kidney and lung. In children, the metastasis to the bone are from neuroblastoma, Wilms' tumor, and osteosarcoma. Morphologically metastasis to the skeleton are multifocal and have a predominance for the extremity of the long bones, where there is a rich capillary network of blood supply. The metastasis could be destructive of the bone (lytic) or forming bone (blastic). *(Cotran et al., p. 1245)*

1096. **(D)** Chondrosarcomas are malignant neoplasms that produce cartilage. According to the location, they could be classified into intramedullary or juxtacortical. Histologically, they can also be classified according to cellular appearance. These mostly affect the elderly and occur more frequently in men than in women. The chondrosarcomas characteristically originate in the central portion of the skeleton, which includes the pelvis, shoulders, and ribs. *(Cotran et al., pp. 1240–1241)*

1097. **(B)** Refer to Answer 1074. *(Cotran et al., p. 1232)*

1098. **(A)** Deposition of pyrophosphate crystals in the joints is known as *chondrocalcinosis*. There is a sporadic and hereditary variant. The crystals develop around the articular matrix, menisci, and intervertebral discs, and they could rupture and release in the joint. *(Cotran et al., p. 1257)*

1099. **(C)** Rhabdomyosarcoma, which most commonly appears in the head and neck, as well as the genitourinary tract, is the most common soft tissue sarcoma of childhood and adolescence. Morphologically, different types have been described: the embryonal, alveolar, and pleomorphic variants. Of these, the most common is the embryonal sarcoma, which accounts for about 60–70% of the cases. On histological sections, it consists of malignant round to spindloid cells in a myxomatous stroma. With special stains, it is possible to see the rhabdomyoblasts with atypical cytoplasmic cross striations. Grossly, it resembles a bunch of grapes; hence, the name "sarcoma botryoides." *(Cotran et al., p. 1265)*

1100. **(A)** Although it has been thought that synovial sarcoma originates in the synovial cells, the origin is still controversial. Sixty to seventy percent of the tumors develop in the lower extremities, in and around the joints. Histologically, the most important characteristic of the synovial sarcoma is the biphasic pattern. Here, the spindle cells, which are arranged in fascicles, are surrounding spaces, which form pseudoglandular structures, giving a pseudoepithelial appearance. Some are composed of spindle cells only, in a monophasic pattern. *(Cotran et al., p. 1266)*

1101. **(B)** This type of tumor, which is characterized by a presence of spindle cells with storiform architecture and interspace atypical pleomorphic cells that, under special stains, are proved to be histiocytes. According to the predominance of the cells, as well as the morphologic appearance of the stroma, they are classified in different categories. *(Cotran et al., p. 1264)*

1102. **(C)** The parathyroid hormone binds to the receptors of the osteoblasts, which in turn, releases mediators that stimulate the osteoclast activity. The osteoclast promotes the bone resorption. *(Cotran et al., p. 1228)*

REFERENCES

Cotran RS, Kumar V, Robbins, SL. *Robbins Pathologic Basis of Disease,* 6th ed. Philadelphia: Saunders, 1999.

Rubin E, Farber JL. *Pathology.* Philadelphia: Lippincott, 1999.

CHAPTER 17

Central Nervous System

The central nervous system is an extremely complex structure. This tissue is in charge of many functions that cover many parts of the body and inter-relates with the surrounding environment. The cerebrum and its different parts, as well as the attached spinal cord, are capable of innumerable functions with rapid interconnections between them. Therefore, the motor functions, the sensory, storage of memory, as well as automatic functions differentiate the neurons from the other tissues of the body. There is also a pathologic selective vulnerability of the neurons, that may produce unique clinical pathologic pictures. The pathologic process that affects the central nervous system will be related to the special topography of the organ enclosed in the bone of the skull and the spinal column, protecting the spinal cord. In addition, the central nervous system has a special blood supply with absence of conventional lymphatic system and the special circulation of cerebrospinal fluid. Another important feature in the central nervous system is that the diseases are related to age. Many diseases affect children, and the degenerative process affects adults and elderly people. The cells that compose the central nervous system are (a) the neurons; their histological characteristics and functions are beyond the scope of this book. (Pathological changes of these neurons are chromatolysis, atrophy, neuronophagia, intraneuronal inclusions (viral or nonviral), and so forth); and (b) the glia, which are derived from the neuroectoderm, the astrocytes, oligodendrocytes, and ependymal cells; however, the microglia is derived from the bone marrow. The astrocytes are characterized by their geographic distribution in the brain, as fibrillary and protoplasmic astrocytes. The pathologic changes show that the astrocytes can multiply and form focus of astrogliosis. Rosenthal fibers are structures typically found in regions of gliosis.

Corpora amylacea are lamellar bodies considered as astrocytic and process. They represent the degenerative change in the astrocytes, most characteristic with advancing age. Glial cytoplasmic inclusions are filamentous structures that characterize degenerative diseases. Alzheimer's type II astrocytes, which despite its name it unrelated to Alzheimer's disease, are seen in chronic liver disease. The most important process of the astrocytes is the malignant transformation with the production of benign and malignant astrocytomas.

The primary function of oligodendrocytes is to produce myelin, and they wrap around the axis of the neuron cells. Injury of oligodendroglial cells is seen in acquired demyelinating disorders. Oligodendroglial cells may contain viral inclusions in such conditions as progressive multifocal leukoencephalopathy. Oligodendrocytes can undergo neoplastic transformation, with the formation of oligodendrogliomas.

Ependymal cells are seen lining the ventricular system. They are closely related to the choroid plexus. Pathologic findings associated with ependymal cells are affected in special infectious agents such as CMV virus. They can also undergo neoplastic transformation.

Microglia is a mesoderm-derived cell, and the primary function is like a fixed macrophage. They contain markers similar to the monocytes/macrophages in the peripheral blood. The pathologic conditions that affect the microglia are seen in small foci of necrosis in which they aggregate in microglial nodules. They are the principal fibrocytic cell in the central nervous system, and they are not known to undergo neoplasia.

Questions

DIRECTIONS (Questions 1103 and 1104): Each of the numbered items in this section is followed by answers. Select the ONE lettered answer that is BEST in each case.

1103. What does transtentorial (uncal) herniation produce?

    (A) one dilated pupil

    (B) nystagmus

    (C) respiratory arrest

    (D) severe lateral headache

    (E) blindness in one eye

1104. The death of oligodendrogliocytes results in which of the following?

    (A) infarction of brain

    (B) degeneration of myelin

    (C) cerebrospinal fluid characteristic changes

    (D) proliferation of fibroblasts

    (E) brain hemorrhage

DIRECTIONS (Questions 1105 through 1109): For each numbered word or phrase, select the ONE lettered option that is most closely associated with it. Each lettered option may be selected once, more than once, or not at all.

    (A) neuron

    (B) astrocytes

    (C) oligodendrogliocyte

    (D) ependymal cell

    (E) microglial cell

1105. Glial fibrillary acidic protein

1106. Fixed macrophage system

1107. Gliomas

1108. Forms myelin

1109. Neurofibrillary tangles

DIRECTIONS (Question 1110): The numbered item in this section is followed by answers. Select the ONE lettered answer that is BEST.

1110. Vitamin B_{12} deficiency results in which of the following?

    (A) hemorrhages in the mamillary bodies

    (B) cerebellar atrophy

    (C) subacute combined degeneration of spinal cord

    (D) necrosis of basal ganglia

    (E) spinal cord compression

DIRECTIONS (Questions 1111 through 1117): For each numbered word or phrase, select the ONE lettered option that is most closely associated with it. Each lettered option may be selected once, more than once, or not at all.

    (A) Alzheimer's disease

    (B) Pick's disease

    (C) Huntington's disease

    (D) progressive multifocal leukoencephalopathy

    (E) HIV-1 meningoencephalitis (subacute encephalitis)

    (F) Parkinson's disease

    (G) subacute combined degeneration (posterolateral sclerosis)

    (H) acute epidural hematoma

    (I) multiple sclerosis

1111. Caused by polyomavirus

1112. Microglial nodules

1113. Neurofibrillary tangles

1114. Active and inactive plaques

1115. Lewy bodies.

1116. Lobar atrophy

1117. Atrophy of the striatum

DIRECTIONS (Questions 1118 through 1136): Each of the numbered items in this section is followed by answers. Select the ONE lettered answer that is BEST in each case.

1118. What is an almost invariable accompaniment of Alzheimer's disease?

(A) fibrosis
(B) necrosis
(C) amyloid angiopathy
(D) calcification
(E) neuronal vacuolization

1119. Multiple sclerosis is a disease of which of the following?

(A) gray matter
(B) basal ganglia
(C) white matter
(D) neurons
(E) astrocytes

1120. What does the multiple sclerosis active plaque usually contain?

(A) necrosis
(B) inflammatory cells and myelin breakdown
(C) cytoplasmic neuronal inclusions
(D) polymorphonuclear cells
(E) perivascular eosinophils

1121. What is Krabbe disease?

(A) a leukodystrophy
(B) an environmental disease
(C) a genetically determined defects of axons

(D) an autosomal dominant disease
(E) a neoplastic process

1122. Where does hypertensive intraparenchymal brain hemorrhage most frequently occur?

(A) frontal lobes
(B) parietal lobes
(C) pons
(D) medulla
(E) putamen

1123. Where are most brain abscesses located?

(A) putamen
(B) frontal lobes
(C) basal ganglia
(D) cerebellum
(E) hippocampus

1124. Where do brain neoplasms in children most commonly occur?

(A) frontal lobes
(B) infratentorial compartment
(C) supratentorial compartment
(D) spinal cord
(E) basal ganglia

1125. What is the tumor that originates in meningothelial cells?

(A) astrocytoma
(B) ependymoma
(C) meningioma
(D) choroid plexus tumor
(E) medulloblastoma

1126. Which statement correctly describes medulloblastomas?

(A) They are mesodermal in origin.
(B) They are derived from primitive neuro-ectodermal cells.
(C) They are benign neoplasms.
(D) They are more frequent in adults.
(E) They are well circumscribed.

1127. Where do brain cells most sensitive to anoxia lie?

(A) basal ganglia

(B) hippocampus

(C) medulla oblongata

(D) pons

(E) occipital lobe

1128. Microscopically glioblastoma multiforme is characterized by which of the following?

(A) pseudopalisading necrosis

(B) frequent mitosis

(C) vascular proliferation

(D) hypercellularity

(E) all of the above

1129. Herpes simplex virus in the central nervous system produces which of the following?

(A) granulomas

(B) eosinophilia

(C) microabscesses

(D) vasculitis

(E) necrosis, hemorrhage, and perivascular inflammation

1130. Which statement correctly describes cytomegalovirus infection of the central nervous system?

(A) It is the most common opportunistic infection of the CNS in patients with AIDS.

(B) It affects the white matter only.

(C) It typically has large intranuclear inclusions.

(D) It usually causes destruction of the basal ganglia.

(E) It is associated with granulomas of the frontal lobes.

1131. Which statement describes herpes simplex virus type I of the central nervous system?

(A) It usually forms intracytoplasmic inclusion bodies.

(B) It shows granulomata.

(C) It usually is limited to the cerebellum.

(D) It shows Cowdry bodies.

(E) It is characterized by abscesses.

1132. Progressive multifocal leukoencephalopathy (PML) is characterized by which of the following?

(A) lesions rarely seen on CT scan and MRI

(B) lesions in the white matter

(C) intranuclear virus seen by EM

(D) effects on the cerebrum, brain stem, cerebellum, and spinal cord

(E) all of the above

1133. Which statement is correct concerning subacute sclerosing panencephalitis (SSPE)?

(A) It is typically asymptomatic.

(B) Intracytoplasmic inclusions are present.

(C) It is caused by cytomegalovirus.

(D) It is seen in elderly patients.

(E) It is characterized by measles virus infections.

1134. Amyotrophic lateral sclerosis (Lou Gehrig's disease) is characterized by which of the following?

(A) a viral infection

(B) loss of upper and lower motor neurons

(C) dementia

(D) vertigo

(E) white matter demyelinization

1135. Which statement is correct concerning Duchenne muscular dystrophy?

(A) It is a progressive X-linked inherited condition.

(B) It is dystrophin-deficient.

(C) It shows necrosis of muscle fibers.

(D) It starts at the muscle of the pelvic and shoulder girdles.

(E) All of the above statements are correct.

1136. What characterizes benign gliomas?

(A) They permit survival of 5–10 years.

(B) They are not encapsulated.

(C) They have no areas of necrosis or hemorrhage.

(D) They are of indolent growth.

(E) All of the above statements are correct.

Answers and Explanations

1103. **(A)** This type of herniation occurs when the medial aspect of the temporal lobe is compressed against the tentorium. The displacement of the temporal lobe produces a cranial nerve compression of the third nerve, resulting in a pupillary dilatation and impairment of ocular movements on the side of the lesion. *(Cotran et al., p. 1298)*

1104. **(B)** The oligodendrocytes surround the axons of the neurons form myelin sheets along the axons, similar to Schwann cells to peripheral nerves. When there is a death of oligodendrocytes, myelin will no longer be produced, and this will result in degeneration of myelin. This process is characteristic of such demyelinating disorders as multiple sclerosis or leukodystrophies. *(Cotran et al., p. 1297)*

1105. **(B)** On immunoperoxidase staining techniques, it is possible to distinguish astrocytes, because they are positive for glial fibrillary acid protein (GFAP). These positive intermediate filaments are seen on electron microscope aggregated in fascicles or disbursed throughout the cytoplasm in the fibrous astrocytes. *(Cotran et al., p. 1296)*

1106. **(E)** The microglial cells, which are mesoderm-derived share the same markers as the peripheral monocytes/macrophages. *(Cotran et al., p. 1297)*

1107. **(B)** The fibrillary astrocytes are prone to develop malignant neoplasms, and they are responsible for the majority of the malignant gliomas of the brain. *(Rubin and Farber, p. 1447)*

1108. **(C)** The oligodendroglia is the glial cells that produce myelin. On regular staining with hematoxylin and eosin, the oligodendroglia have lymphocytic-like nucleus with abundant cytoplasm. Oligodendroglia in the brain is distributed in close proximity with the neurons to provide myelin for the axons. *(Cotran et al., p. 1295)*

1109. **(A)** Neurofibrillary tangles are present in the cytoplasm of the pyramidal neurons. With silver stains and in light microscopy there appear to be irregular bundles filling out the cytoplasm of the neurons. Although they are not pathognomonic of Alzheimer's disease, they are among the most common histologic features. *(Rubin and Farber, pp. 1512–1513)*

1110. **(C)** Deficiency of vitamin B_{12} could progress from numbness and tingling of the lower extremities to complete paraplegia. The anatomic pathologic changes of the B_{12} deficiency is located in the spinal cord in which axons of both the ascending and descending tracts of the posterior column are degenerated. This combined degeneration, which is characteristic of vitamin B_{12} deficiency, has been designated *subacute combined degeneration of the spinal cord*. *(Cotran et al., p. 1341)*

1111. **(D)** Progressive multifocal leukoencephalopathy is a viral encephalitis caused by polyomavirus. This virus has a special affinity for oligodendrocytes, therefore, demyelination is the most common change. Characteristically, this disease affects immunocompromised hosts who have AIDS or another type of debilitating illness. Clinically, patients develop progressive neurologic deficits that can be seen on MRI or CT. Pathologically, on light microscopy, the lesions consist of patches of destruction of the white matter in various sizes. The brain, brain stem, and cerebellum can be affected. The spinal cord may be involved. The virus can be seen on electron microscopy *(Cotran et al., p. 1321)*

1112. **(E)** Clinical pictures of patients affected with this disease present with dementia. This is also accompanied by abnormalities of the motor system as well as seizures. On light microscopy, it shows a characteristic process of the microglial nodules. Occasionally, these microglial nodules can be accompanied by necrosis and reactive gliosis. In the microglial nodule, multinucleated giant cells can be found. The virus can be detected in the microglia, as well as the multinucleated macrophages by immunoperoxidase or electron microscopy. *(Cotran et al., p. 1320)*

1113. **(A)** Refer to Answer 1109. *(Rubin and Farber, pp. 1512–1513)*

1114. **(I)** The pathology of multiple sclerosis, a white matter disease, is composed of multiple and well-circumscribed plaques. Two different microscopic features can be described. In the first or early plaque (active), there is a myelin breakdown surrounded by abundant macrophages. The inflammatory cells, which are monocytes and lymphocytes, are present mostly surrounding the small vascular channels. If special stains are obtained, the axons show that they are relatively intact with a depletion of myelin. As the lesion progresses, they become inactive, no myelin is found, and the number of oligodendrocytes is markedly decreased. In old plaques, the inflammatory component is smaller, and there is a greater proliferation of astrocytes. *(Cotran et al., pp. 1326–1327)*

1115. **(F)** Parkinson's disease is a syndrome characterized by involuntary movements, rigidity, and tremors that have a common anatomic pathologic substrate affecting the substantia nigra and locus ceruleus. On light

microscopy and hematoxylin and eosin stain, the neurons in these regions are associated with gliosis. Lewy bodies can be found in some of the neurons. These are either single or multiple intracytoplasmic spherical eosinophilic inclusions, surrounded by a pale halo. On electron microscopy, Lewy bodies are composed of neurofilaments. *(Cotran et al., pp. 1333–1334)*

1116. **(B)** Pick's disease is one of the rarest cortical dementias. It differs from Alzheimer's disease, because it is usually localized in the frontal or temporal lobes. In addition to cortical atrophy, there also could be atrophy of the basal ganglia. On light microscopy, an extensive severe loss of the cortical lobe of the brain is seen, and the surviving neurons show a characteristic swelling (Pick cells). These cells contain cytoplasmic inclusions that are oval and composed of filaments. These structures are called Pick bodies. *(Cotran et al., p. 1333)*

1117. **(C)** This autosomal dominant inherited disease is characterized by dementia and involuntary movements. The anatomic pathologic changes on light microscopy show a degeneration of the striatal neurons. The most important histologic changes are found in the caudate nucleus, especially near the ventricle. Loss of the small and large neurons is noted, and fibrillary gliosis is present. *(Cotran et al., pp. 1335–1336)*

1118. **(C)** Alzheimer's disease, which is the most common cause of dementia in the elderly population, shows many characteristic morphologic changes in light microscopy. These are neurofibrillary tangles, senile (neuritic) plaques, and amyloid angiopathy. Angiopathy is an almost invariable accompaniment to Alzheimer's disease, and the amyloid is derived from the same precursor as the amyloid core plaques. On regular H&E stains, the small vessels appears to have a homogenous deep eosinophilic wall. With special stains such as Congo Red, it shows that they are positive for amyloid deposition. *(Cotran et al., pp. 1329–1331)*

1119. **(C)** Multiple sclerosis, a demyelinating disorder, is histologically characterized by well-circumscribed lesions with so-called plaques. There is an active and an inactive plaque. These plaques are composed by a breakdown of myelin surrounded by abundant macrophages and occasional lymphocytes. The lesions are localized in the white matter. *(Cotran et al., pp. 1326–1327)*

1120. **(B)** Refer to Answer 1119. *(Cotran et al., pp. 1326–1327)*

1121. **(A)** Leukodystrophy is a disease that selectively involves the myelin with no evidence of neuronal storage defect. They diffusely involve the white matter, which leads to a deterioration of the motor neurons leading to spasticity and hypertonia or ataxia. Krabbe disease is an autosomal recessive leukodystrophy resulting from a deficiency of an enzyme that acts in the catabolism of galactocerebroside to ceramide and galactose. The clinical course is rapidly progressive, with an onset of symptoms between the ages of 3–6 months. Survival beyond the age of 2 is uncommon. On histological examination, there is a loss of myelin and oligodendrocytes. Not only do these also extend, to the central nervous system, but also to the peripheral nerves. *(Cotran et al., pp. 1339–1340)*

1122. **(E)** Fifty to sixty percent of the cases of hypertensive intraparenchymal hemorrhage originate in the putamen. When they originate in the putamen, as well as in other basal ganglia, the hemorrhage is called ganglionic hemorrhage. Those that occur in the cerebral hemisphere are called lobar hemorrhages. The hemorrhage destroys the cerebral matter by compression, and it could also invade the ventricles. *(Cotran et al., p. 1310)*

1123. **(B)** Brain abscesses are secondary to either local extension from mastoiditis or sinusitis or are spread hematogenously from such primary sites as heart, lungs, or bones. Commonly, bacterial endocarditis seems to be the etiology of brain abscesses. The most common organisms are *Streptococcus* and *Staphy-*

lococci. On microscopic examination, there is a central area of liquefactive necrosis surrounded by gliosis and edema. Inflammatory cells are also present in the wall of the abscess. *(Cotran et al., p. 1316)*

1124. **(B)** According to the location in the brain, the tumors can be divided into a supra or a infratentorial. This division is very important, because the topographic location and patient's age are needed for differential diagnosis of the histologic type of neoplasm. Children usually present with a neoplasm in the infratentorial compartment. *(Chandrasoma and Taylor, pp. 939–940)*

1125. **(C)** Meningiomas are benign tumors that originate in the meningothelial cells of the arachnoid, and they are attached to the dura. On histologic examination, there is a variegated pattern from syncytial to fibroblastic, transitional, psammomatous, etc. By special stains these cells are positive for epithelial membrane antigen and carcinoembryogenic antigen. Malignant meningiomas, which are extremely rare, are very difficult to recognize histologically. Cellularity, abundant mitosis, and foci of necrosis are helpful, although the most important feature is invasion of the underlying brain tissue. *(Cotran et al., p. 1350)*

1126. **(B)** Medulloblastoma is a malignant tumor of the central nervous system common in children. Generally, it is located in the midline of the cerebellum, but in adults, can be in other locations. Because of the area it involves, it can lead to hydrocephalus. On microscopic examination, the tumor is composed of small rather anaplastic cells with a deeply hyperchromatic small nucleus. The cytoplasm is undiscernible. Mitotic activity is conspicuous. On immunohistochemistry studies, neurosecretory granules can be detected in the cytoplasm. Dissemination through the cerebrospinal fluid is common. *(Cotran et al., pp. 1348–1349)*

1127. **(B)** Neurons are vulnerable to oxygen deficiency more than glial cells. The gray matter of the spinal matter and the adult brain stem may be damaged by lack of oxygen when there is almost total destruction of the cerebral cortex. When an episode of hypoxia occurs, damage may be limited to only the neurons. If hypoxia persists or affects the glial tissue, an infarct will result. This selective neuron sensitivity to hypoxia is seen in the hippocampus and also in the Purkinje cells of the cerebellum. *(Rubin and Farber, pp. 1470–1471)*

1128.   **(E)** Glioblastoma multiforme is the most aggressive of all of the malignant glial tumors of the brain. Grossly, it infiltrates the brain parenchyma and shows extensive areas of hemorrhage and necrosis. Microscopically, it is composed of pleomorphic astrocytes, which show frequent mitosis. The tumors are highly cellular, and vascular proliferation is noted. Characteristically, they show areas of necrosis with peripheral palisading of the surrounding surviving cells. The prognosis has a median survival rate of 1 year after the diagnosis. *(Chandrasoma and Taylor, p. 941)*

1129.   **(E)** The encephalitis caused by herpes simplex virus type I on microscopic examination shows areas of necrosis and hemorrhage. The surrounding area is severely affected, and perivascular infiltrates are usual. Glial tissue, as well as the neurons, show intranuclear inclusion bodies called Cowdry inclusions. *(Cotran et al., pp. 1318–1319)*

1130.   **(A)** Cytomegalovirus most commonly occurs in patients with immunosuppression as an opportunistic viral pathogen in patients with acquired immunodeficiency syndrome. It is also seen in fetuses that develop encephalitis localized in the ependymal cells some of the regions of the brain. This results in periventricular calcification. Any type of cell, including the neurons and glial tissue, as well as the ependymal, can be infected by CMV. Microscopically, the cells contain cytomegalic inclusions that are intracytoplasmic and intranuclear. With immunohistochemistry and in situ hybridization it can also be demonstrated. *(Cotran et al., p. 1319)*

1131.   **(D)** Refer to Answer 1129. *(Cotran et al., pp. 1318–1319)*

1132.   **(E)** PML is a viral encephalitis caused by the polyomavirus. The virus affects the oligodendrocytes and demyelination occurs. This disease happens in immunodeficient individuals, as well as myelo or lymphoproliferative disorders and AIDS. The lesions are rarely seen in CT and MRI. These lesions, which mainly affect the cerebrum, brain stem, cerebellum and rarely the spinal cord, show viral nuclear inclusions that can be seen on electron microscopy. *(Cotran et al., p. 1321)*

1133.   **(E)** Subacute sclerosing panencephalitis is a rare, progressive clinical syndrome characterized by the spasticity of the arms and legs and convulsions. It usually occurs in children or young adults. This disease occurs at the early age after acute infection with measles. This disease is thought to be secondary to persistent, but nonproductive infection of the central nervous system by altered measles virus. *(Cotran et al., pp. 1321–1322)*

1134.   **(B)** Amyotrophic lateral sclerosis is the most common disease of motor neuron disease entities. It is characterized by degeneration of the corticospinal tracts (lateral sclerosis) in the spinal cord, which results in upper motor neuron paralysis in the extremities. Clinically, this disease is characterized by muscle atrophy and hyperflexia. Five to ten percent of the cases are familial without autosomal dominance inheritance. The etiology and pathogenesis are unknown. On light microscopy, there is a demonstrable reduction of the number of anterior horn cells with associated reactive gliosis and loss of the anterior root myelinated fibers. Similar histologic findings are seen in the hypoglossal, motor trigeminal cranial nerve nuclei. *(Chandrasoma and Taylor, pp. 936–937; Cotran et al., p. 1338)*

1135.   **(E)** Duchenne muscular dystrophy is an X-linked, progressive, inherited condition. It is characterized by degeneration of the muscles of the pelvic and shoulder girdles. This is the most common myopathy in children. Duchenne muscular dystrophy is caused by mutations of a large gene on the short arm of the X chromosome. This gene encodes for dystrophin, a protein that is localized on the inner surface of the sarcolemma. The dystrophin links the subsarcolemma cytoskeleton to the exterior of the cell, and when dystrophin is absent or greatly reduced, the muscle fibers lack normal interaction. On pathology of the fibers, it shows that there is necrosis of the muscles with reparation and progressive fibrosis. *(Chandrasoma and Taylor, pp. 954–955)*

1136. **(E)** Although some glial tumors are considered benign they, however, are not encapsulated. The well-differentiated astrocytomas show an infiltrative pattern through the surrounding brain tissue. The only reason for the term *benign* being applied is because of the indolent growth that permits survival of 5–10 years. *(Rubin and Farber, p. 1514)*

REFERENCES

Chandrasoma P, Taylor CR. *Concise Pathology*, 3rd ed. Norwalk, CT: Appleton & Lange, 1998.

Cotran RS, Kumar V, Robbins SL. *Robbins Pathologic Basis of Disease*, 6th ed. Philadelphia: Saunders, 1999.

Rubin E, Farber JL. *Pathology*. Philadelphia: Lippincott, 1999.

CHAPTER 18

Transplantation Pathology

This chapter is dedicated to the study of the pathology of solid organ transplantation, which has increased dramatically in the last two decades. The availability of solid organs; however, far from being ideal, has dramatically changed the focus of the study of the pathology of transplantation, because it has become so frequent. Transplantation of solid organs is now viewed as a team effort in which surgeons insert the organs, and they must be followed by a medical team of specialists. For pathologists, new books and new chapters have been produced to cover the most important changes in transplanted organs, as well as the hosts, in the more detail. In addition, extraordinary considerations must be given to new drugs under development. Modern drugs for immunosuppression have brought a guarantee, up to 90%, of successful transplant over 1 year.

Experience from kidney transplants, one of the most common, oldest, and frequently performed, has been extended to many other organs, such as heart, liver, lung, bone marrow, skin, and pancreas. Statistics show that there is a better, long-term survival for these patients, and this success is secondary to a more careful understanding of the immunologic and pathologic mechanisms involved in organ rejection. Improvement is secondary to the development of new immunosuppressive agents, combination therapy, and better selection of the organ matching to recipient. Moreover, there is now a better control of the opportunistic infectious diseases that so frequently affect the immunosuppressed patients. Shortage of organ donors has led to a search for organs in different species (xenotransplantation).

The questions in this chapter deal with transplantation, rejection, immunologic aspects, and pathologic effects in the organs. Most opportunistic infections in immunosuppressed patients have been addressed in other chapters.

Questions

DIRECTIONS (Questions 1137 through 1139): For each numbered word or phrase, select the ONE lettered option that is most closely associated with it. Each lettered option may be selected once, more than once, or not at all.

(A) suppresses T cell-mediated immunity
(B) adrenomedullary insufficiency
(C) induces donor-specific tolerance
(D) highest incidence of pancreatitis
(E) renal insufficiency

1137. Cyclosporine

1138. Azathioprine

1139. Antibodies to CD28

DIRECTIONS (Questions 1140 through 1144): Each of the numbered items in this section is followed by answers. Select the ONE lettered answer that is BEST in each case.

1140. Graft versus host disease develops when which of the following is (are) present?

(A) immunocompetent T cells in the graft
(B) antibodies in the host
(C) monocytes in the graft
(D) vascular endothelial cells
(E) necrosis in the graft

1141. Which is the major action of cyclosporine A?

(A) to activate B cells
(B) to suppress T cell-mediated immunity
(C) to activate complement
(D) to activate neutrophils
(E) to inhibit IgG production

1142. Interferon (IFN-γ) action in delayed-type hypersensitive reaction (transplant rejection) occurs by which of the following?

(A) stimulation of T cells
(B) epithelial membrane binding receptors
(C) increase in immunoglobulins
(D) activation of monocytes/macrophages
(E) B cell activation

1143. Bone marrow transplants are more useful in which of the following?

(A) aplastic anemia
(B) leukemia
(C) metastatic breast cancer
(D) immunodeficiency states
(E) all of the above

1144. In transplantation of the liver and heart, what is most important?

(A) high platelet count
(B) minor histocompatibility antigen matching
(C) activation of recipient T cells
(D) size and availability of the organs
(E) HLA compatibility testing

DIRECTIONS (Questions 1145 through 1152): Each group of items in this section consists of a list of lettered options followed by a set of numbered words or phrases. For each numbered word or phrase, select the ONE lettered option that is most closely associated with it. Each lettered option may be selected once, more than once, or not at all.

Questions 1145 through 1148

    (A) anaphylaxis
    (B) chronic rejection
    (C) hyperacute rejection
    (D) delayed-type hypersensitivity
    (E) acute rejection vasculitis

1145. Vascular endothelium

1146. Granulomas

1147. Necrotizing vasculitis

1148. Dense intimal fibrosis

Questions 1149 through 1152

    (A) an isograft
    (B) a xenograft
    (C) an autograft
    (D) an allograft
    (E) a syngraft

1149. Identical twin graft

1150. Hosts' own tissue

1151. Same species

1152. Different species

DIRECTIONS (Questions 1153 and 1154): Each of the numbered items in this section is followed by answers. Select the ONE lettered answer that is BEST in each case.

1153. The mechanism involved in the tuberculin reaction is triggered by which of the following?

    (A) sensitized T lymphocytes
    (B) humoral immunity
    (C) immunoglobulins
    (D) local immune complex disease
    (E) anaphylaxia

1154. After bone marrow transplantation, activation of donor lymphocytes can cause which of the following?

    (A) acute rejection
    (B) chronic cellular rejection
    (C) Arthur's reaction
    (D) anaphylaxis
    (E) graft versus host disease

DIRECTIONS (Questions 1155 through 1160): For each numbered word or phrase, select the ONE lettered option that is most closely associated with it. Each lettered option may be selected once, more than once, or not at all.

    (A) immediate hyperacute rejection
    (B) acute rejection vasculitis
    (C) chronic rejection
    (D) opportunistic infection
    (E) graft versus host disease

1155. Endothelial cells

1156. Produces progressive intimal fibrosis and organ ischemia

1157. Nonpathogenic organisms

1158. Results from activation of donor lymphocytes

1159. Associated with intimal fibrosis and proliferation

1160. Antidonor antibodies

DIRECTIONS (Questions 1161 through 1163): Each of the numbered items in this section is followed by answers. Select the ONE lettered answer that is BEST in each case.

1161. In kidney transplant, arterial thickening is characteristic of which of the following?

    (A) acute cellular rejection
    (B) hyperacute rejection
    (C) prednisone toxicity
    (D) azathioprine toxicity
    (E) chronic rejection

1162. In cardiac transplant, what diagnostic test is required for evaluation?

(A) right ventricular endomyocardial biopsy

(B) heart size

(C) coronary artery angiography

(D) opportunistic infections in the myocardium

(E) all of the above

1163. How soon after transplantation does hyperacute rejection of a transplanted organ occur?

(A) minutes to hours

(B) 2 days

(C) 1 week

(D) 3 weeks to 1 year

(E) 2–5 years

DIRECTIONS (Questions 1164 through 1167): For each numbered word or phrase, select the ONE lettered option that is most closely associated with it. Each lettered option may be selected once, more than once, or not at all.

(A) acute cellular rejection

(B) acute humoral rejection

(C) accelerated rejection

(D) chronic rejection

(E) hyperacute rejection

1164. Arterial intimal fibrosis

1165. Perivascular and interstitial mononuclear cell infiltration

1166. Occurs minutes after transplantation

1167. Antidonor antibodies present in the circulation of the recipient

Answers and Explanations

1137. **(A)** Cyclosporine is a drug that suppresses T cell-mediated immunity by inhibiting activation of cytokine genes (the gene for interleukin-2). Before cyclosporine was available, only corticosteroids and azathioprine were used; therefore, only 50% of the grafts had a survival of 1 year. Now with the use of cyclosporine, the expectation for a solid organ transplant success ranges from 80–90% after 1 year. This figure drops to 50 and 60% if we consider 10 years after transplantation; therefore, the development of new drugs is very important to improve these numbers. *(Cotran et al., p. 210)*

1138. **(D)** Therapeutic drugs such as, azathioprine, which is used for rejection of transplanted organs, as well as mercaptourine, are drugs incriminated as causing acute pancreatitis. *(Rubin and Farber, p. 847)*

1139. **(C)** Immunosuppression of the patient in order to receive an organ transplant successfully puts the patient at risk of high susceptibility to opportunistic pathogens that cause fungal and viral infections. To minimize the immunosuppression effects, much effort has been focused on induced donor-specific tolerance in host T cells. This tolerance can be accomplished by interrupting the interaction of the B7 molecules of the dendritic cells of the graft donor with the CD28 receptor on the host T cells. This is accomplished by administration of antibodies that bind to CD28 receptors. *(Cotran et al., p. 210)*

1140. **(A)** Graft versus host disease (GVH) develops when immunocompetent cells are transplanted into a patient who is immunologically crippled. For example, a recipient of a bone marrow is immunodeficient either because of the primary disease or the previous treatment. When the patient receives normal allogeneic cells, the immunocompetent T lymphocytes from the donor recognize the recipients' antigens as foreign tissue and react against them. *(Cotran et al., p. 210)*

1141. **(B)** Refer to Answer 1137. *(Cotran et al., p. 210)*

1142. **(D)** IFN-γ is very important in the mediated delayed-type of hypersensitivity. It stimulates the macrophages and causes further secretion of interleukin-12. The response of the macrophages is increased fibrocytosis, and they express more class II molecules on the surface, facilitating antigen presentation. *(Cotran et al., p. 205)*

1143. **(E)** Bone marrow transplantation has been progressively broadening the spectrum of therapeutic modalities for different diseases. Leukemias, lymphoproliferative neoplasias, immunodeficiency states, and aplastic anemias are a few examples in which bone marrow transplantation has been used. The stem cells could be obtained either from the bone marrow or harvesting stem cells from the peripheral blood. *(Cotran et al., p. 210)*

1144. **(D)** Transplantations such as liver or heart are regarded in a different way than those of kidney and other organs. Because the liver and heart must fit into the space of the host, the size and availability of the organs take precedent over HLA matching. Also, the donor liver and heart cannot remain for a long period of time outside of the donor to routinely wait for HLA matching. *(Cotran et al., p. 210)*

1145. **(C)** Hyperacute rejection occurs only a few minutes after the transplantation has taken place. On light microscopy, the histology lesions consist of an accumulation of neutrophils in the small vessels and immunoglobulin complement are deposited in the walls of these vessels. The early lesions point to an antigen–antibody reaction at the level of the vascular endothelium. *(Cotran et al., pp. 207–208)*

1146. **(D)** This type of hypersensitivity is initiated by specifically sensitized T lymphocytes. The classic examples of delayed-type hypersensitivity is the tuberculin reaction. On microscopic examination, epithelioid cells are present, which aggregate to form epithelioid granulomas. These granulomas are surrounded by lymphocytes and, for the most part, do not contain a necrotic center. *(Cotran et al., p. 204)*

1147. **(E)** Acute rejection vasculitis is primarily mediated by antidonor–antibodies. It is manifested by damage of the blood vessels. Often it takes the form of necrotizing vasculitis with endothelial cell necrosis. This is accompanied by infiltration of polymorphonuclear cells and deposition of immunoglobulins, complement, and fibrin. *(Cotran et al., p. 209)*

1148. **(B)** Chronic rejection is present in transplanted tissues as a progressive degeneration of the organ over a period of months or years. In general, the patients have a history of rejection that has been controlled by immunosuppression. Microscopically, the vascular changes consist of dense intimal fibrosis, the wall of the vessel is thickened and the lumen extremely narrow. This is probably the result of secondary proliferative arteritis, which is controlled with immunosuppression. *(Cotran et al., p. 210)*

1149. **(A)** When transplants are between genetically identical twins (monozygotic), they are called *isografts*. *(Chandrasoma and Taylor, pp. 116–117)*

1150. **(C)** An autograft is the transplantation of the host's tissue from one part of the body to another or bone marrow transplantation, such as in some type of leukemias and other disease. *(Chandrasoma and Taylor, pp. 116–117)*

1151. **(D)** An allograft is the transplantation between genetically different members of the same species. *(Chandrasoma and Taylor, pp. 116–117)*

1152. **(B)** This graft is done when tissues are obtained from a different species, (such as baboon or swine). Much research is being done on this, because the shortage of human organs has led to an intensive search for new available organs. *(Chandrasoma and Taylor, pp. 116–117)*

1153. **(A)** Refer to Answer 1142. *(Cotran et al., p. 204)*

1154. **(A)** Acute rejection consists of two major problems originating in bone marrow transplant—the graft versus host (GVH) disease and transplant rejection. The mechanism for rejection of allogeneic bone marrow transplant is poorly understood; however, it is believed that T cells are responsible for this rejection. *(Cotran et al., p. 210)*

1155. **(A)** Hyperacute rejection, which is a form of reaction that occurs immediately after transplantation, is characterized by severe necrotizing vasculitis. The beginning of this lesion appears to be in damage to the endothelial cells. *(Cotran et al., pp. 207–209)*

1156. **(C)** Chronic rejection is seen months or years after the transplant has been performed. In general, the patient has had previous episodes of rejection that have been controlled by immunosuppressive therapy. Microscopically, the vascular changes consist of dense intimal fibrosis, and there is also a narrowing of the lumen and fibrosis of the entire wall of the vessel, which leads to ischemia of the transplanted organ. *(Cotran et al., pp. 207–209)*

1157. **(D)** Nonpathogenic opportunistic organisms are life threatening in many cases in immuno-suppressed patients who are undergoing or have received transplanted organs. *(Cotran et al., 207–209)*

1158. **(E)** Refer to Answer 1154. *(Cotran et al., pp. 207–209)*

1159. **(C)** Refer to Answer 1156. *(Cotran et al., pp. 207–209)*

1160. **(B)** It is mediated by antidonor antibodies and is expressed by damage of the blood vessels. The histological changes are characterized by a necrotizing vasculitis with endothelial cell necrosis and infiltration of polymorphonuclear cells. In addition, on immunofluorescence studies, immunoglobulins, complement, and fibrin can be detected. *(Cotran et al., pp. 207–209)*

1161. **(E)** Refer to Answer 1156. *(Cotran et al., pp. 207–209)*

1162. **(E)** Evaluation of the transplanted heart requires multiple and special techniques to determine the rejection or the histologic changes that can happen to the organ. Repeated and sequential biopsies of the endomyocardium of the right ventricle are very important for evaluating the possible rejection, and systemic grading has been proposed for the evaluating these changes. In addition, in the same biopsy, evaluation for infections with virus or other organisms can be detected. The size of the heart is evaluated for the possibility of congestive heart failure, as well as coronary artery disease. Last, but probably one of the most important evaluations, is the coronary artery angiography, to evaluate the patency of the coronary arteries. This is not a segmental type of narrowing of the lumen, as in cases of atherosclerosis, because the rejection phenomenon produces vascular changes that are usually generalized and sometimes very severe. *(Thiru and Waldman, pp. 301–312)*

1163. **(A)** Refer to Answer 1145. *(Cotran et al., pp. 207–208)*

1164. **(D)** Refer to Answer 1156. *(Cotran et al., pp. 207–209)*

1165. **(A)** This type of rejection occurs days or months after transplantation. Histologically, it shows an infiltration of mononuclear cells in the vessels that may also be seen with areas of necrosis. The vascular damage seems to be limited to the endothelium and is antibody-mediated vasculitis. The wall of the vessels are swollen, and occasional lymphocytes may be seen. These patients usually quickly respond to immunosuppressive therapy. *(Cotran et al., p. 209)*

1166. **(E)** Refer to Answer 1145. *(Cotran et al., pp. 207–208)*

1167. **(B)** Refer to Answer 1160. *(Cotran et al., pp. 207–209)*

REFERENCES

Chandrasoma P, Taylor CR. *Concise Pathology,* 3rd ed. Norwalk, CT: Appleton & Lange, 1998.

Cotran RS, Kumar V, Robbins SL. *Robbins Pathologic Basis of Disease,* 6th ed. Philadelphia: Saunders, 1999.

Rubin E, Farber JL. *Pathology.* Philadelphia: Lippincott, 1999.

Thiru S, Waldmann H. *Pathology and Immunology of Transplantation and Rejection.* London: Blackwell Science Ltd., 2001.

CHAPTER 19

Practice Test
Questions

Carefully read the following instructions before taking the Practice Test.

1. This examination consists of questions covering the subject areas listed in the Table of Contents.
2. The Practice Test simulates an actual examination in question types and integration of subject areas.
3. You should set aside 2 hours and 10 minutes of *uninterrupted,* distraction-free time to take the Practice Test. This averages out to 50 seconds per question.
4. Be sure you have a clock (to time and pace yourself).
5. Be sure to answer all questions.
6. Use any remaining time to review your answers.
7. After completing the Practice Test, you can check all of your answers on pages 327 to 334. A score of 75% or higher should be considered as a passing score (115 correct answers).

DIRECTIONS (Questions 1 through 73): Each of the numbered items or incomplete statements in this section is followed by answers or by completions of the statement. Select the ONE lettered answer or completion that is BEST in each case.

1. In diphtheria, systemic reactions are caused by which of the following?

   (A) anaerobic spore formation within visceral abscesses
   (B) antihistone autoantibodies
   (C) localized upper respiratory tract infection with release of exotoxin
   (D) overwhelming bacterial septicemia
   (E) viral septicemia

2. Which is the correct statement concerning leprosy?

   (A) It can be found in wild armadillos.
   (B) It is caused by *Mycobacterium leprae.*
   (C) It occurs in lepromatous and tuberculoid forms.
   (D) Organisms show acid-fast staining.
   (E) All of the above are correct.

3. What type of rejection is due to the presence in the recipient's serum of high levels of preformed antibodies against antigens on the transplanted cells?

   (A) acute rejection
   (B) chronic rejection
   (C) graft versus host disease
   (D) hyperacute rejection
   (E) successful transplantation

4. Which is the correct statement about cell membranes?

    (A) Portions may be coated by glycocalyx.
    (B) Membrane-associated particles can include ABO blood groups.
    (C) Morphologic pattern is termed "unit membrane."
    (D) They are composed of complex mixture of lipids, proteins, and carbohydrates.
    (E) All of the above are correct.

5. What is the major intracellular cation?

    (A) bicarbonate
    (B) calcium
    (C) magnesium
    (D) potassium
    (E) sodium

6. How would you define phagocytosis?

    (A) abnormal mitotic figures in malignancy
    (B) collagen deposition in a wound
    (C) engulfment of particulate matter by cells
    (D) enzyme found in ribosomes
    (E) tight junctions on the cell membrane

7. What is the correct statement concerning hydropericardium?

    (A) It is associated with myxedema.
    (B) It can produce cardiac tamponade.
    (C) It is seen with congestive heart failure.
    (D) It usually is a transudate.
    (E) All of the above are correct.

8. A Langhans' giant cell would be an expected finding in which of the following?

    (A) suppurative inflammation
    (B) granulomatous inflammation
    (C) serous inflammation
    (D) fibrinous inflammation
    (E) purulent inflammation

9. Acetaminophen combined with alcohol will result in damage of what cell type?

    (A) alveolar macrophage
    (B) fibroblast

    (C) hepatocyte
    (D) neuron
    (E) smooth muscle

10. Type I hypersensitivity reactions are mediated by which immunoglobulin?

    (A) IgA
    (B) IgD
    (C) IgE
    (D) IgG
    (E) IgM

11. Which is the correct statement concerning B lymphocytes?

    (A) They do not express surface immunoglobulin.
    (B) They do not have a receptor for complement 3b (C3b).
    (C) They have a receptor for Fc.
    (D) They have receptors for sheep erythrocytes.
    (E) They can mature into histiocytes.

12. In Gaucher's disease, what is the enzyme defect?

    (A) sphingomyelin
    (B) beta-glucosidase
    (C) ceramide trihexoside
    (D) sulfatide
    (E) GMs-ganglioside

13. Which is the correct statement about respiratory distress in newborns?

    (A) Prematurity increases risk.
    (B) Newborns may have hyaline pulmonary membranes.
    (C) A major cause is lack of pulmonary surfactant.
    (D) There may be increased risk with diabetic mothers.
    (E) All of the above are correct.

14. What is the most common place in which fatty tissue undergoes necrosis?

    (A) heart

(B) ovary

(C) pancreas

(D) skeletal muscle

(E) testicle

15. Which cells are highly sensitive to radiation?

(A) chondrocytes

(B) fibroblast

(C) lymphocytes

(D) osteocyte

(E) skeletal muscle cell

16. What is the microorganism most commonly associated with gas gangrene?

(A) clostridial infections

(B) fibroblast

(C) lymphocyte

(D) osteocyte

(E) skeletal muscle cell

17. Which is the correct statement about acute cyanide poisoning?

(A) Less than 0.1 g ingested may be lethal.

(B) At death, blood is cherry red.

(C) It kills by cellular asphyxiation.

(D) It binds to cytochrome oxidase.

(E) All of the above are correct.

18. Which is the correct statement about chromomycosis?

(A) It is caused by several pigmented fungi.

(B) It involves caseous necrosis.

(C) It is also called "tinea capitis."

(D) It usually occurs in the trunk.

(E) It exhibits painful deep abscess.

19. Which is the fat-soluble vitamin?

(A) vitamin B_6

(B) vitamin B_{12}

(C) niacin

(D) vitamin E

(E) riboflavin

20. A patient with fever, bradycardia, leukopenia, diarrhea, and lymphoid hyperplasia most likely has which of the following?

(A) staphylococcal meningitis

(B) typhoid fever

(C) staphylococcal myelitis

(D) gonococcal meningitis

(E) pneumococcal pneumonia

21. If we are only judging the cancer behavior for the grade, which would be the worst?

(A) All have the same prognosis.

(B) Cancers are not graded.

(C) Grade I is the worst.

(D) Grade II is the worst.

(E) Grade III is the worst.

22. Which is the malignant neoplasm in which the neoplastic cells contain keratin and form keratin pearls?

(A) adenocarcinoma

(B) choriocarcinoma

(C) epidermoid carcinoma

(D) fibroadenoma

(E) melanocarcinoma

23. Which is the infection that *Haemophilus influenzae* is likely to produce?

(A) urinary tract infection

(B) cellulitis

(C) abscess

(D) diarrhea

(E) acute epiglottitis

24. Which of the following bacterial pathogens have toxin production as the major component of its pathogenicity?

(A) *Corynebacterium diphtheriae*

(B) *Clostridium perfringens*

(C) *Vibrio cholerae*

(D) *Bacillus anthracis*

(E) All of the above

25. A focal, often circumscribed, overgrowth in improper proportions of tissues normally present in that part of the body is termed what?

   (A) hyperdiploid
   (B) metastasis
   (C) hamartoma
   (D) inflammatory response
   (E) abscess cavity

26. Which is the correct statement about phenylketonuria?

   (A) Untreated patients will suffer mental retardation.
   (B) It is usually caused by lack of phenylalanine hydroxylase.
   (C) Treatment includes a phenylalanine-free diet.
   (D) Cerebral changes include demyelination.
   (E) All of the above are correct.

27. An alcoholic is found to have lobar pneumonia. The sputum is purulent and contains abundant pairs of lance-shaped, gram-positive cocci with prominent capsules. What is the causative organism?

   (A) *Streptococcus pneumoniae*
   (B) *Klebsiella pneumoniae*
   (C) *Neisseria meningitidis*
   (D) *Haemophilus influenzae*
   (E) *Enterobacter aerogenes*

28. A short-term dose of 1,000 rad acute whole body irradiation would be expected to produce which of the following?

   (A) severe nausea, 20% fatality rate
   (B) 100% fatality rate
   (C) mild nausea, 5% fatality rate
   (D) loss of hair, 35% fatality rate
   (E) only minor blood changes, 0% fatality rate

29. Which is the correct statement about carbon monoxide poisoning?

   (A) Carbon monoxide poisons by acting as a systemic asphyxiant.

   (B) Toxic effects can include mental confusion, unconsciousness, and death.
   (C) Chronic poisoning may result in degeneration of basal nuclei.
   (D) Hemoglobin's affinity for carbon monoxide is 200% greater than that of oxygen.
   (E) All of the above are correct.

30. Which vitamin is required for synthesis of collagen, ground substance, and osteoid?

   (A) iron
   (B) niacin
   (C) thiamine
   (D) vitamin C
   (E) vitamin D

31. What is the most common organism causing respiratory infections and meningitis?

   (A) *Campylobacter jejuni*
   (B) *Haemophilus influenzae*
   (C) *Salmonella sp.*
   (D) *Shigella sp.*
   (E) *Vibrio cholerae*

32. Accumulation of fluid in the pleural cavity is known as which of the following?

   (A) anasarca
   (B) ascites
   (C) hydropericardium
   (D) hydrothorax
   (E) pericardial effusion

33. Which is the eosinophilic, acellular substance that stains positive for Congo Red with apple green birefringence?

   (A) amyloid
   (B) bilirubin
   (C) hematin
   (D) hemosiderin
   (E) urate

34. Which of the following are possible features of herpes simplex type 1, viral infections?

   (A) intranuclear inclusions
   (B) keratoconjunctivitis

(C) latency period in neural ganglia

(D) encephalitis

(E) all of the above

35. Infections transmitted to humans from an animal host or reservoir are termed what?

(A) vertical transmission

(B) zoonotic

(C) horizontal transmission

(D) commensalism

(E) fomites

36. The process by which the information contained in a molecule of messenger RNA is converted to a protein is known as what?

(A) transcription

(B) translation

(C) organization

(D) granulation

(E) first intention

37. Which is an unexpected finding in an occlusive coronary thrombosis?

(A) coronary arterial atherosclerosis

(B) ischemic necrosis

(C) myocardial infarct

(D) thrombocytopenia

(E) thrombus at the site of abnormal vessel wall

38. The occurrence of scrotal carcinoma in chimney sweeps supports which theory for carcinogenesis?

(A) radiation carcinogenesis

(B) genetic carcinogenesis

(C) viral carcinogenesis

(D) chemical carcinogenesis

(E) asbestos carcinogenesis

39. Immunoperoxidase as well as flow cytometric studies of a lymph node showed that they contain monoclonal kappa chains. What is the most likely diagnosis?

(A) hepatoma

(B) lymphoma

(C) melanoma

(D) metastatic adenocarcinoma

(E) metastatic squamous cell carcinoma

40. Which is the most common fatal malignancy in childhood?

(A) bone cancer

(B) central nervous system cancer

(C) connective tissue cancer

(D) kidney cancer

(E) leukemia

41. Which is the most frequent fatal malignancy for males in North America?

(A) bladder cancer

(B) breast cancer

(C) lung cancer

(D) lymphomas

(E) prostate cancer

42. Which is the cause of the organism of the immunodeficiency syndrome (AIDS)?

(A) cytomegalovirus

(B) Epstein–Barr virus

(C) herpes simplex virus

(D) human immunodeficiency virus (HIV)

(E) Kaposi's sarcoma

43. In systemic lupus erythematosus (SLE), which finding(s) would you expect?

(A) antibodies against DNA

(B) glomerulonephritis

(C) a positive fluorescent antinuclear antibody test

(D) lesion in skin, joints and heart

(E) all of the above

44. Which is the major chromosomal abnormality in cat's cry syndrome?

(A) trisomy 18

(B) deletion of the short arm of chromosome 5

(C) trisomy 21

(D) trisomy 13

(E) 47,XXY

45. Which statement below is an example of hyper-trophy?

    (A) A clot in the femoral artery causes gangrene of toes.
    (B) Fibrosis occurs in the pancreas after parenchymal loss.
    (C) A low-protein diet causes ascites.
    (D) The left cardiac ventricle increases in thickness in systemic hypertension.
    (E) Vitamin K deficiency predisposes to bleeding.

46. Which is the brown granular pigment composed of iron-ferritin complexes present in heart failure macrophages?

    (A) melanin
    (B) hemosiderin
    (C) lipofuscin
    (D) bilirubin
    (E) ceroid

47. Common tumors of infancy and childhood include which of the following?

    (A) hepatoblastoma
    (B) Wilms' tumor
    (C) neuroblastoma
    (D) retinoblastoma
    (E) all of the above

48. Electron microscopy of brain cells from a deaf infant with rapid mental deterioration reveals abundant whorled membranous bodies in neuronal lysosomes. Which statement is correct?

    (A) The disease does not have a genetic basis.
    (B) The disease is probably a sex linked chromosomal abnormality.
    (C) An enzyme that degrades the membranes may be missing.
    (D) The cells will not have any DNA.
    (E) The infant's prognosis is good.

49. Which is a likely consequence of a staphylococcal infection?

    (A) furuncle
    (B) caseous necrosis
    (C) gangrene
    (D) thrombophlebitis
    (E) erysipelas

50. Which is the true statement concerning rickettsial diseases?

    (A) Rickettsiae are obligate intracellular parasites.
    (B) Rickettsiae usually produce no rash or eschar.
    (C) Rickettsiae usually have no insect vectors.
    (D) Rickettsiae cause yaws and pinta.
    (E) Rickettsiae lack DNA and RNA.

51. Which is a malignant neoplasm that forms a glandular pattern?

    (A) adenocarcinoma
    (B) lymphoma
    (C) melanoma
    (D) squamous cell carcinoma
    (E) teratoma

52. What disease is caused by arbovirus?

    (A) yellow fever
    (B) diphtheria
    (C) cytomegalic inclusion disease
    (D) scarlet fever
    (E) impetigo

53. Which is the correct statement about mumps?

    (A) Parotid gland swelling is unusual.
    (B) It usually causes diarrhea.
    (C) It causes pneumonia.
    (D) It is caused by paramyxovirus.
    (E) It may cause lymphadenitis.

54. Which characteristic is likely to be seen in malignancy?

    (A) encapsulation
    (B) slow growth
    (C) lack of mitotic figures
    (D) metastasis
    (E) euploidy

55. Chlamydial diseases include which of the following?

(A) nonspecific urethritis
(B) inclusion conjunctivitis
(C) lymphogranuloma venereum
(D) psittacosis
(E) all of the above

56. Bruton's agammaglobulinemia includes which of the following?

(A) X-linked inheritance
(B) markedly reduced B lymphocytes
(C) relatively normal delayed hypersensitivity
(D) increased incidence of autoimmune disorders
(E) all of the above

57. Antibodies against microsomal antigens are commonly seen with which of the following?

(A) scleroderma
(B) mixed connective tissue disease
(C) Hashimoto's thyroiditis
(D) dermatomyositis
(E) systemic lupus erythematosus

58. Type I hypersensitivity reactions usually involve which of the following?

(A) anaphylaxis
(B) cell-mediated reactions
(C) complement-mediated cytotoxicity
(D) circulating immune complexes
(E) delayed hypersensitivity

59. Sphingolipidoses include which of the following?

(A) Tay–Sachs disease
(B) Fabry's disease
(C) Krabbe's disease
(D) Niemann–Pick disease
(E) all of the above

60. Granulomatous lesions that are composed of a central area of coagulative necrosis known as "gummas" are associated with which of the following?

(A) all forms of meningitis
(B) anthrax
(C) cholera
(D) primary syphilis
(E) tertiary syphilis

61. Idiopathic arterial medionecrosis is characteristically seen in which of the following diseases?

(A) Marfan's syndrome
(B) polycystic kidney disease
(C) sickle cell anemia
(D) thalassemia
(E) von Willebrand's disease

62. Which is the expected karyotype of Klinefelter's syndrome?

(A) 45,XO
(B) 46,XX
(C) 47,XYY
(D) 46,XY
(E) 47,XXY

63. A hemorrhagic venous infarct would be most likely in which site?

(A) small intestine
(B) heart
(C) kidney
(D) spleen
(E) distal leg

64. Wound healing occurs because of the production of which of the following?

(A) actin
(B) chemotactic factors
(C) collagen
(D) kinins
(E) myosin

65. What is a localized collection of pus termed?

(A) abscess
(B) ascites
(C) caseous necrosis
(D) fibrinous exudate
(E) pseudomembrane

66. Which is a pathologic change in which an adult cell type is replaced by another adult cell type?

    (A) atrophy
    (B) dysplasia
    (C) hyperplasia
    (D) hypoplasia
    (E) metaplasia

67. Intermediate filaments of the cytoskeleton and membrane skeleton include which of the following?

    (A) desmin
    (B) keratins
    (C) neural filaments
    (D) vimentin
    (E) all of the above

68. Which of the following cell changes are seen in necrosis?

    (A) cellular swelling
    (B) fatty change
    (C) hydropic change
    (D) karyorrhexis
    (E) vacuolar degeneration

69. The microscopic appearance of an occlusive arterial infarct of the spleen is which of the following?

    (A) coagulative necrosis
    (B) liquefaction necrosis
    (C) enzymatic fat necrosis
    (D) caseous necrosis
    (E) giant cell inflammation

70. Gas embolism is most likely to result from which of the following?

    (A) hypercoagulable states
    (B) fracture of the femur
    (C) low protein states
    (D) venous stasis
    (E) rapid decompression

71. Which is the factor most likely to oppose thrombus formation?

    (A) exposed collagen
    (B) hypercoagulable states
    (C) plasmin
    (D) vascular stasis
    (E) endothelial injury

72. Common causes of edema include which of the following?

    (A) increased endothelial permeability
    (B) increased vascular hydrostatic pressure
    (C) lymphatic obstruction
    (D) reduced plasma oncotic pressure
    (E) all of the above

73. Which is the largest compartment in the body?

    (A) extracellular fluid compartment
    (B) whole blood fluid compartment
    (C) interstitial fluid compartment
    (D) intracellular fluid compartment
    (E) plasma fluid compartment

DIRECTIONS (Questions 74 through 153): Each group of items in this section consists of a list of lettered options followed by a set of numbered words or phrases. For each numbered word or phrase, select the ONE lettered option that is most closely associated with it. Each lettered option may be selected once, more than once, or not at all.

Questions 74 through 77

    (A) rhabdomyosarcoma
    (B) leiomyoma
    (C) hidradenoma
    (D) choriocarcinoma
    (E) lipoma

74. Malignant tumor of trophoblastic cells

75. Malignant tumor of skeletal muscle cells

76. Benign tumor of smooth muscle cells

77. Benign tumor of sweat gland cells

Question 78 through 81

    (A) *Mycoplasma pneumoniae*
    (B) *Bartonella bacilliformis*

(C) *Yersinia pestis*

(D) *Calymmatobacterium donovani*

(E) *Mycobacterium tuberculosis*

78. Carrion's disease

79. Granuloma inguinale

80. Primary atypical pneumonia

81. Bubonic plague

Questions 82 through 85

(A) *Diphyllobothrium latum*

(B) *Echinococcus granulosus*

(C) *Necator americanus*

(D) *Trichinella spiralis*

(E) *Trichuris trichiura*

82. Hydatid disease

83. Whipworm

84. Raw pork

85. Megaloblastic anemia

Questions 86 through 89

(A) silicosis

(B) asbestosis

(C) byssinosis

(D) anthracosis

(E) amyloidosis

86. Coal worker's pneumoconiosis

87. Multiple fibrotic pulmonary nodules

88. Pleural mesothelioma

89. Cotton fibers

Questions 90 through 93

(A) ribosomes

(B) cell membrane

(C) mitochondria

(D) nucleus

(E) centrioles

90. Site of cellular antigens and glycocalyx

91. Site of translation and protein manufacture

92. Important in cellular division

93. Contains euchromatin

Questions 94 through 97

(A) hemophilia A

(B) albinism

(C) achondroplasia

(D) Tay–Sachs disease

(E) phenylketonuria

94. Autosomal recessive lack of phenylalanine hydroxylase

95. Autosomal dominant dwarfism

96. Autosomal recessive lack of hexosaminidase A

97. Sex-linked deficiency of factor VIII

Questions 98 through 101

(A) Hashimoto's thyroiditis

(B) primary biliary cirrhosis

(C) Goodpasture's syndrome

(D) Addison's disease

(E) vitiligo

98. Anti-adrenal cell antibodies

99. Antimitochondrial antibodies

100. Antithyroglobulin antibodies

101. Antibasement membrane antibodies

Questions 102 through 105

(A) alpha-fetoprotein

(B) acid phosphatase

(C) serotonin

(D) CA 125

(E) cortisol

102. May be elevated with metastatic prostatic carcinoma

103. May be elevated with metastatic ovarian carcinoma

104. May be elevated with carcinoid tumors

105. May be elevated with hepatocellular carcinoma

Questions 106 through 109

(A) gummatous inflammation
(B) foreign body inflammation
(C) acute suppurative inflammation
(D) granulomatous inflammation
(E) coagulative inflammation

106.   Usually seen with tuberculosis

107.   Usually seen with syphilis

108.   Usually seen with staphylococcal infections

109.   Usually seen as a reaction to suture material

Questions 110 through 113

(A) IgA
(B) IgG
(C) IgE
(D) IgD
(E) IgM

110.   Delta heavy chain

111.   Most often found as dimers in mucosal secretions

112.   Usually constructed as pentamers

113.   Serum level frequently elevated with asthma or allergy

Questions 114 through 117

(A) hydrothorax
(B) hydroperitoneum
(C) hematosalpinx
(D) pyarthrosis
(E) hematopericardium

114.   Ascites

115.   Pus in a joint space

116.   Watery fluid accumulation in the pleural cavity

117.   Collection of blood in the fallopian tube

Questions 118 through 121

(A) metaplasia
(B) dysplasia
(C) atrophy
(D) karyorrhexis
(E) hyperplasia

118.   Enlargement of individual cells

119.   Reversible change of one adult cell type for another

120.   Shrinkage in the size of individual cells

121.   Irreversible dissolution of the cell nucleus

Questions 122 through 125

(A) vitamin A
(B) niacin
(C) vitamin C
(D) vitamin D
(E) vitamin K

122.   Deficiency results in scurvy

123.   Deficiency results in rickets

124.   Deficiency results in pellagra

125.   Deficiency results in hypoprothrombinemia

Questions 126 through 129

(A) plasma cell
(B) thrombocyte
(C) neutrophil
(D) eosinophil
(E) basophil

126.   Often seen with parasitic infections or asthma

127.   Secretes immunoglobulin

128.   Vital component of thrombosis and coagulation

129.   Cell's basophilic granules are rich in histamine

Questions 130 through 133

(A) granulomas of tuberculosis
(B) red infarct
(C) autoimmune hemolytic anemia
(D) serum sickness
(E) anaphylaxis

130.   Type I hypersensitivity reaction

131.   Type II hypersensitivity reaction

132. Type III hypersensitivity reaction

133. Type IV hypersensitivity reaction

Questions 134 through 137

    (A) interleukin-1
    (B) bradykinin
    (C) platelet-activating factor
    (D) myeloperoxidase
    (E) prostacyclin

134. Plasma protease that produces local pain at site of injection

135. Cyclooxygenase pathway member with vaso-dilatory and antiplatelet aggregating properties

136. Neutrophilic enzyme used for bacterial killing in lysosomes

137. Lymphokine

Questions 138 through 141

    (A) Edwards' syndrome
    (B) Down syndrome
    (C) Klinefelter's syndrome
    (D) cat's cry syndrome
    (E) Turner's syndrome

138. 45,X

139. 47,XXY

140. 47,XX, +21

141. 47,XY, +18

Questions 142 through 145

    (A) adenoma
    (B) teratoma
    (C) hemangioma
    (D) lipoma
    (E) adenocarcinoma
    (F) squamous cell carcinoma
    (G) malignant lymphoma
    (H) malignant melanoma

142. A 54-year-old woman has noticed a small reddish nodule on her arm for about a year. The nodule blanches with pressure. After surgical excision, the nodule is examined microscopically and found to be composed entirely of benign blood vessels. What term most correctly defines this tumor?

143. A 34-year-old woman has an ovary removed. Grossly, the ovary has been replaced by a solid and cystic tumor composed of hair, teeth, skin, and other benign elements. Microscopically, there are organoid constructions of various benign ectodermal, endodermal, and mesenchymal elements. What term most correctly describes this tumor?

144. A 77-year-old man has an enlarged lymph node removed. Grossly, the nodal architecture is effaced by a solid tan "fish flesh" tumor. Microscopically, there is a monomorphic population of large malignant lymphoid cells. What term most correctly defines this tumor?

145. A 65-year-old man complains to his doctor of increasing fatigue. On examination, the man is found to be anemic and to have a mass in his right colon. The colonic tumor is excised and found to be composed of malignant cells that form numerous gland-like structures. What term most correctly identifies this tumor?

Questions 146 through 149

    (A) anaerobic bacteria
    (B) aerobic bacteria
    (C) spirochete
    (D) mycobacterium
    (E) rickettsia
    (F) virus
    (G) protozoan
    (H) nematode

146. A 13-year-old male with sore throat, fever, and enlarged tonsils has a throat culture performed. The laboratory reports that *Streptococcus pyogenes* has been isolated. What type of organism has been isolated?

147. A 23-year-old sexually active male suddenly develops painful vesicles on his penis. A culture of vesicle fluid is reported as containing herpes simplex. What kind of organism is this?

148. A 34-year-old female camper develops diarrhea. An examination of her feces reveals *Giardia lamblia.* What type of organism is this?

149. A 43-year-old male hiker develops a rash, headache, and malaise. A diagnosis of Rocky Mountain spotted fever is made. What type of organism causes this disease?

Questions 150 through 153

   (A) tophus
   (B) ceroid
   (C) borate
   (D) bilirubin
   (E) amyloid
   (F) cholesterol
   (G) carbon
   (H) asbestos

150. A 55-year-old female with chronic osteomyelitis develops congestive heart failure. A rectal biopsy demonstrates abundant eosinophilic acellular material that has apple green birefringence after Congo red staining. What is this material?

151. A hilar lymph node is removed from an urban dweller who also smokes. The nodal macrophages contain abundant black particulate material. What is this material most likely to be?

152. An end-stage alcoholic is admitted to the hospital. He is jaundiced, and, in particular, his sclerae have a yellowish discoloration. What is this yellowish pigment?

153. A 47-year-old male with gout notices numerous subcutaneous nodules along the extensor tendons of his arm. One of these nodules is removed and demonstrates abundant positively birefringent needle-shaped crystals. What are these nodules?

Answers and Explanations

1. **(C)** Diphtheria is caused by *Clostridium diphtheriae*, an organism that causes a localized upper respiratory tract infection. The release of exotoxin produces the severe systemic changes that accompany the disease. *(Cotran et al., p. 343)*

2. **(E)** Leprosy is caused by *M. leprae*, an acid-fast bacillus. Clinically, the disease is divided into tuberculoid and lepromatous forms. Armadillos in the wild can harbor leprosy. The peripheral nerves are almost always involved in leprosy. *(Cotran et al., pp. 385, 386)*

3. **(D)** Hyperacute rejection involves preformed circulating antibodies, such as the blood group O recipient's anti-A and anti-B. Kidney cells will contain the donor's B antigen, and a hyperacute rejection will occur. *(Chandrasoma and Taylor, pp. 115–121)*

4. **(E)** The site of oxidative phosphorylation is mitochondria. All statements about cell membranes are true. *(Chandrasoma and Taylor, pp. 6–7)*

5. **(D)** Cations are positively charged ions and include all the listed choices except bicarbonate (anion). The major intracellular cation is potassium. Sodium is the major extracellular cation. *(Chandrasoma and Taylor, p. 28)*

6. **(C)** Phagocytosis is the engulfment of particulate matter by cells. These cells can be of two classes, fixed tissue cells (Kupffer cells in liver) and migrating cells (neutrophils). *(Rubin and Farber, pp. 25–27)*

7. **(E)** The normal pericardial sac contains about 5–50 mL of fluid. Accumulation of 100 mL or more of transudative fluid is a hydropericardium. The term "hydropericardium" is not applied to exudative expansions of the pericardium as seen in pericarditis. Hydropericardium can occur in most edematous states, including heart failure and myxedema. An accumulation of fluid can distend the pericardial sac to as great as 1,000 mL if there is no associated pericardial disease offering resistance to gradual expansion. *(Cotran et al., pp. 587–589)*

8. **(B)** Langhans' giant cells are the hallmarks of granulomatous inflammation. *(Cotran et al., pp. 83, 84)*

9. **(C)** Acetaminophen is a hepatotoxin. Toxic metabolites bind to the macromolecules of hepatocellular protein, with resultant coagulative necrosis of hepatocytes. *(Cotran et al., p. 46)*

10. **(C)** Type I hypersensitivity reactions are anaphylactic and require IgE (cytotropic antibody) to trigger release of vasoactive amines from basophils and mast cells. *(Chandrasoma and Taylor, pp. 106, 107)*

11. **(C)** B lymphocytes have receptors for FC. They express immunoglobulin and mature to plasma cells. *(Cotran et al., p. 190)*

12. **(B)** The enzyme defect in Gaucher's disease is beta-glucosidase. The diseases in which sphingomyelin, ceramide trihexoside, sulfatide, and

GM-s ganglioside accumulate are Niemann–Pick, Fabry's, metachromatic leukodystrophy and Tay–Sachs, respectively. *(Chandrasoma and Taylor, pp. 237, 238)*

13. **(E)** Respiratory distress in newborns results in large part from lack of pulmonary surfactant. Diabetic mothers and prematurity increase the risk. Pulmonary histopathologic changes usually include hyaline membranes. Survivors have an increased risk of patent ductus arteriosus, intraventricular hemorrhage and necrotizing enterocolitis. *(Chandrasoma and Taylor, pp. 242, 512–513)*

14. **(C)** Fat necrosis is common in adipose tissue contiguous to the pancreas as a result of leakage of lipase after acute injury to pancreatic acinar tissue. Grossly, minute firm yellowish-white deposits occur. Microscopically, the necrotic fat cells have pale outlines and are filled with fine basophilic soap material. *(Chandrasoma and Taylor, pp. 15–16)*

15. **(C)** The more radiosensitive a cell is, the more likely it is that the cell will be damaged or killed by a given dose of radiation. Lymphocytes are highly radiosensitive. The other listed choices have low radiosensitivity. *(Chandrasoma and Taylor, pp. 171, 172)*

16. **(A)** In gas gangrene, the tissues become discolored and foul, with microscopic evidence of cellular disruption. Leukocytes are scarce. This pattern of necrosis is seen in association with clostridial toxins and infections. *(Cotran et al., pp. 368, 369)*

17. **(E)** Acute cyanide poisoning is caused by cyanide's ability to bind to cytochrome oxidase and produce cellular asphyxia. Less than 0.1 g of ingested inorganic salt may be fatal. At death, the blood is cherry red, and a pungent bitter-almond smell may be present. *(Chandrasoma and Taylor, p. 187)*

18. **(A)** Tinea capitis is a superficial fungal infection of the hair of the scalp, eyebrows, and eyelashes. *(Rubin and Farber, p. 444)*

19. **(D)** Of the listed choices, only vitamin E is fat-soluble. The other choices are water-soluble vitamins. *(Chandrasoma and Taylor, p. 158)*

20. **(B)** The triad of fever, leukopenia, and bradycardia should suggest the diagnosis of typhoid fever, particularly in association with diarrhea and lymphoid hyperplasia. Typhoid fever is caused by *Salmonella typhi. (Cotran et al., pp. 356, 357)*

21. **(E)** Cancers are graded into three or four grades by their microscopic appearance. Increasing anaplasia and dedifferentiation are seen with increasing grades from I (well differentiated) to grade III or IV (poorly differentiated). With most tumors, the highest grades are associated with the poorest prognoses. *(Cotran et al., pp. 321, 322)*

22. **(C)** Epidermoid carcinoma, alternatively called "squamous cell carcinoma," usually produces keratin products, including keratin pearls. None of the other listed choices routinely produces keratin. The fibroadenoma is a benign tumor. *(Rubin and Farber, p. 158)*

23. **(E)** All of the listed choices, except for acute epiglottitis are not seen with *H. influenzae* infection. *(Cotran et al., pp. 348, 349)*

24. **(E)** All choices listed produce exotoxins. *(Cotran et al., pp. 343, 344)*

25. **(C)** A hamartoma is a focal, often circumscribed overgrowth in improper proportions of tissue normally present in that part of the body. Hamartomas arise in many organs and locations. One of the most common sites for hamartomas is the lungs. *(Cotran et al., p. 263)*

26. **(E)** Phenylketonuria is an autosomal recessive disorder that produces all the changes listed. *(Cotran et al., pp. 475, 476)*

27. **(A)** The only organism of the five listed that is gram-positive is *S. pneumoniae. K. pneumoniae* and *E. aerogenes* pneumonias also occur in alcoholics but are caused by gram-negative, rod-shaped bacteria. *(Rubin and Farber, p. 374)*

28. **(B)** A 1,000-rad acute whole body irradiation is a devastating amount of radiation, and after a few days, the fatality rate would be 100%. *(Chandrasoma and Taylor, pp. 171–174)*

29. **(E)** All of the other statements are true in carbon monoxide poisoning. *(Chandrasoma and Taylor, pp. 186, 187)*

30. **(D)** Vitamin C produces alterations in the synthesis of collagen, ground substance, and osteoid. The clinical picture is known as scurvy. Lack of iron, thiamine, niacin, and vitamin D result in microcytic anemia, beriberi, pellagra, and rickets, respectively. *(Chandrasoma and Taylor, pp. 158, 159)*

31. **(B)** *H. influenzae* usually causes meningitis and respiratory infections. The other choices classically produce acute gastroenterocolitis with diarrhea. *(Rubin and Farber, pp. 381, 382)*

32. **(D)** Edema fluid that accumulates in the pleural cavity is hydrothorax. Ascites are edema fluid collections in the abdominal cavity. Anasarca is severe generalized edema, particularly noticeable in the subcutaneous tissues. Hydropericardium is a pericardial effusion. *(Cotran et al., p. 750)*

33. **(A)** The positive Congo red stain is characteristic of amyloid deposition. Hemosiderin, hematin, and bilirubin are brownish pigments. Urate is eosinophilic but does not have Congo red birefringence. *(Cotran et al., pp. 42, 43, 255)*

34. **(E)** Herpes simplex type I (HSV 1) infections are caused by a DNA virus. The most common infection is the fever blister or cold sore. Less common infections include keratoconjunctivitis, aphthous stomatitis, and a latency of virus in ganglia. *(Cotran et al., pp. 1318, 1362)*

35. **(B)** Zoonotic infections are transmitted to humans from animal hosts or reservoirs. Examples include arboviruses and rickettsial diseases. *(Cotran et al., pp. 383–385)*

36. **(B)** Translation involves the production of protein molecules from messenger RNA. Transcription is the production of RNA from DNA. Organization, first intention, and granulation are terms used with wounds and healing. *(Chandrasoma and Taylor, pp. 7, 8)*

37. **(D)** An occlusive arterial thrombus, such as coronary thrombosis, is almost always at the site of a vessel abnormality. The most common abnormality is atherosclerosis. Rarer abnormalities would include arteritis and trauma. An expected finding in coronary thrombosis is infarction of the myocardium with ischemic (coagulative) necrosis. Thrombocytopenia is not expected in coronary thrombosis, because platelets must be present in adequate numbers and function to initiate a thrombus. A low platelet count would make thrombus formation unlikely. *(Cotran et al., pp. 132–137)*

38. **(D)** Sir Percival Pott astutely related an increased incidence of scrotal skin cancer in chimney sweeps to chronic exposure to soot. After institution of the practice of daily bathing, the rate of cancer dropped dramatically. Many polycyclic and heterocyclic aromatic hydrocarbons are chemical carcinogens and are present in high concentration in soot. *(Chandrasoma and Taylor, pp. 283–286)*

39. **(B)** The malignant tumor is derived from lymphocytes, resulting from an immunologic kappa-chain marker. Malignant tumors of lymphocytes are termed "lymphoma." The other choices do not contain kappa light chains. *(Rubin and Farber, pp. 1130–1132)*

40. **(E)** Leukemia is the most common fatal malignancy in children 15 years old and younger. The other choices are the four next most common causes of childhood fatal cancers. *(Rubin and Farber, pp. 1117–1119)*

41. **(C)** After fatal skin cancer, lung carcinoma is the most frequent cancer in North American males. Lung cancer is followed in frequency by prostate cancer, colorectal cancer, bladder cancer, and lymphomas, respectively. *(Cotran et al., p. 741)*

42. **(D)** AIDS is caused by HIV, formerly called HTLV III. The other listed choices are commonly

found with AIDS but are not the direct cause of the disease. *(Cotran et al., pp. 236–251)*

43. **(E)** SLE is an autoimmune disorder characterized by autoantibodies against numerous nuclear components. *(Cotran et al., pp. 217, 218)*

44. **(B)** Cat's cry syndrome involves the deletion of the short arm of chromosome 5. Trisomy 18, trisomy 21, trisomy 13, and 47,XXY are Edward's syndrome, Down's syndrome, Patau's syndrome, and Klinefelter's syndrome, respectively. *(Cotran et al., pp. 233, 234)*

45. **(D)** Hypertrophy is an increase in the size of cells and, with such a change, an increase in the size of the organ. A classic example of hypertrophy is left ventricular cardiac hypertrophy seen in systemic hypertension. *(Cotran et al., pp. 32–35)*

46. **(B)** Hemosiderin is the iron–ferritin complexes seen in heart failure macrophages. The other listed choices have black to brown coloration but are not composed of iron–ferritin complexes. *(Cotran et al., pp. 42–43)*

47. **(E)** All choices are common malignant neoplasms of childhood and infancy. *(Cotran et al., pp. 485–487, 880, 1373)*

48. **(C)** The electron microscope pattern describes a lysosomal storage disease. These are genetic and usually result from an absence of a specific degradative enzyme. The infant's prognosis is poor. DNA is still present in the affected cells, however. *(Rubin and Farber, pp. 249–257)*

49. **(A)** Most staphylococcal infections result in abundant pus formation, termed "suppuration." Staphylococcal skin infections include furuncles, carbuncles, surgical wounds, and impetigo. *(Cotran et al., pp. 365–367)*

50. **(A)** Rickettsiae are obligate intracellular parasites that contain DNA and RNA and usually produce rashes and eschars. Insect vectors are necessary for transmission of all the rickettsial diseases except Q fever. Spirochetes cause yaws and pinta. *(Cotran et al., pp. 383–385)*

51. **(A)** Gland-forming carcinomas are called "adenocarcinomas." Squamous cell carcinoma, melanoma, and lymphoma are malignant tumors derived from squamous cells, melanocytes, and lymphocytes, respectively. *(Cotran et al., p. 262)*

52. **(A)** Cytomegalic inclusion disease is caused by a herpes family double-strand DNA virus. Yellow fever is arthropod-borne virus (arbovirus) of the single-strand RNA type. Scarlet fever and impetigo are secondary to bacteria. *(Rubin and Farber, pp. 378–380)*

53. **(D)** Mumps is an acute contagious childhood disease caused by a paramyxovirus that usually is acquired by respiratory droplet infection. Parotitis, orchitis, and encephalitis occur. Diarrhea is unusual. *(Cotran et al., pp. 370, 371)*

54. **(D)** Common features of malignancy include invasiveness, metastases, aneuploidy, elevated mitotic rate, abnormal mitoses and anaplasia. Encapsulation, slow growth, euploidy and low mitosis usually are seen with benign tumors. *(Chandrasoma and Taylor, pp. 260, 261)*

55. **(E)** All the diseases listed are produced by chlamydial organisms. *(Cotran et al., pp. 361, 362, 1361)*

56. **(E)** Bruton's agammaglobulinemia is a sex-linked disorder characterized by virtual absence of B cells. Antibody production is, therefore, essentially nil. The T cell functions, such as delayed hypersensitivity, are normal. An increased incidence of autoimmune disorders occurs with Bruton's agammaglobulinemia. *(Cotran et al., pp. 232, 233)*

57. **(C)** Antimicrosomal and antithyroglobulin antibodies characterize Hashimoto's thyroiditis. The other listed autoimmune diseases principally have antibodies against nuclear fractions. *(Chandrasoma and Taylor, pp. 846, 847)*

58. **(A)** Type I hypersensitivity reactions are anaphylactic. Complement-mediated cytotoxicity and circulating immune complexes are type II and III hypersensitivity reactions, respectively. Type IV reactions are those of cell-mediated or

delayed hypersensitivity. (*Chandrasoma and Taylor, pp. 106, 107*)

59. **(E)** All the choices are sphingolipidoses caused by an inherited inability to degrade sphingolipids. (*Cotran et al., pp. 155–157*)

60. **(E)** Gummas are circumscribed, rubbery lesions measuring from a few millimeters to several centimeters in diameter. Microscopically, the central portion has coagulative necrosis, which is surrounded by a peripheral wall of epithelial cells, lymphocytes, and plasma cells. Gummas are the characteristic lesion of tertiary syphilis. (*Rubin and Farber, pp. 410–412*)

61. **(A)** Marfan's syndrome (arachnodactyly) usually has cardiovascular dissolution termed "cystic medionecrosis." The other choices are also hereditary diseases but are not associated with cystic medionecrosis. (*Rubin and Farber, pp. 241, 242*)

62. **(E)** Klinefelter's syndrome (testicular atrophy, eunuchoid habitus, mental retardation, gynecomastia) usually has a 47,XXY karyotype. The 46,XX and 46,XY karyotypes are normal female and male karyotypes, respectively. Turner's syndrome is 45,XO. The double-Y male is 47,XYY. (*Rubin and Farber, pp. 235, 236*)

63. **(A)** Hemorrhagic venous infarcts are most likely to occur with occlusive venous thromboses, in loose tissues, tissues with a double circulation, and tissues previously congested. These criteria usually are present in the small intestine. The other choices usually experience pale arterial infarcts. (*Cotran et al., pp. 820, 821*)

64. **(C)** Collagen provides the critical framework for wound healing. Actin and myosin are contractile proteins. Chemotactic factors and kinins are important in acute inflammatory reactions but are not critical components of wound healing. (*Cotran et al., pp. 108, 109*)

65. **(A)** An abscess is a localized collection of pus. (*Cotran et al., p. 85*)

66. **(E)** Metaplasia is the reversible change in which one adult cell type is replaced by another. (*Cotran et al., p. 31*)

67. **(E)** Intermediate filaments include keratins, desmin, vimentin, glial filaments, and neural filaments. Actin (6–8 nm) is a thin contractile protein, not an intermediate filament. Identification of intermediate filaments in a tumor tissues permits more precise histologic diagnoses. (*Cotran et al., pp. 27, 28*)

68. **(D)** Cell death, necrosis, is best identified by nuclear changes, such as karyorrhexis, the dissolution of the nucleus. Vacuolar degeneration, hydropic change, and cellular swelling are interchangeable terms describing nonlethal, reversible intracellular water accumulation. Fatty change is a nonlethal, reversible change, usually occurring in hepatocytes. (*Cotran et al., pp. 16, 17*)

69. **(A)** The hallmark of ischemic infarcts is coagulative necrosis. Liquefaction necrosis, enzymatic necrosis, and caseous necrosis are seen with brain infarcts, acute pancreatitis, and tuberculosis, respectively. Giant cells are seen in a number of nonspecific reactions and with tumors. They are not usually associated with ischemic necrosis. (*Cotran et al., pp. 16, 17*)

70. **(E)** Gas embolism (caisson disease) usually results from rapid decompression; e.g., scuba divers who ascend too rapidly to the surface. Less common causes include traumatic pneumothorax or uterine manipulation. The other choices have no relation to gas embolism. (*Cotran et al., p. 131*)

71. **(C)** Thrombus formation is most likely with endothelial damage (exposure of collagen), hypercoagulable states, and alterations in blood flow, such as stasis. Activated plasmin is a key component of the fibrinolytic system and is likely to oppose thrombus formation. (*Cotran et al., pp. 118, 119*)

72. **(E)** Edema can be caused by increased vascular hydrostatic pressure, reduced oncotic plasma

pressure, lymphatic obstruction, increased sodium retention, or increased endothelial permeability. *(Cotran et al., pp. 113–116)*

73. **(D)** The body is about 65% water. Of that, two-thirds is intracellular water, and one-third is extracellular water. The extracellular compartment is further subdivided as 80% interstitial water and 20% plasma water. Whole blood volume is only about twice the plasma volume. *(Rubin and Farber, pp. 300, 301)*

74–77. **(74-D, 75-A, 76-B, 77-C)** The nomenclature of tumors is complex. The suffix *oma* implies a tumor. Benign tumors usually are named by adding the suffix to the name of the cell type involved, such as leiomyoma (smooth muscle cells) and hidradenoma (sweat gland cells). Malignant tumors of mesenchyme are sarcomas. This suffix can be added to the cell type [e.g., rhabdomyosarcoma (skeletal muscle cells)]. Malignant tumors of epithelium are called "carcinomas," which can be added as a suffix to the cell type [e.g., choriocarcinoma (trophoblastic cells)]. *(Cotran et al., pp. 261–263)*

78–81. **(78-B, 79-D, 80-A, 81-C)** Each of the listed diseases has only one causative organism. *(Rubin and Farber, pp. 359–478)*

82–85. **(82-B, 83-E, 84-D, 85-A)** All of the organisms listed are helminths. *(Rubin and Farber, pp. 370–478)*

86–89. **(86-D, 87-A, 88-B, 89-C)** The four disease states are all pneumoconioses, pulmonary diseases caused by inhaled substances. Inhaled cotton fibers and coal dust characterize byssinosis and coal workers' pneumoconiosis, respectively. Pleural mesotheliomas occur with increased frequency with exposure to asbestos. Inhaled silica particles characteristically caused nodular pulmonary fibrosis. *(Cotran et al., pp. 727–734)*

90–93. **(90-B, 91-A, 92-E, 93-D)** The nucleus of the cell contains interphase chromosomes that are relatively uncoiled, called "euchromatin." The cell membrane, a unit membrane, is the site of glycocalyx and numerous cellular antigens. The centrioles direct cellular division.

The ribosomes, either free or attached to the endoplasmic reticulum, are the site of protein synthesis, or translation. *(Rubin and Farber, pp. 2–5)*

94–97. **(94-E, 95-C, 96-D, 97-A)** Phenylketonuria is an autosomal recessive disorder caused by a hereditary lack of the enzyme phenylalanine hydroxylase. Affected neonates suffer from mental retardation unless fed a diet deficient in phenylalanine. Dwarfism, also termed "achondroplasia," is an autosomal dominant disorder of abnormal cartilage growth with resultant short stature. A genetic absence of the enzyme hexosaminidase A produces Tay–Sachs disease. Mental retardation and blindness occur because of an accumulation of ganglioside in lysosomes. Hemophilia A is a sex-linked hemorrhagic disorder due to a lack of factor VIII. *(Rubin and Farber, pp. 245, 252, 257–259, 262, 263)*

98–101. **(98-D, 99-B, 100-A, 101-C)** Autoantibodies characterize a number of diseases. In Addison's disease, there are usually antibodies directed against adrenal cells. Antimitochondrial antibodies are seen in primary biliary cirrhosis. Antibodies against thyroglobulin and basement membrane material are seen with Hashimoto's thyroiditis and Goodpasture's syndrome, respectively. With vitiligo there may be autoantibodies against melanocytes. *(Chandrasoma and Taylor, pp. 121–124)*

102–105. **(102-B, 103-D, 104-C, 105-A)** A number of tumor cell products are manufactured by neoplasms. The detection of these products may assist in diagnosis and in directing therapy. Metastatic prostate cancer may produce elevations of serum-acid phosphatase and prostate-specific antigen. Ovarian carcinomas may secrete CA 125. Carcinoid tumors can be associated with elevations of serotonin and its urinary metabolite, 5-HIAA. Elevations in serum alpha-fetoprotein can be seen with hepatocellular carcinoma and with gonadal germ cell tumors. *(Chandrasoma and Taylor, pp. 295–298)*

106–109. **(106-D, 107-A, 108-C, 109-B)** The specific pattern of inflammation is orchestrated by both the immune state of the host and the type of challenge presented to it. With tubercle bacilli a granulomatous reaction characteristically develops. In chronic syphilitic infections, a gummatous reaction is seen. Staphylococcal infections produce acute suppuration and abscess formation. Suture material usually causes a foreign body inflammatory reaction. *(Rubin and Farber, pp. 65–74)*

110–113. (110-D, 111-A, 112-E, 113-C) The delta heavy chain is present in IgD immunoglobulin molecules. IgA is most frequently encountered as dimers in mucosal secretions. The pentameric form of IgM is the most common variant of the IgM molecule. Elevated serum levels of IgE may be seen with asthma or with other allergic states. *(Chandrasoma and Taylor, pp. 59–67)*

114–117. (114-B, 115-D, 116-A, 117-C) Watery accumulations of fluid in the peritoneum and pleural cavities are termed "hydroperitoneum" (ascites) and "hydrothorax," respectively. An accumulation of pus in a joint space is called a "pyarthrosis." A dilated, blood-filled fallopian tube is called a "hematosalpinx." *(Chandrasoma and Taylor, pp. 39–41)*

118–121. (118-E, 119-A, 120-C, 121-D) Hyperplasia is an enlargement of individual cells, such as cardiac ventricular hyperplasia due to essential hypertension. The reversible change of one adult cell type for another is metaplasia. Metaplasia is usually a protective adaptation of cells to noxious environmental stresses. Atrophy can be defined as the shrinkage of individual cells. Karyorrhexis is the irreversible dissolution of the cell nucleus associated with cell death. *(Cotran et al., pp. 31–35)*

122–125. (122-C, 123-D, 124-B, 125-E) Deficiencies of vitamin C and vitamin D produce scurvy and rickets, respectively. Niacin-deficient diets can produce a disease state termed "pellagra" characterized by diarrhea, dermatitis, and dementia. Deficiency of vitamin K, a fat-soluble vitamin, can result in a hemorrhagic diathesis due to an inability of the liver to

synthesize sufficient prothrombin and other vitamin K-dependent blood-clotting factors. *(Chandrasoma and Taylor, pp. 153–161)*

126–129. (126-D, 127-A, 128-B, 129-E) Eosinophils may be seen in increased numbers in parasitic and allergic reactions. Plasma cells manufacture and secrete immunoglobulins. Platelets, also called "thrombocytes," are an integral part of coagulation and thrombosis. The basophil has abundant histamine containing granules that are strikingly basophilic when stained with the routinely employed hematology dyes. *(Rubin and Farber, pp. 39–61)*

130–133. (130-E, 131-C, 132-D, 133-A) Anaphylaxis is an example of a type I hypersensitivity reaction. Autoimmune hemolytic anemia is an example of a cytotoxic hypersensitivity reaction (type II). Serum sickness serves as an example of generalized immune complex disease. Immune complex reactions with or without complement activation are type III hypersensitivity reactions. Granulomatous inflammation with tuberculosis is a type IV hypersensitivity reaction of the cell-mediated variety. *(Cotran et al., pp. 195–206)*

134–137. (134-B, 135-E, 136-D, 137-A) Bradykinin is a plasma protease that produces local pain if injected into the skin and elicits reversible edema. Prostacyclin is a cyclooxygenase-derived prostaglandin with vasodilatory and antiplatelet aggregating properties. Myeloperoxidase is an enzyme manufactured by neutrophils. It is used for bacterial killing in phagolysosomes. Interleukin-1 is a lymphokine with the ability to produce fever and stimulate prostaglandin synthesis. *(Rubin and Farber, pp. 50, 51, 55, 62, 63, 66, 111, 483)*

138–141. (138-E, 139-C, 140-B, 141-A) Turner's syndrome may include short stature, web neck, cardiac abnormalities, and streak gonads. The karyotype is 45,X or a mosaic 45,X/46,XX. The karyotype for Klinefelter's syndrome is 47,XXY. Down syndrome and Edward's syndrome are trisomies of chromosomes 21 and 18, respectively. *(Chandrasoma and Taylor, pp. 231–233)*

142–145. (142-C, 143-B, 144-G, 145-E) Hemangiomas are benign tumors composed of blood vessels. A benign teratoma of the ovary, also called a "dermoid," is usually constructed by organoid ectoderm, endoderm, and mesenchyme. Malignant lymphomas are composed of clonal proliferations of lymphoid cells. The degree of cellular anaplasia and differentiation vary from case to case. Malignant tumors of glandular epithelium are termed "adenocarcinomas." *(Cotran et al., pp. 261–264)*

146–149. (146-B, 147-F, 148-G, 149-E) The organism, *Streptococcus pyogenes*, is an aerobic bacterium. It is the usual cause of strep throat. Infection with herpes simplex, a virus, may result in painful genital vesicles. *Giardia lamblia* is a protozoan organism that frequently causes diarrhea. The infectious agent of Rocky Mountain spotted fever is a rickettsial organism. *(Cotran et al., pp. 355–385)*

150–153. (150-E, 151-G, 152-D, 153-A) Amyloid is acellular eosinophilic material that may accumulate throughout the body. It is seen with chronic infections and lymphoproliferative disorders. Amyloid material demonstrates apple green birefringence after staining with Congo red. Carbon particles, also termed "anthracotic pigment," are commonly seen in the hilar lymph nodes of smokers, urban dwellers, and coal miners. The yellowish pigment that causes jaundice is bilirubin. Uric acid crystals form tophi in many individuals with chronic gout. *(Cotran et al., pp. 42, 43, 251–257, 989, 990)*

REFERENCES

Chandrasoma P, Taylor CR. *Concise Pathology*, 3rd ed. Norwalk, CT: Appleton & Lange, 1998.

Cotran RS, Kumar V, Robbins SL. *Robbins Pathologic Basis of Disease*, 6th ed. Philadelphia: Saunders, 1999.

Rubin E, Farber JL. *Pathology*. Philadelphia: Lippincott, 1999.

Notes

Notes

Notes

Notes

Notes

Notes

Notes

Notes